NEUROPSYCHOLOGICAL EVALUATION OF THE OLDER ADULT

A Clinician's Guidebook

NEUROPSYCHOLOGICAL EVALUATION OF THE OLDER ADULT

A Clinician's Guidebook

Joanne Green

Department of Neurology and Wesley Woods Geriatric Center
Emory University School of Medicine

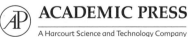

ACADEMIC PRESS
A Harcourt Science and Technology Company

San Diego   San Francisco   New York   Boston   London   Sydney   Tokyo

Academic Press
A Harcourt Science and Technology Company
525 B Street, Suite 1900, San Diego, California 92101-4495, U.S.A.
http://www.academicpress.com

Academic Press
Harcourt Place, 32 Jamestown Road, London NW1 7BY, UK
http://www.hbuk.co.uk/ap/

Library of Congress Catalog Card Number: 99-68194

International Standard Book Number: 0-12-298190-1

PRINTED IN THE UNITED STATES OF AMERICA
00   01   02   03   04   05   SB   9   8   7   6   5   4   3   2   1

CONTENTS

6 Neuropsychological Profiles of Common Disorders Affecting Older Adults I: Alzheimer's Disease, Frontotemporal Lobar Degeneration

7 Neuropsychological Profiles II: Vascular Disease, Dementia with Lewy Bodies

8 Neuropsychological Profiles III: Parkinsonian Disorders, Corticobasal Degeneration, Huntington's Disease

9 Neuropsychological Profiles IV: Traumatic Brain Injury, Substance-Related Disorders, Normal Pressure Hydrocephalus, Metabolic and Toxic Disorders

13 Providing Feedback and Planning Follow-up Services

PREFACE

This guidebook summarizes an approach for providing efficient, effective, and humane neuropsychological evaluation of older individuals. Neuropsychological evaluation is important in determining whether an individual has experienced abnormal intellectual or behavioral decline and whether that decline is related to underlying disease of the central nervous system. It is a major clinical procedure used in diagnosing memory dysfunction and the cause of that dysfunction. Neuropsychological evaluation is required for the diagnosis of Alzheimer's disease (McKhann et al., 1984).

A number of factors motivated the development of this book. As a larger proportion of our population becomes elderly, there will be increased demand for neuropsychological evaluation. It has been estimated that by the year 2030, between 17 and 20% of the population of the United States will be over the age of 65 (Schoenberg, 1986). The prevalence of dementia among those over age 65 has been reported to be as high as 25% worldwide (Ineichen, 1987). These figures suggest that dementia will constitute a major public health burden.

The detection and treatment of dementing illnesses are important for medical, social, and financial reasons and thus are likely to become an increasingly large focus of health care services. Early detection of the most common dementing illness, Alzheimer's disease (Erkinjuntti, Sulkava, Kovanen, & Palo, 1987;

Thal, Grundman, & Klauber, 1988), will allow treatments to be offered before the individual has declined sufficiently to require expensive health care and social support services. Early detection of dementia, regardless of the etiology, can represent a preventive measure in that it may deter an individual's involvement in unsafe or unwise behaviors, such as continued driving when confused, poor financial decision making, and forgetfulness while using a stove, which may lead to fires. Identification of significant cognitive decline may encourage compensatory changes that reduce the likelihood of behaviors harmful to the patient or to others and may allow some patients to remain independent longer. Determination that a patient is demented often reduces family stress by clarifying the reason for unusual behaviors, such as paranoia, loss of interest in usual activities, confusion, or poor judgment, and by facilitating neuropsychiatric treatment.

In addition, neuropsychological evaluation provides information on the specific nature of strengths and weaknesses in intellectual function that can be helpful in identifying the etiology of a dementing syndrome and in developing recommendations for the treatment and management of behavioral problems. Treatment alternatives vary for different dementing illnesses, and neuropsychological evaluation contributes to the accuracy of identifying the underlying disorder and treatment options that are most likely to be effective. The findings of neuropsychological evaluation can provide a baseline measure that can be used to monitor disease progression and the effectiveness of selected treatments.

However, the increased demand for neuropsychological evaluation is likely to be accompanied by even greater emphasis on the cost effectiveness of these services. Neuropsychological evaluation is a time-intensive procedure, and only psychologists who are highly efficient and effective in their practice will be able to survive professionally. Since specialized training in the needs and characteristics of older individuals increases the efficiency of service providers, there has already been dramatic growth in geriatric training and specialties. Application of the principles and procedures described in this guidebook will help psychologists to become more efficient practitioners and thus more responsive to social and health care needs.

The book describes a framework in which the basic phases of a standard clinical neuropsychological evaluation can be conducted, as well as the principles and knowledge integral to each of these phases, as outlined in Figure P. Chapter 1 describes activities occurring once a patient has been referred but before the patient has arrived for the scheduled appointment. Completion of these activities provides an initial focus for the evaluation and increases its efficiency. Chapter 2 describes the first part of the formal evaluation, the clinical interview. This interview provides initial exposure to the patient and is critical for engaging the patient's cooperation, for gathering initial data, and for tailoring the formal testing. In Chapter 3, principles that are fundamental to psychometric assessment are briefly reviewed, including the screening of sensory abilities, optimization of the testing environment, orientation of the patient to formal testing, use of psychometrists, concepts of test reliability and validity, choice of normative data, and selection of the test battery. In Chapter 4, tests useful for

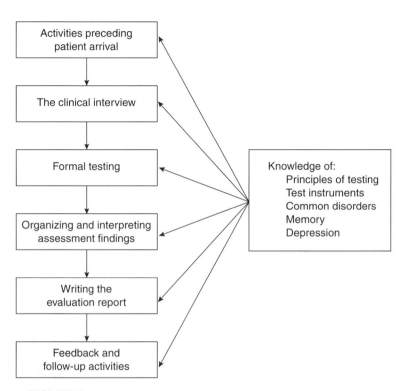

FIGURE P. Framework for neuropsychological evaluation of older adults.

evaluating the neuropsychological domains of general intellectual function, attention, executive function, verbal abilities, and visuospatial and visuoconstructive abilities are described. Because assessment of memory is often critical, Chapter 5 presents a conceptual framework for the clinical evaluation of memory and reviews tests useful for evaluating the memory of older adults. Chapters 6 through 9 outline common disorders affecting older individuals and their neuropsychological characteristics, including Alzheimer's disease, frontotemporal lobar degeneration, vascular disease, dementia with Lewy bodies, Parkinson's disease, other Parkinsonian disorders, Huntington's disease, traumatic brain injury, substance-related disorders, normal pressure hydrocephalus, and metabolic and toxic disorders. Chapter 10 describes the assessment of depression during the neuropsychological evaluation. In Chapter 11, an approach to organizing and interpreting test findings is introduced, including steps leading to compilation of the data summary sheet, estimation of premorbid ability, and guidelines for interpreting test findings. Recommendations for writing the evaluation report are included in Chapter 11, focusing on a style and organization that easily communicate the psychologist's findings and impression to other professionals. Finally, Chapter 12 outlines feedback and follow-up services that may be provided after completion of the formal evaluation, including an approach to organizing and conducting the feedback session, clinical issues related to delivery of feedback, and planning of treatment alternatives. The appendixes include forms useful to the clinician (for example, a clinical interview form) and patient cases illustrating specific disorders. A unique feature of the book is the inclusion of patient cases for which the final diagnosis has been confirmed with neuropathological evaluation of brain tissue.

The book was designed to contribute to the training of graduate students in clinical psychology as well as to the continuing education of practicing psychologists who are seeking specialized training in the neuropsychological evaluation of older individuals. It may also be informative to physicians, nurses, social workers, and other professionals who wish to better understand the nature and meaning of the neuropsychological evaluations their patients may be receiving. The book is designed to be concise and clinician-oriented, with research references cited to direct the interested clinician to source material. To facilitate the clarity of the writing, it is assumed that the psychologist is female, the patient is male, and the patient is accompanied to the evaluation by other family members.

It must be emphasized that the book is intended as a *supplement* to formal training and supervision in neuropsychological assessment and should not be used as a substitute for this training. For the psychologist or graduate student who is undergoing specialized training in the evaluation of older adults, it is critical that initial work with·this population be supervised by a professional experienced in this field. The combination of didactic training together with supervised clinical practice will increase the likelihood that our older population is provided with efficient, effective, and humane services.

A variety of individuals made important contributions to this book. My husband, Craig Zimring, provided the earliest encouragement when this project was first conceptualized and has remained very patient and enthusiastic during the several years required to complete the book. My in-laws, Fred Zimring, Lois Zimring, Jane Zimring, and Arnold and Donna Yellin, have been supportive and interested throughout the writing process.

A number of colleagues and students have reviewed chapters and made helpful comments, including Felicia Goldstein, Ph.D., Nancy Kriseman, M.S.W., Randi Jones, Ph.D., Frank Haist, Ph.D., Marian Evatt, M.D., Kenneth Graap, M.Ed., Rebecca Bone, M.A., and Lucy MacIntyre, M.A. The preparation of the manuscript benefited from the help of Jessica S. Brown, B.A., Helena M. Wood, M.A., and Marlene Goldman, B.A. I also acknowledge the encouragement and expertise provided by mentors early in my career, Edith Kaplan, Ph.D., David Freides, Ph.D., Roberta F. White, Ph.D., and Robin Morris, Ph.D.

I dedicate this book to the individuals who first inspired my love for adults older than I am as well as my enthusiasm for learning—to my parents, Nancy and Julius Green; to my grandparents, Rebecca and Joseph Shapiro and Jacob and Edna Green; and to my aunts and uncles, Ruth and Bernard Green, Miriam and Martin Goldstein, and Beatrice and David Wallas.

ACTIVITIES PRECEDING PATIENT ARRIVAL

A number of activities can be performed before the patient arrives for a scheduled appointment in order to facilitate the focus and efficiency of the evaluation. These include clarifying why the patient was referred, anticipating what services may be needed, sending advance information to the patient about the evaluation, including the informed consent to treatment form, and obtaining and reviewing medical records.

CLARIFYING THE REFERRAL QUESTION

Most patients are referred for neuropsychological evaluation by another professional who has treated them, most commonly an internist, psychiatrist, neurologist, or social worker. An important first step involves clarifying why the patient was referred and that the psychologist is able to provide the requested services.

Certain referral questions occur most commonly, including the following:

- Is there evidence that the patient has experienced significant decline in general intellectual function or in specific abilities, either from the characteristic level or since the previous evaluation?
- What is the likely etiology of the patient's neuropsychological decline? Most commonly, is the pattern of results consistent with Alzheimer's disease or suggestive of another disorder?

- To what extent might depression be contributing to the patient's decline? Is treatment for depression likely to result in significant improvement in cognitive status?
- Is the patient demented?
- Is the patient able to function independently in a safe and comfortable manner? If not, what level of functional support is recommended?
- What are the patient's specific cognitive strengths and weaknesses that should be considered in choosing treatments and designing rehabilitation programs?

These questions can often be addressed within the context of a standard neuropsychological evaluation.

In some cases, however, the patient may require help with other issues, and the psychologist who is specialized in evaluating older adults must decide whether to provide these services or to refer the patient to someone who is more expert in this area. For example, patients are sometimes referred for evaluation of disorders that are not a focus of geriatric neuropsychology. It is increasingly common for adults to be referred for evaluation of possible attention deficit disorder. Evaluation of this disorder may involve the use of specialized test instruments and evaluation procedures that are not typically included in an evaluation focused on detecting cognitive decline in older individuals, and such patients might be better referred to a clinician who specializes in attention deficit disorder. Some referral sources may make specific requests for tests and services that are not typically included in a neuropsychological evaluation, for example, "evaluate possible personality disorder using the Rorschach test." The patient may be referred for treatment services that a psychologist may not provide, for example, psychotherapy, behavior modification, or cognitive rehabilitation. Many older patients and their families are interested in information about assisted living facilities, personal care homes, or nursing homes, which may be better provided by other sources such as social service agencies or social workers.

Thus, reviewing upcoming referrals and clarifying both what is expected and what can be provided will ensure that both the patient and the referral source will be satisfied with the outcome of the evaluation. An experienced secretary may be invaluable in screening referrals to identify those that require clarification. As referral sources become more familiar with the primary interests and expertise of the psychologist, the likelihood increases that most patients will be referred for appropriate services.

THE PREEVALUATION LETTER

When referred for neuropsychological evaluation, some older individuals become somewhat anxious or confused about what is involved. Patients often have some awareness that the evaluation may have significant implications for their health and future independence. The purposes of neuropsychological evaluation are unfamiliar to most people, and they may be concerned about whether the evaluation is physically painful. Since neuropsychological evaluation often takes at least several hours, longer than most medical evaluations, patients must be prepared to spend sufficient time.

Sending patients a brief preevaluation letter, including an informed consent form, may alleviate these concerns and ensure informed participation in the evaluation. Most importantly, since many patients are referred for evaluation of possible memory dysfunction, the provision of written information about the evaluation may help ensure that the patient will actually remember to attend the appointment.

A sample preevaluation letter is included as Appendix A. The letter indicates the date, time, location, and anticipated length of the evaluation and the phone number to call if the appointment must be changed or canceled. It may be helpful to include a map clarifying the exact location of the evaluation. The letter briefly describes the purposes, procedures, and prerequisites for the evaluation. Since an evaluation lasting several hours may feel intimidating to a prospective patient, it is important to mention that short rest breaks will be allowed as they are needed. Clarifying that the evaluation involves "interesting pencil and paper tests and some other activities" may reduce concerns about physical discomfort. Patients should be encouraged to arrive well rested and well fed, having taken their usual medications. They should be requested to bring necessary eyeglasses and hearing aides. Since the patient's memory or awareness of deficits may be questionable, the patient should be strongly encouraged to bring along a knowledgeable informant, typically a close family member or a friend.

Finally, the preevaluation letter may include an informed consent form, which the patient is asked to review before the appointment. This letter informs the patient that the evaluation results will be held confidential but also requests permission to share the findings with other professionals involved in the patient's care as well as with health insurance providers, if necessary. The patient is provided with information concerning the approximate cost of the evaluation and policies concerning billing, payment, and cancellation of appointments. Clarifying financial obligations is particularly important for older patients who may have fixed budgets or limited resources. Many older patients are insured by Medicare, and the psychologist's policy for accepting Medicare reimbursement should be stated. Regardless of patients' health insurance, they should be encouraged to clarify their coverage so that they will not be unhappily surprised to discover that they have become personally encumbered by the financial obligation of a large bill for neuropsychological services. Some clinicians also ask their secretary to inform the patient about the billing and payment policy when the appointment is initially scheduled. However this information is communicated, it is instrumental in ensuring both the patient's satisfaction and the psychologist's financial security.

Ideally, the preevaluation letter should be mailed as soon as the referral question has been reviewed and determined to be appropriate. The letter should be followed with a confirmatory phone call several days prior to the appointment. For patients suspected to have memory deficits, the confirmatory phone call serves as an important reminder about the appointment time. If the patient is suspected to have a moderate to severe memory deficit and the appointment was arranged by a family member, it is advisable to contact that family member to remind him or her of the appointment.

REVIEWING RECORDS OF PREVIOUS HISTORY

Older patients may have a voluminous medical history, and scanning these records before the patient is interviewed can help tailor the evaluation and clarify the services that may be needed. From a practical point of view, it does not make sense to invest a lot of time reviewing records until the patient's intention to attend the appointment is confirmed. Some psychologists prefer to review the records just before the clinical interview once the patient has arrived for the appointment.

The advance review of records can focus the clinical interview and increase the efficiency with which formal testing is performed. For example, knowledge of the patient's history allows the psychologist to evaluate the accuracy of the information provided by the patient during the clinical interview. Assuming that the records are accurate, a discrepancy between the patient's report and information in the records may raise questions about the patient's memory. The review of medical records may also suggest variables, such as medical conditions, neurologic disorders, or family characteristics that may place the patient at increased risk for neuropsychological dysfunction. Variables associated with increasing the risk of specific disorders are described in Chapters 6 through 10. Identification of variables that increase the patient's risk for neuropsychological dysfunction alerts the psychologist to obtain detailed information about these variables. Examples of the types of questions that may be used to obtain this information are included in Chapter 2 as part of the discussion of the clinical interview.

The review of medical records can also be used to determine the nature and findings of recent medical and neurologic evaluations that may have relevance in determining the etiology of neuropsychological dysfunction. Laboratory tests can be helpful in determining whether metabolic or toxic conditions may be contributing to neuropsychological dysfunction, such as vitamin deficiencies or thyroid dysfunction (see Chapter 9). Brain electrophysiological function can be evaluated through use of electroencephalography or evoked potentials. The findings from structural and dynamic neuroimaging of the brain (by computed tomography, magnetic resonance imaging, position emission tomography, or single-photon emission computed tomography) may be helpful in differentiating between different disorders causing neuropsychological dysfunction.

2

THE CLINICAL INTERVIEW

This chapter will describe the major phases of the clinical interview conducted during neuropsychological evaluation. These phases include introducing the purpose and nature of the evaluation to the patient and establishing initial rapport, obtaining the history of concerns that motivated the evaluation, reviewing the patient's medical, educational, social, and family history, and concluding the interview and transitioning to formal testing. The clinical interview provides the first opportunity for the psychologist to observe the patient, and behaviors that may be particularly informative are outlined in this chapter. The suggested framework can be adapted and modified as the interview proceeds, depending on the needs of the patient, the accompanying persons, and the interpersonal dynamics. Appendix C includes a form that can be used to organize and record information during the clinical interview. Most interviews take between 30 and 45 minutes.

The clinical interview sets the stage for subsequent phases of the evaluation, both for the patient and for the psychologist. It is recommended that the clinical interview occur before formal testing because this can help accomplish several important purposes. The clinical interview offers the psychologist the first opportunity to interact directly with the patient, and the quality of the interview is critical in determining the patient's motivation in fully participating in the evaluation and exerting his best effort to perform well. Patients who develop positive feelings about the psychologist and the evaluation process during the interview are more likely to be fully cooperative during formal testing. For the psychologist, the review of background records probably provided some hypotheses about the nature of the patient's difficulties, and these hypotheses can be further explored during the interview. These hypotheses are used to tailor the formal testing to the patient's needs and thus to increase the efficiency of the evaluation.

The interview should be conducted in a relaxed and conversational but structured manner. The patient and accompanying persons should be allowed the opportunity to express their concerns as fully as possible, particularly early in the interview, when they are gaining an initial impression of the psychologist. The psychologist's ability to listen carefully and express empathy are critical. However, it is also important to acknowledge that the evaluation has some structure and limits, and that the psychologist retains control over the course of the interview. If the psychologist feels that discussion of a particular issue is becoming too extended in a nonproductive fashion, a comment such as the following may be made: "This discussion has been very helpful, and I think I understand your concerns. I wish we had more time, but we still have a lot to do today, so I'd like to move on to the next part of the interview. If we have time at the end, I'd be glad to talk about any additional concerns or comments you may have."

INTRODUCING THE EVALUATION AND ESTABLISHING RAPPORT

Establishing rapport with patients is critical for increasing the likelihood that they will benefit from any psychological service, either assessment or psychotherapy. This is particularly important in the neuropsychological evaluation of older individuals, many of whom have significant anxiety about developing debilitating neurodegenerative disorders or may be resistant to evaluation because they have felt pressured into receiving evaluation. Especially when the patient's evaluation was motived by the concerns of others, older individuals may be angry or resentful because they perceive a loss of control over their lives.

Training in clinical psychology emphasizes the sanctity of the psychologist–patient relationship and the responsibility of the psychologist to represent the patient's best interests (American Psychological Association, 1992). Adherence to these principles is particularly important in evaluating older individuals, who may be sensitive to being treated as less than fully responsible and independent adults. The psychologist is an advocate for the patient, and the more quickly this can be conveyed to the patient, the more likely it is that the patient will fully cooperate with the evaluation. Although the outcome of the evaluation may determine that the patient is incompetent to make his own decisions, it is important not to assume or imply this at the beginning of the evaluation. In some cases, the psychologist may, in fact, decide that the best interests of the patient will be served if there is significant communication with family members, but this should not be assumed on the basis of the patient's history alone.

The first few moments of the clinical interview are used to affirm that the patient is respected and has some control over the course and outcome of the evaluation. This begins during the initial greeting of the patient. A patient who has been accompanied by family members is greeted first ("Hello, I'm glad to meet you, Mr. Jones") and is then asked who has accompanied him ("Who came with you today?"). This allows the patient to the opportunity to introduce the psychologist to the others and to gain a sense of control in this interaction. If the psychologist greets the patient in a waiting area, she can engage the patient in conversational questions as they walk to the interview room, such as "How long did it take for you to get here?" or "How do you like the weather we're having?" If the patient is unsteady on his feet, the psychologist can offer an arm for balance. This initial physical contact can be very reassuring to patients. Once in the interview room, the psychologist can sit closer to the patient than to other family members, again trying to establish an alliance.

The psychologist begins the formal interview by asking the patient about his understanding of the nature of the evaluation ("What is your understanding of why you are here today?"). His response often provides highly valuable information. For example, if the patient clearly states the purpose of the evaluation, this suggests that neuropsychological function is better preserved than if he appears confused or uncertain. Regardless of the patient response, it is important to clarify the purpose and structure of the evaluation. A statement such as the following may be useful.

> We're going to be doing a neuropsychological evaluation today. We'll be asking you to perform tests and activities that will accomplish a checkup of your memory, concentration and some other abilities. These tests are not painful or uncomfortable, and most people find them interesting. The tests will identify both your strengths and weaknesses. They may identify some problem areas, and then we can discuss treatments that may help you. In any case, we'll have a baseline measurement that can be used to track your intellectual functioning should you develop any concerns in the future.
>
> I'd like to start with an interview so that I can get to know you better and address any of your concerns, and then we'll do the testing. The testing will take some time, but we'd be glad to take rest breaks so that you can use the rest room, get a drink of water, or just stretch. We won't know the test results today, but I will make arrangements to have you informed of them either by meeting with me or with another professional involved in your care. Do you have any questions before we start the interview?

This explanation concerning the nature of the evaluation often alleviates many of the patient's concerns. Many patients are anxious that the testing may be long and uncomfortable, and they are relieved by comments assuring them that efforts will be made to keep them as comfortable as is possible. At the beginning of the formal testing, the commitment to the patient's comfort can be demonstrated by asking if he is comfortable with starting and by providing a cup of water in case he gets thirsty. Describing the outcomes of the evaluation will also help increase the patient's involvement. Although some patients may initially resist participation in the evaluation, surprisingly few resist communication of results to concerned family members, particularly if the psychologist succeeds in establishing rapport with the patient.

The discussion of the purpose, nature, and outcomes of the evaluation typically requires about 15 minutes and ends by asking if the patient has any additional concerns about the evaluation. The patient can be asked, "How does this sound to you?" The great majority of patients, even those who are initially most resistant, are agreeable to continuing. They have sensed the psychologist's respect and concern and have some appreciation that the evaluation may be useful.

If the patient has not already signed the informed consent form signifying his agreement to participate in treatment, then he should be asked to do this before the evaluation proceeds further (see Appendix B). In rare cases, the patient refuses to sign the form, and then the psychologist must begin considering the reasons for this refusal and whether the patient is competent to make decisions in his own best interests. Although the patient may express adequate reasons for refusing to participate in the evaluation, such refusal may be suggestive of significant cognitive or affective dysfunction. If there is substantial data suggesting that the patient is incompetent, such as reported or observed instances of consistent confusion or unwise behavior, then the psychologist may recommend that the patient receive a separate competency evaluation (Appelbaum & Grisso, 1988; Grisso, 1994).

IDENTIFYING CONCERNS ABOUT THE PATIENT

The review of the background records is the initial step in gathering information about the patient's concerns and those of the family. These records may provide a rich source of information and form the basis of initial hypotheses concerning the source of the patient's difficulties. During the second phase of the clinical interview, the psychologist performs a detailed and systematic investigation of the patient and family's concerns, beginning with a general inquiry about these concerns followed by specific questions to obtain further details.

The General Inquiry

An effective strategy is to begin by asking the patient a general question about his concerns, followed by a request for concrete examples of these concerns. For example, the psychologist could ask, "Have you been concerned about any changes in your intellectual functioning or how you feel? Can you tell me about them?" Beginning with a general question such as this gives the patient more freedom to express concerns in his own words rather than in terms of categories provided by the examiner. If the patient responds vaguely, he can be further prompted by asking, "For example, have you been concerned about changes in your memory, concentration, reasoning, or mood?"

The patient's response often falls into one of the following categories:

- The patient is quite aware that he is having intellectual or behavioral problems.
- The patient admits to some difficulties, for example, mild decline in memory, but believes this is age-appropriate and feels that family members are exaggerating the extent of the problems.
- The patient denies any difficulties and is confused, and perhaps irritated, about the family's concerns.

In the latter two cases, the psychologist's rapport with the patient can be strengthened if she makes an empathetic comment, perhaps about how differences of opinion between the patient and family can be distressing. If the patient appears resistant to the evaluation, it may be useful to stress the similarity between this check-up and other yearly check-ups recommended for older adults. The psychologist can mention that the findings of the evaluation may help resolve the differences in opinion. It is important that the psychologist maintain a neutral position and not be perceived as taking the family's side in the disagreement.

If the patient's initial response suggests some awareness of change, it is important to obtain concrete examples of what he has found difficult. These examples can help clarify the patient's concerns and are often very useful in suggesting major areas of neuropsychological dysfunction. For example, if a patient says, "I often feel confused," the psychologist can ask, "Can you give me some examples of when you've felt confused?" Some common responses and their implications are indicated below:

- "I was driving to my daughter's house and couldn't figure out how to get there." This suggests dysfunction of visual memory or a visuospatial deficit.
- "I was listening to my neighbor, and lost track of what she was saying." This suggests a problem with sustaining attention.
- "I have trouble getting my hand to do what I want it to do." This suggests *apraxia*.
- "I can't find the words to say what I mean." This suggests *dysnomia*.

It is common for patients with some awareness of deficit to report, "I can't remember things." Asking for examples of forgetfulness may clarify the nature of the memory problem. Obtaining information about whether the memory dysfunction primarily affects recent memory, remote memory, or both may be diagnostically useful. For example, difficulty remembering information such as the day of the week, new phone numbers, or upcoming appointments is more symptomatic of a recent memory deficit, while difficulty remembering oft-repeated details of familiar family stories is more consistent with a remote memory deficit. A conceptual framework for developing specific questions about memory is presented in Chapter 5.

After the patient has been queried concerning his concerns, similar questions may be addressed to family members who accompany the patient. They can be asked about general concerns and to provide specific examples of when the patient has exhibited unusual behaviors. Interviewing family members has some potential for disrupting the psychologist's rapport with the patient, particularly if the patient does not report concerns about dysfunction, and the psychologist suspects that the family has serious concerns. However, rapport with the patient can usually be maintained and the family's opinion elicited in the presence of the patient if the patient is queried first, and it is acknowledged that the family member may have a different opinion. The patient can be gently informed that to make the evaluation most useful, and perhaps to resolve differences of opinion, it is best if information is collected from several involved family members. The psychologist may choose to address the patient with a comment such as the following before querying the family:

> I think I understand some of your concerns. Now I'm going to ask your family about their concerns. They may have a different opinion, and I'd like to hear your thoughts concerning their comments. Your family member is here because the family is concerned about you. Since you're here together, it makes sense to gather information from everyone, and perhaps we can help resolve any differences in opinion concerning your health.

This comment reinforces the allegiance of the psychologist to the patient by letting him know that his opinion is respected and that he will be allowed to respond to comments with which he disagrees.

If the psychologist senses that the patient is likely to become very upset or that family members are reluctant to fully air their concerns in the patient's presence, the psychologist may choose to interview the family separately. In most cases, if a technician is assisting with the testing, the psychologist can suggest that additional information will be gathered from the family during the testing, and few patients object to this.

As behavioral changes are mentioned by either the patient or an accompanying person, it is important to obtain a detailed description concerning each symptom of concern. This description should include events surrounding the change, the progression of the change, and subsequent areas of change. If multiple changes have occurred, the chronology of these should be explored. Questions such as the following may be particularly useful:

- When was the initial change observed?
- What was the nature of this change?
- Did this change occur suddenly or did it appear slowly and progressively?
- Were there other symptoms or significant life events surrounding the change? For example, were there other symptoms suggestive of a stroke, such as motor weakness or slurred speech? Were the changes noted only after a personal loss, such as the death of a spouse or the patient's reluctant move into a retirement facility? If this is the case, the role of depression in contributing to cognitive change must be considered. On the other

hand, some patients with mild dementia are able to manage well in a familiar environment or with the support of a spouse, but their deficits become more apparent when they must adapt to a new setting or when their spouse is no longer available to help them.

- Has the initial problem worsened, remained stable, or improved over time? If the patient's problem initially seemed related to a personal loss, did it continue to worsen even after any depression was relieved? It is not uncommon for family members to become concerned about a patient's competence only after a spouse has died because the spouse had been compensating for the patient's impairments, and this support is no longer available.

- Have other behavioral changes occurred subsequent to the initial problem? What was the nature of these changes and surrounding events? For example, does it appear that the patient has consistently had only one difficulty, for example, difficulty remembering appointments, or have additional problems developed, for example, difficulty recognizing familiar faces? This clarification can be helpful to the diagnostic process since progression of neuropsychological dysfunction is more characteristic of some disorders than of others. For example, the spreading and progression of impairment is more suggestive of a progressive neurodegenerative disorder such as Alzheimer's disease or frontotemporal lobar degeneration than of a potentially less progressive disorder such as a single stroke.

The Specific Inquiry

After the patient and family have expressed their concerns, a more structured interview is conducted to check on a wider range of possible symptoms and to obtain a more detailed history. The Neuropsychological Interview form in Appendix C includes an outline that can be used to guide this part of the interview. The outline suggests a wide range of possible questions, although it is rarely necessary for all of these to be asked.

One approach to starting the specific inquiry is, "Now that we've gone over some of your concerns, I'd like to ask some more specific questions. I'd appreciate responses from everyone. Have you noticed any changes in Mr. _____'s concentration (word finding, writing, etc.)"

This introduction avoids separately querying the patient and the family member, which can be very time-consuming. The psychologist phrases the inquiry about each behavior in a manner that is comprehensible to the patient and family and is sensitive to confusion about what is being asked. Examples of the behavior being queried may be helpful. ("Do you have any difficulty with your sense of direction? For example, do you find yourself getting easily lost in the shopping mall or even confused about where you are in your home?") If the patient or a family member endorses concerns about a particular behavior, then details should be elicited concerning the symptom onset, surrounding events, and the progression of the change.

The specific inquiry is used to investigate not only the possibility of cognitive change but also whether there has been any change in psychiatric status. As is detailed in Chapter 10, the clinical interview plays a critical role in determining whether the patient is depressed and the extent to which this may be contributing to behavioral change. Patients are often reluctant to admit spontaneously that they may be experiencing depression but are, in fact, willing to discuss this possibility when it is raised during the specific inquiry. Patients can be queried as to whether they feel sad and hopeless, whether they have experienced episodes of tearfulness, and whether there are other vegetative symptoms of depression such as poor appetite or insomnia. The presence of persistent, anxious thoughts can be explored. If a patient endorses feelings of depression or anxiety, the bases for these feelings should be explored to help determine whether the depression is reactive to a personal loss.

Whether or not the patient endorses depressive symptoms, family members frequently believe that depression is fundamental to the patient's unusual behaviors. Although it is possible that behaviors such as confusion or loss of interest in usual activities may be symptoms of depression, they may also reflect early symptoms of dementia. Therefore, it is important to obtain specific descriptions concerning the nature of the behaviors believed to reflect depression.

While less common than affective disorder, the presence of psychotic symptoms, such as hallucinations or thought disorder, should also be examined. It is important to distinguish between true psychotic symptoms and symptoms more closely associated with neurologic disorders. For example, family members may describe the patient's difficulty in expressing himself in words as "crazy talk," when this behavior, in fact, reflects dysnomia or expressive aphasia.

If there is evidence of current psychiatric disorder, then it is important to determine whether there is a past history of similar symptoms. As will be discussed in Chapter 7, the onset of psychiatric disorder in later life alerts the psychologist to the possibility of subtle underlying cerebrovascular disease (Coffey, Figiel, Djang, & Weiner, 1990; Cummings, Miller, Hill, & Neshkes, 1987; Miller et al., 1989).

If there has not been recent evaluation by a neurologist, the patient and family should be briefly queried concerning the presence of motor abnormalities. A variety of disorders causing neuropsychological dysfunction are associated with these abnormalities, including Parkinson's disease, Parkinson's plus syndromes, Huntington's disease, cerebrovascular disease, normal pressure hydrocephalus, and sometimes even Alzheimer's disease. Motor abnormalities of interest include low-frequency tremor, bradykinesia (slowed movement), unexpected falls, unstable balance, shuffling gait while walking, dysarthria (slurred speech), masked facial expression, micrographia (small writing), and supranuclear paresis of gaze (limitation in vertical eye movement).

If motor symptoms are endorsed, the onset of these symptoms and their relationship to cognitive changes should be noted because these may have both diagnostic and prognostic implications, as is detailed in Chapter 8. For example, if recent memory dysfunction and dysnomia were initially noted and the patient later began to exhibit tremor, this may suggest the overlay of an extrapyramidal motor syndrome on top of Alzheimer's disease (Funkenstein et al., 1993). Patients with Alzheimer's disease who also exhibit motor symptoms often experience more rapidly progressive and severe cognitive and psychiatric dysfunction than those without motor symptoms (Chui, Lyness, Sobel, & Schneider, 1994; Richards et al., 1993a; Stern et al., 1996). In contrast, if the initial symptoms included tremor and micrographia, and more pronounced memory problems emerged later, then the patient may be experiencing the cognitive changes sometimes associated with Parkinson's disease (Bondi, Kaszniak, Bayles, & Vance, 1993; Cummings & Huber, 1992; Taylor, Saint-Cyr, & Lang, 1990). It is important that patients endorsing or exhibiting motor symptoms receive neurologic evaluation to help determine the etiology of these symptoms.

OBTAINING THE BACKGROUND HISTORY

After the inquiry concerning behavioral changes, the patient's medical, educational, occupational, and family history are reviewed. This review provides a more general context within which the meaning and etiology of the behavioral changes can be understood and interpreted.

Medical History

Although extensive records may be available, it is advisable for the psychologist to briefly review the patient's medical history with him and his family, particularly focusing on disorders that may compromise neuropsychological function. As during the inquiry about behavioral changes, the inquiry about medical history can begin with a general question (e.g., "Have you experienced any significant medical problems, particularly in the last ten years?") and then move on to more specific questions. The patient's ability to recall details concerning recent, documented medical problems serves as an informal test of recent memory.

After a general discussion, the inquiry focuses on disorders that may compromise brain function. The most common disorders affecting older adults are discussed in Chapters 6 through 10. Even if extensive medical records are available, it is important that the presence and extent of these disorders be reviewed, particularly if the patient has not been previously seen by a physician.

If the presence of a disorder with possible neurobehavioral implications is endorsed, then specific follow-up questions are used to determine the nature and previous treatment of that disorder. The nature of the disorder determines the follow-up questions that are needed. To illustrate possible follow-up questions, the following sections outline some questions relevant to selected disorders along with the implications of some possible responses. The detailed review of specific disorders in Chapters 6 through 10 will suggest additional issues that may need to be addressed.

Vascular Disease (see Chapter 7)

• Has the patient been diagnosed with hypertension, and has this been well controlled with medication or otherwise? Is there evidence that the patient has been regularly taking medication to treat hypertension? Patients with memory problems may have difficulty remembering and following their medication regimen, thus placing them at greater risk for a vascular event. Patients with uncontrolled hypertension are at increased risk for mild neuropsychological deficits, particularly on tests of memory, attention, and abstract reasoning (Waldstein, Manuck, Ryan, & Muldoon, 1991). In addition, hypertensive individuals experience an increased frequency of small vascular lesions in deep periventricular white matter and subcortical brain regions (Schmidt et al., 1991), which may be related to behavioral abnormalities. The accumulation of periventricular white matter lesions has been associated with a dementia that has been termed *senile dementia of the Binswanger type* (Roman, 1987).

• Is the patient diabetic? Diabetes is associated with increased risk of atherosclerotic vascular disease (Colwell, Lopes-Virella, & Halushka, 1981), which may contribute to the development of Binswanger's dementia (Roman, 1987). Patients with a history of diabetes, particularly adult-onset diabetes, are at increased risk for neuropsychological deficits (Franceschi et al., 1984; Lawson et al., 1984), especially if they have experienced frequent hypoglycemic episodes (Pramming, Thorsteinsson, Theilgaard, Pinner, & Binder, 1986). Has the patient experienced symptoms of peripheral neuropathy, such as retinopathy or loss of sensation in the extremities? Peripheral neuropathy suggests the presence of more severe vascular disease and associated neuropsychological deficits. What treatment has been prescribed for the diabetes (e.g., diet- or medication-controlled), and has the patient been following the prescribed treatment regimen? Patients who are forgetful may have greater difficulty remembering and following a treatment plan, thereby increasing their risk of hypoglycemic episodes and diabetes-related vascular disease.

• Has the patient ever experienced a stroke or behaviors suggestive of a transient ischemic attack, such as an unexplained brief episode of confusion or motor weakness? If a stroke or vascular disease is suspected, it is recommended that the interview be expanded to include questions based on those used to obtain the Hachinski Ischemia Score (Hachinski et al., 1975), as described in Chapter 7.

• What symptoms were displayed before, during, and after the possible or documented vascular event (e.g., expressive or receptive aphasia, loss of consciousness, proactive or retroactive amnesia, motor weakness)? Comparison of current behavioral abnormalities with those surrounding a previous vascular event suggests whether the present symptoms are related to that event or reflect a different disease process. Data from a previous neuropsychological evaluation can often facilitate this comparison.

• What is the temporal relationship between the occurrence of the vascular event and the current problems? Did the current behaviors begin immediately following the vascular event or at some later time? If significant dysfunction did not occur either preceding or following the vascular event but only at a later time, this raises the possibility of an additional disease process.

• Did the patient receive hospitalization or rehabilitation? For what purpose and for how long? How successful was the rehabilitation? This information can shed further light on the nature and severity of cognitive deficits related to the stroke.

Parkinson's Disease (see Chapter 8)

• What are the patient's primary parkinsonian symptoms (e.g., tremor, bradykinesia, rigidity?) Cognitive dysfunction is more likely to be increased in patients who experience Parkinsonian motor symptoms of rigidity and bradykinesia rather than tremor (Levin, Tomer, & Rey, 1992).

• What medications are currently being used to treat his Parkinson's disease? Certain medications, particularly anticholinergic agents, can have adverse effects upon memory and behavior (Saint-Cyr, Taylor, & Lang, 1993).

• Does the patient appear to be depressed? Parkinson's patients with depression are more likely to exhibit cognitive dysfunction (Troster et al., 1995a).

• Has the patient exhibited hallucinations, particularly nonthreatening visual hallucinations? In patients with Parkinson's disease, visual hallucinations and other neuropsychiatric symptoms are sometimes related to toxic levels of medication (Cummings, 1992b), and adjustment of medications may relieve the symptoms.

Head Injury (see Chapter 9)

• When did and how did the head injury occur (e.g., as a consequence of a car accident or a fall)? What were the circumstances (e.g., was the patient responsible for a driving accident, was a fall due to stumbling over an object or without apparent cause)? If a recent auto accident is described, the patient's responsibility in causing the accident should be determined since this may reflect on his intellectual competence and his continued ability to drive safely. For example, if it appears that a recent car accident occurred because the patient was confused, this supports the presence of cognitive dysfunction, and it is advisable that the patient refrain from driving until the results of the neuropsychological evaluation are available. On the other hand, if the patient sustained a concussion because the rear end of his car was hit while he was stopped at a red light, this may not imply impairment in cognitive status prior to the accident.

• Did the patient suffer a concussion, appear confused following the accident, and/or lose consciousness? If he was unconscious or confused, what was the duration of this? Does he have difficulty remembering the events preceding and following the accident? The presence of confusion, loss of consciousness, or amnesia for the events surrounding the accident suggests the possibility of a closed head injury with associated cognitive dysfunction (Kay et al., 1993). Police and hospital reports about the accident may be useful in determining the presence and extent of confusion or loss of consciousness. Since a past history of head injury is associated with increased risk of developing Alzheimer's disease

(Schofield et al., 1997), it is important to query concerning both recent and past history of head injury.

• What was the temporal relationship between the memory or cognitive problems and the accident? Were these problems noted before the accident? Did they start immediately following the accident or at some later time? The onset of cognitive difficulties subsequent to a head injury suggests a causal relationship, but onset at a time either preceding or some extended time after the accident suggests the possibility of a different underlying disorder. It is, however, important to recognize that if physical injuries were the focus of attention immediately following the accident, more subtle cognitive deficits may not be noticed until some time after the accident when the importance of physical injuries has subsided.

• Did the patient require hospitalization and/or rehabilitation and if so, for what purpose? This information can indicate the severity and nature of cognitive deficits related to the accident.

Substance Abuse (see Chapter 9)

• Does the patient consume alcohol? If yes, of what kind, how often, and under what circumstances (e.g., during social occasions only, daily before dinner, when alone during the evening)?

• Does the patient or the family have any concern about the extent of the patient's alcohol consumption? For how long have they been concerned? Does the patient ever become intoxicated? Older individuals who overuse alcohol are particularly vulnerable to nutritional deficiencies, particularly of thiamine, that may compromise intellectual function (Victor & Adams, 1985). If the patient abstains from alcohol consumption, these mild abnormalities may be somewhat reversible (Brandt, Butters, Ryan, & Bayog, 1983). However, continued alcohol abuse may result in more wide-ranging and severe deficits (Cutting, 1978; Ryan & Butters, 1986; Salmon, Butters, & Heindel, 1993).

• Has the patient ever received treatment for alcohol abuse? If yes, what was the nature of this treatment? Has the patient experienced delirium tremens and seizures related to withdrawal from alcohol use? Such complications during alcohol withdrawal are sometimes associated with cognitive deficits.

• Is there any evidence that the patient may be overusing medications prescribed for psychiatric disturbance, particularly anxiolytic agents? Long-term abuse of certain psychoactive medications can compromise cognitive function (Learoyd, 1972; Ouslander, 1981).

Previous Psychiatric History (see Chapter 10)

• Has the patient ever experienced psychiatric disorder, particularly depression, anxiety, hallucinations, or delusional thought? When did this occur? A period of depression or anxiety following a major personal loss, such as death of a spouse or moving from a long-time home, may be reactive and not reflective of neurologic dysfunction. However, the initial onset of psychiatric disorder in later life without apparent cause may be associated with cerebrovascular disease (Coffey et al., 1990; Cummings et al., 1987; Miller et al., 1989).

• Has the patient been prescribed medication to treat psychiatric disorder, and has this been taken as prescribed? If the patient has been violating a prescribed medication regime, then it is possible that unusual behaviors may normalize once the regimen is resumed.

• If the patient had been previously treated for depression, did he receive electroconvulsive therapy (ECT)? If so, what type of therapy was administered (e.g., unilateral or bilateral), and for how many trials? Was the patient evaluated for dementia before this therapy began? Some patients treated with bilateral ECT experience subsequent mild memory problems (Abrams, 1992), although these are generally transient. Unilateral ECT involving the right brain hemisphere is least likely to be associated with memory dysfunction (Abrams, Swartz, & Vedak, 1991). However, in patients with preexisting dementia, the risk of more permanent confusion after ECT is increased (Sobin et al., 1995).

Similar questions may be useful for evaluating the contributions of other conditions to neuropsychological status.

Educational, Occupational, and Family History

The patient's education and occupational history should be reviewed. This information is useful in estimating the patient's characteristic level of functioning, known as the patient's *premorbid ability*. Specific procedures for estimating premorbid ability are described in Chapter 11. For individuals who did not complete high school, the reasons for leaving school should be further explored. Older individuals who grew up during times of economic depression may have left school for financial reasons, so failure to complete high school may be less predictive of academic level or premorbid ability. Patients should be asked if they believe they suffered from learning disabilities, hyperactivity, or attention deficit disorder. However, since evaluation procedures for diagnosing these disorders have only recently become available, retrospective diagnosis in older individuals must be tentative and cautious. Patients should be asked to describe the kind of work they have done and whether they believe that this exposed them to potential neurotoxins such as solvents or heavy metals.

It is often useful to ask patients for information concerning the education and occupation of their spouses and children. An older individual is likely to have premorbid ability similar to that of his immediate family. So, for example, if an older individual completed only high school but has several children involved in intellectually demanding occupations, one might predict that the older individual has also been characteristically highly functioning. This may be particularly helpful in estimating the premorbid ability of older women, for whom educational and occupational opportunities have historically been more limited.

It is becoming increasingly well established that a family history of certain neurodegenerative disorders may place individuals at increased risk for developing these disorders. A family history of Alzheimer's disease places an individual at increased risk for developing this disorder (Breitner, Silverman, Mohs, & Davis, 1988; Mayeux, Sano, Chen, Tatemichi, & Stern, 1991). It is well established that Huntington's disease involves autosomal dominant inheritance (Gusella et al., 1983), and thus individuals having a parent with this disorder have a 50% chance of developing this disease. Genetic variables may also play a role in a minority of Parkinson's disease cases (Tanner, Hubble, & Chan, 1997).

Therefore, a review of the health history of the patient's family may be useful in suggesting neurobehavioral disorders for which the patient is at increased risk. Information concerning the patient's siblings and older relatives (parents, grandparents, aunts, uncles) is particularly relevant. A general question such as the following can be asked: "In your family, is there a history of memory problems, dementia, Alzheimer's disease, strokes, or Huntington's disease? Have these disorders been diagnosed in your parents, grandparents, aunts, uncles, brothers, or sisters?"

If a positive family history is endorsed, more specific follow-up questions can be used to better determine the nature of the family member's illness and its similarity to the patient's current symptoms.

USING THE INTERVIEW TO EVALUATE THE PATIENT

Observations of the patient's behavior during the clinical interview can be invaluable in refining hypotheses concerning the patient's difficulties and in tailoring testing to meet the indicated needs. The following behaviors may be particularly informative.

Awareness of Cognitive Change or Other Unusual Behaviors

Failure to fully appreciate the extent of cognitive change, particularly deficits in recent memory, is a fascinating characteristic of some patients and may be diagnostically useful. The medical records may indicate that some patients have a history of unusual behaviors suggesting a memory problem, yet the patients may report their memory as age-appropriate. Patients may make defensive comments to excuse memory lapses, such as, "I'm just getting older" or "I'm not interested in remembering that." If the patient appears unaware of a memory problem, even when there is substantial contrary evidence from other sources, the psychologist must take care to reflect appreciation of the patient's point of view in order to maintain rapport.

Unawareness of cognitive deficit is one form of *anosognosia* (Prigatano & Schacter, 1991), and there is considerable evidence that this behavioral phenomena reflects brain dysfunction rather than a psychological defense mechanism.

Such unawareness has been associated with prominent dysfunction in the frontal lobes (Goldberg & Barr, 1991; Michon, Deweer, Pillon, Agid, & Dubois, 1992) and in right hemisphere brain systems (Auchus, Goldstein, & Green, 1992; Reed, Jagust, & Coulter, 1993; Starkstein et al., 1995). Unawareness is commonly observed in patients with Alzheimer's disease (Feher, Mahurin, Inbody, Crook, & Pirozzolo, 1991; Green, Goldstein, Sirockman, & Green, 1993; McGlynn & Kaszniak, 1991) and in other dementias believed to involve prominent dysfunction of the frontal lobe, including certain forms of frontotemporal lobar degeneration and alcohol-induced dementias (Ryan & Butters, 1986; Victor, Adams, & Collins, 1989). Although cognitive deficits in Parkinson's disease have been related to dysfunction in dorsolateral prefrontal regions (Taylor et al., 1990), awareness of deficit is often preserved in these patients (Danielczyk, 1983) unless they become demented.

Affect

The patient's affect during the clinical interview may provide useful diagnostic information. Tearfulness, particularly when talking about cognitive dysfunction or personal losses (death of a spouse, moving from their familiar home) may signal depression. Inappropriate tearfulness during discussion of an apparently neutral issue may reflect *pseudobulbar behavior*, a symptom of neurologic disease often associated with dysfunction in pathways connecting the frontal lobes and subcortical brain structures (Heilman, Bowers, & Valenstein, 1993a). The absence of concerned affect in the presence of significant neuropsychological deficit may suggest unawareness of deficit (Prigatano & Schacter, 1991).

Expressive and Receptive Language

It is important to observe the quality of expressive speech, particularly whether the patient exhibits dysnomia, dysarthria, or slowness. Dysnomia is characteristic of the early phases of Alzheimer's disease (Hodges, Salmon, & Butters, 1991; Jacobs et al., 1995b; Shuttleworth & Huber, 1988) and is generally more severe than that associated with other dementing disorders, even in the intermediate phase (Hodges et al., 1991; Huber, Shuttleworth, & Freidenberg, 1989b). Dysarthria is often associated with dysfunction in subcortical structures involved in speech production (Colombo, Sorgato, & Scarpa, 1989) and is common in disorders affecting the basal ganglia (Ackeman & Hertrick, 1997) and cerebellum (Lechtenberg & Gilman, 1978), including Parkinson's disease, cerebrovascular disease, and alcoholism.

The quality of responses to questions also provides useful information. If responses are focused and well organized and include accurate detail of recent medical or personal history, this suggests relatively preserved cognition. If responses are loose and poorly organized or become tangential to the question asked, this may suggest the presence of a thought disorder or of frontal lobe dysfunction (Damasio, 1995; Stuss & Benson, 1986). Difficulty in accurately remembering sequences of events within personal history, for example, the sequence of jobs held since high school, may also suggest frontal lobe dysfunction.

If the patient often requires that questions be repeated, this suggests several potential problems. One possibility is a hearing deficit. If this is suspected, the patient and family can be queried as to whether the patient typically uses or needs a hearing aide, and an audiologic evaluation might be recommended. If the patient's hearing is not defective, frequent requests for questions to be repeated suggest that the patient may be having difficulty remembering or concentrating during the interview. Less common is the likelihood that the patient has a receptive aphasia and truly has impaired ability to comprehend spoken language. However, if this is suspected, a more comprehensive aphasia evaluation might be included in the formal testing.

Memory for Personal History

The manner in which the patient relates past and recent personal history may suggest the nature of memory deficits. Before the patient is seen, it is useful to use available medical records to formulate some specific questions about the patient's history that can be used to "test" the patient during the clinical interview. For example, the patient can be asked about his date of retirement from full-time employment, his recent medical problems, where he has lived in the past and recently, and the number and occupations of his children. If the patient is able to provide a detailed, focused, and accurate description about both past and recent history, this suggests that verbal memory dysfunction is mild or absent. However, difficulty remembering or describing past history is suggestive of cognitive dysfunction. Ability to clearly describe past personal history but not more recent personal history is suggestive of a recent memory deficit.

A patient who acknowledges some forgetfulness can be asked to describe episodes of forgetfulness ("Can you give me some examples of times when you've been forgetful or confused?"). Some patients will acknowledge forgetfulness or confusion but look to family members for help in describing episodes of difficulty. A patient's tendency to rely on accompanying persons for help in answering these questions suggests that the patient may have a serious memory problem but retains some awareness of this problem.

CONCLUDING THE INTERVIEW AND TRANSITIONING TO FORMAL TESTING

Based on the review of records, the patient's presentation during the clinical interview, and family members' report of their concerns, the clinician has developed initial hypotheses concerning the patient's overall level of general intellectual functioning, possible neuropsychological strengths and weaknesses, and the disorder underlying this pattern. In addition, the clinician has developed a sense of how much testing the patient will be able to tolerate. A patient who has appeared alert, pleasant, and motivated to receive evaluation is likely to have little difficulty completing at least 2 hours of testing. However, an appearance of irritability, uncooperativeness, or physical frailty suggests that the patient may have difficulty participating in even 2 hours of testing.

Both the initial hypotheses and the patient's presentation are instrumental in tailoring the test battery. If the patient appeared high functioning during the clinical interview, a more challenging and more intensive test battery may be required to detect subtle deficits. At the other extreme, patients who exhibit obvious and widespread deficits during the clinical interview may experience considerable frustration and have difficulty cooperating with a challenging battery, so less demanding tests may be preferable. Options for test selection are suggested in Chapter 3. If the patient appears irritable or easily fatigued during the clinical interview, the test battery can be designed so that on the basis of initial hypotheses about the patient, critical tests are administered early in the battery when the patient's level of cooperation and energy are likely to be maximal.

In addition, on the basis of the clinical interview, many patients sense that the clinician is sympathetic to their concerns and has the expertise to provide some help. Even patients who may be intellectually compromised often develop an intuitive sense of this. The patient's perception of the clinician's empathy with his or her concerns heavily determines whether rapport is established and facilitates the patient's cooperation with the formal testing.

To help determine whether cooperation is likely and to reinforce the patient's feeling of having control over his participation in the evaluation, the patient can be queried at the end of the interview as to whether he feels ready to start the testing. The interview might be ended with a statement such as, "Now we've gone through your history and discussed your concerns and those of your family, I have a better idea of the testing that is necessary. Do you have any additional questions you'd like to ask me? If not, I'd like to start the testing now. Are you ready?"

If the patient has any concerns, these should be addressed before formal testing begins. When the patient appears comfortable to start, accompanying family members can be asked to leave the testing room.

3

GENERAL PRINCIPLES AND GUIDELINES FOR FORMAL TESTING

This chapter reviews some practical general principles and guidelines for formal testing. These include screening the patient's sensory abilities, optimizing the testing environment, orienting the patient to formal testing, and using psychometrists in test administration. The importance of test reliability and validity, issues in choosing normative data for evaluating older adults, and considerations and recommendations for choosing a test battery are also discussed. A 2-hour test battery that can be used to address many common referral issues is outlined.

SCREENING SENSORY ABILITIES

It is well established that visual and auditory abilities decline with normal aging (Kline & Scialfa, 1996). Older adults have reduced sensitivity to light (poorer dark adaptation, contrast discrimination, and color discrimination), spatial vision (poorer visual acuity and contrast sensitivity), and ability to detect and track visual motion. Cataracts, glaucoma, and even difficulty using corrective lenses may further disrupt vision. The hearing of older individuals is compromised by decreased sensitivity to auditory frequencies, particularly high frequencies, and poorer temporal resolution of auditory stimuli.

Difficulty in seeing visual stimuli or hearing questions asked by the examiner can compromise the findings of neuropsychological evaluation and may invalidate the findings of formal testing of nonsensory abilities such as memory. At the extreme, if the patient cannot clearly see visual material or hear verbal material presented during memory testing, poor memory test scores may, in fact, reflect impairment in sensory abilities rather than in memory. In preevaluation materials that the patient receives prior to the evaluation, the importance of bringing hearing aids and eyeglasses is stressed, but even with these aids patients may still have difficulty in perceiving stimulus materials.

The clinical interview is typically the first occasion during which the psychologist may observe whether the patient has a hearing deficit. If the patient frequently requests that questions be repeated or provides responses that do not directly address the question, these behaviors raise the possibility that he may have deficient hearing. As discussed in Chapter 2, these behaviors also raise the possibility that the patient may be experiencing neuropsychological deficits such as receptive or expressive aphasia, attentional inconsistency, or a memory deficit. However, if the patient responds more easily when the volume of the examiner's voice is raised, this suggests that auditory acuity is problematic, and it becomes particularly important that both the psychologist and the psychometrist speak loudly and clearly throughout the remainder of the evaluation. Alternative explanations for difficulty in responding to questions can also be differentiated by consideration of other data gathered during the evaluation, particularly the nature of errors made during formal testing.

Initial screening of vision may also occur during the clinical interview. The patient is specifically asked whether he sees clearly and whether he has ever experienced periods of disrupted vision, such as sudden blurring, double vision *(diplopia)*, or symptoms of an optic migraine. Further screening of visual acuity during the evaluation may be performed prior to formal testing with a near-vision card, in which the patient is asked to read letters and numbers of decreasing size. This card can be purchased at most medical supply stores. Visual acuity below 20/50 may compromise performance on neuropsychological tests.

Performance on the near-vision screening test is useful not only for examining visual acuity but also for suggesting neuropsychological abilities that require further evaluation. For example, if the patient skips items on a given line, this may suggest impairment in attention or in visual scanning. Failure to read items either on the left or right end of each line might suggest hemispatial inattention or neglect. Repetition of items within a line might suggest either double vision or perseverative tendencies. Each of these possibilities can be further evaluated during formal testing.

OPTIMIZING THE TEST ENVIRONMENT

Since the sensory abilities of older adults may already be compromised, it is important that testing be performed in a room that is quiet and well lit. Patients should be seated so that they look at the examiner against a neutral, nondistract-ing visual background. It is undesirable for the examiner to sit with her back to a window because the patient may be distracted by outdoor activities or his eyes may be taxed by accommodating to differences in light levels between the indoor and outdoor environments. It is important that the testing be conducted in quiet conditions with minimal auditory distraction, particularly for patients with hear-ing impairments. Ideally, the room's climate control (heating, air conditioning) should be adjustable to ensure the patient's comfort.

Although an informal seating arrangement is desirable during the clinical interview, once formal testing begins, the patient should be seated in a comfort-able chair across a table from the examiner. The furniture should be chosen so that the patient can easily manipulate test materials placed on the table. To avoid distracting the patient, test materials that are not currently in use can be placed on an adjacent desk or table.

Instructions should be read to the patient in a clear voice with adequate vol-ume and in a conversational style, emphazing important phrases and maintaining natural eye contact with the patient. Because the examiner is highly familiar with test instructions, she may tend to speak quickly, and this should be avoided. If the patient appears confused about instructions, these may be repeated where the test allows this. Initially, instructions should be repeated verbatim, but paraphrasing may be necessary if the patient remains confused after reinstruction. When instructions are repeated, this should be noted in the test protocol.

ORIENTING THE PATIENT TO TESTING

Before formal testing begins, general instructions are provided to orient the patient to the general characteristics of the testing and what will be expected. These instructions facilitate continued development of rapport and promote the patient's cooperation and motivation. Instructions such as the following are effec-tive in accomplishing these purposes:

> We're going to be asking you some questions and to do some activities. Some of the questions are easier, and some are more difficult. The most important thing is to just try to do your best. You won't be able to do everything perfectly—no one can. So please try not to get frustrated or upset if you miss some of the items. Some of the tests will start out easy and then get harder and harder until you miss some of the items—that's the way some tests are designed. Everyone has some strengths and some weaknesses. Please just try to do your best.
>
> The testing will take some time, but we think you'll find it interesting. When you would like a short break, just let us know. If you need a drink of water, to use a rest room, or to just stand up and stretch, please let us know. We want you to be as comfortable as possible.
>
> Are you ready to start?

These instructions both inoculate the patient against frustration when he makes errors and also give him some sense of control. Warning the patient that he will make some errors reduces the negative emotional impact when this occurs.

As the testing proceeds, when the patient has difficulty with test items, the examiner can comment that the patient is exerting good effort, thus stressing the positive aspect of the patient's response and deemphasizing the negative impact of an incorrect response. Many patients will express displeasure when they are informed that the testing may last several hours, and this may be relieved when they are informed that their comfort is of concern and that they are able ask for rest breaks if they feel uncomfortable. In fact, once patients understand the scope of the evaluation, most are motivated to finish it efficiently and are able to persist through several hours of testing with only a brief pause to use the rest room.

GUIDELINES FOR USE OF PSYCHOMETRISTS

It is common for psychologists to employ psychometrists in their clinical practice. The psychometrist is responsible for administering formal tests, scoring test data, converting the raw data into standardized scores using normative data designated by the psychologist, and compiling the data in a summary sheet. In addition, the psychometrist plays an important role in maintaining the patient's motivation and level of effort, so that assessment of the optimal level of performance is obtained.

Use of an experienced psychometrist has the additional advantage of providing another perspective on the patient's behavior. The patient may behave somewhat differently with the psychometrist than in the presence of the psychologist, and the psychometrist's observations can frequently contribute to the overall assessment. The psychometrist can be instructed to note behaviors observed during the testing. The inexperienced psychometrist may be supplied with an outline of behaviors to be observed. A sample of a behavioral observation form is included in Appendix D.

Guidelines for the education and training of psychometrists have been delineated by the American Psychological Association's Division 40 (Division of Clinical Neuropsychology) (American Psychological Association, 1989; American Psychological Association, 1991). The major qualifications for psychometrists include:

- A Bachelor's degree, preferably with course work in clinical psychology, assessment, and statistics
- Training in ethical issues related to patient assessment, particularly the importance of confidentiality
- Expertise in administering tests according to standardized practice
- Knowledge of the specific role of the psychometrist in the evaluation
- Knowledge of institutional procedures for dealing with medical emergencies or unusual patient behaviors (agitation, suicidal or homocidal threats, inappropriate behavior)

The guidelines stress that even when an experienced psychometrist participates in the evaluation, her role must be clearly defined and well understood.

Although an experienced psychometrist can make major contributions to the evaluation, the ultimate responsibility for the quality of the evaluation, including the accuracy of the data, lies in the hands of the licensed psychologist.

It is recommended that the psychologist initially interview the patient, orient him to the testing, and perform some initial testing, even if a psychometrist administers most of the formal tests. This allows the psychologist to observe how the patient reacts to the testing and to develop additional hypotheses for tailoring the testing. The testing performed by the psychologist can be very brief. For example, administration of the Information and Orientation and Mental Control tests of the Wechsler Memory Scale, Third Edition (WMS-III) may be sufficient for gaining an initial impression of the patient's neuropsychological functioning and his attitude toward testing. For patients who are highly disoriented or who display impaired mental control, it is probably unnecessary to obtain a comprehensive assessment of general intellectual function through a complete intelligence test. Patients displaying irritability during this initial testing may not be able to tolerate several hours of additional testing. In such cases, the psychologist may decide to place critical tests at the beginning of the battery to increase the likelihood that they will be completed. On the other hand, unimpaired performance on these initial WMS-III tests may signal that more challenging evaluation of memory and attention is required.

It is recommended that the psychometrist be present during the clinical interview and during the brief testing administered by the psychologist. This approach allows her to begin establishing rapport with the patient, thus facilitating the formal testing. Especially for patients who are anxious or irritable, the sudden arrival of an unfamiliar psychometrist after the interview has begun can seem disruptive. To enhance the psychometrist's credibility, the psychologist may want to conclude the interview by asking her whether she can think of other issues that should be pursued before formal testing begins. This reinforces the patient's impression that the psychometrist has an expertise that will contribute to the evaluation.

PRINCIPLES OF TEST DESIGN: RELIABILITY AND VALIDITY

An important qualification for performing psychological assessment, including neuropsychological assessment, is basic understanding of the principles of test construction, administration, and interpretation. Understanding of these principles helps to ensure that test are performed as designed. This section will briefly review the concepts of test reliability, test validity, and the related notions of sensitivity and specificity, particularly with respect to their implications for conducting clinical evaluation. More detailed discussions are provided by Anastasi and Urbina (1997).

Reliability refers to the extent to which a test score is consistent, assuming that the phenomenon being assessed remains constant. If the phenomenon being measured is unchanging, then, in theory, identical values should be obtained each time it is measured. Reliability can be assessed in a number of different ways (Anastasi & Urbina, 1997), but from the perspective of neuropsychological assessment, test–retest reliability is critical. A test is said to have test–retest reliability if, when it is administered to the same individual at two different times, the critical test scores do not change significantly, assuming that the individual has remained stable. For example, if a test is purported to assess memory, and the patient's memory has not, in fact, changed between two successive assessments, then the same memory score should be obtained during each assessment.

In reality, it is unlikely that measures taken at different times will be identical. Even if the underlying phenomenon is stable, changes in random variables that cannot be completely controlled contribute to test score variability. This *random error* will be reduced to the extent that the patient, examiner, test administration, and testing environment are identical in different sessions. Administration of tests using prescribed instructions in a well-controlled environment makes a major contribution to reducing random error in test scores.

However, some variation is unavoidable. For example, on two successive assessments, it is likely that there will be subtle variation in patient characteristics such as his energy or motivation, as well as environmental distractions from ambient noise. Minor variations in test administration may cause scores to fluctuate somewhat. Such random variation may cause test–retest scores to vary, even in the absence of significant change in the phenomenon being measured.

Thus, each obtained test score can be considered as a sum of two scores, the true test score and a random error score. If the test is highly reliable, the true test score will make a much greater contribution than the random error score. When some tests are developed, calculations are performed to quantify the *standard error of measurement* (SEM), the amount of variability in a test score that is related to the impact of uncontrolled random variables. For example, age-stratified SEMs and reliability data for test scores derived from the WMS-III and the Wechsler Adult Intelligence Scale, Third Edition (WAIS-III) are published in the *WAIS-III-WMS-III Technical Manual* (1997). When these data are available, it is possible to calculate a confidence interval for an obtained test score. This is most commonly done for IQ scores. The *confidence interval* is a range of scores around the observed score within which the true score lies with some known probability. Confidence intervals having probabilities of 90% or 95% are typically used in clinical practice. The formula for constructing the confidence interval around an observed score is indicated in Table 3.1.

In order for a test to be useful, the test must not only be reliable, but must also have *validity* for the purpose to which it is applied. A test is described as valid if it truly measures the phenomenon it is purported to measure. Within the context of neuropsychological evaluation, validity most often refers to whether the test is able to produce measures reflecting the integrity of the behavior of interest or of the brain region of interest. For example, if a test is designed to measure immediate verbal memory, to what extent does that test actually measure

TABLE 3.1 Computation of the Confidence Interval around an Observed Score

Confidence interval = Observed score ± z (SEM)
　where z = z-value corresponding to the desired probability, for example,
　　z = 1.96 for a probability of 95%, z = 1.65 for a probability of 90%,
　SEM = the SEM for the test score.

this ability? If a test is intended to measure the functioning of the frontal lobe, to what extent do test measures actually change with variation in the functioning of this brain region?

It is important to note that a test can be reliable without being valid for its intended purpose. That is, a test can produce highly consistent measures, but these may be unrelated to the underlying phenomenon. For example, measures of a person's height may be reliable, but these are clearly invalid for assessing memory.

It is also critical to recognize that, although many neuropsychological measures are labeled as measuring a specific domain (e.g., memory) or brain region (e.g., the frontal lobe), these measures are most valid for assessing the functioning of cognitive systems (e.g., the memory system) and brain networks (e.g., a frontal lobe system). This is because the brain is organized in distributed neural systems, with each brain region participating in a complex network linking a number of different neural regions. For example, the frontal lobe participates in several complex systems, including a system linking it to subcortical structures important to movement, notably the basal ganglia and thalamus (Alexander, DeLong, & Strick, 1986) and another linking it with more posterior parietal regions involved in the control of visuospatial attention (Mesulam, 1985).

Thus, most, if not all, neuropsychological measures have the greatest validity for assessing neuropsychological and brain systems rather than focal abilities or brain regions. For example, the Wisconsin Card Sorting Test (WCST) has been described as a measure of dorsolateral prefrontal function, based on its analogy to the delayed response paradigm used to study dorsolateral prefrontal function in animals (Milner, 1963). However, the validity of this interpretation has been questioned by reports of impaired performance, not only in patients with dorsolateral prefrontal lesions but also in those with lesions in nonprefrontal and more posterior brain lesions (Anderson, Damasio, Jones, & Tranel, 1991). These findings can be understood as reflecting the common participation of these brain regions in neural systems including the dorsolateral prefrontal lobe, and suggest that the WCST is better described as a measure of prefrontal system integrity than as a measure of focal prefrontal function. Thus, the WCST can be used to detect dysfunction in the frontal lobes as well as in other brain regions closely linked with the frontal lobe. Similarly, most neuropsychological tests are valid for assessing the function of cognitive or brain systems rather than of focal abilities or brain regions.

Because neuropsychological measures assess brain systems, each test score becomes most useful when viewed within the context of the other scores obtained during the evaluation. The overall pattern of test scores, rather than a single test score, is often most informative in identifying brain systems that are dysfunctional, as well as in suggesting focal regions within that system that are most compromised. As will be discussed in Chapters 6 through 10, different neurobehavioral disorders affecting older adults are associated with different patterns of neuropsychological findings. It is the similarity between an observed pattern and that associated with a particular disorder that often makes the greatest contribution to diagnostic issues. An approach to identifying neuropsychological patterns is discussed in Chapter 11.

Related to the concept of validity are the notions of *sensitivity* and *specificity*. These terms are used to describe the accuracy of a measure for providing correct categorizations of the underlying phenomena using a specified test cutoff score. They are generally applied to describing diagnostic accuracy. The sensitivity of a measure refers to the percentage of individuals who are correctly diagnosed as having an illness on the basis of the test score; the specificity refers to the percentage of healthy individuals who are correctly diagnosed on the basis of the same cutoff score.

For example, the Beck Depression Inventory (BDI), an instrument commonly used to assess depression, has a cutoff score of 10, such that individuals obtaining 10 or more points may be classified as depressed. A number of studies have examined the sensitivity and specificity of the BDI for classifying patients who have already been diagnosed as depressed or not depressed by other assessment procedures. Several have observed sensitivity exceeding 80% and specificity exceeding 65% (Norris, Gallagher, Wilson, & Winograd, 1987; Rapp, Parisi, Walsh, & Wallace, 1988). These findings suggest that the BDI is useful for diagnosing depression and support the validity of this test.

CHOOSING NORMATIVE DATA FOR OLDER INDIVIDUALS

In neuropsychological evaluation, each of the obtained test scores is compared with a normative data set to determine if the patient's score falls within normal limits. If the patient's score is considerably lower than the mean of the normative sample, then the patient's score may be interpreted as impaired (see Chapter 11). Thus, the availability of appropriate normative data is critical to the quality of the evaluation.

Several issues must be carefully considered when choosing normative data for evaluating older individuals. The first is the *screening procedure* applied to select individuals for the normative sample, particularly the information that was used to confirm that the individuals were healthy and without significant cognitive dysfunction. Ideally, normative data should be based on performance of individuals who are well functioning and who do not have a current or past history of significant cognitive dysfunction.

In reality, however, this standard is rarely met. Many sets of normative data are based on the performance of active, community-dwelling individuals whose health history has been evaluated through interview and review of medical records to exclude those with obvious medical or other conditions likely to compromise neuropsychological function. This approach is efficient, relatively inexpensive, and widely used by test developers. However, it may not exclude individuals with subtle but significant neurologic or cognitive dysfunction (Green, Woodard, & Green, 1995). A better approach would be to perform more intensive neurologic (e.g., electroencephalographic, magnetic resonance imaging), medical, and psychiatric evaluation to identify and exclude individuals with mild disease, but this approach is rarely possible because of the time and expense required.

When interpreting a patient's data, it is therefore important to bear in mind the screening procedures that were used in recruiting the normative sample. When the normative sample has received less stringent screening, this increases the likelihood that mean test scores will be abnormally low because of the inclusion of individuals with mild neuropsychological dysfunction. In addition, the inclusion of individuals with both healthy and mildly compromised brain functioning may result in a greater range or variation of test scores, resulting in a larger standard deviation around the mean scores. Thus, the use of a normative data set based on less stringent screening procedures increases the likelihood that a given patient's score will be interpreted as being within normal limits when he is, in fact, experiencing mild neuropsychological dysfunction.

A second issue important in choosing and applying normative data is the *adjustment for significant individual characteristics* that may impact test scores, such as age, education, or socioeconomic group. For example, scores on tests of attention, memory, and mental speed decline somewhat with normal aging. Scores derived from tests dependent on verbal ability often vary as a function of patient education, with lower scores being observed in less well educated individuals. The impact of socioeconomic class on test scores is less well understood but important to examine in future research.

For test scores that vary with individual characteristics, it is best if a patient's test score is compared with that of a normative sample having characteristics similar to those of the patient. The discussion of individual tests in Chapter 4 indicates the characteristics affecting specific tests and the availability of normative data sets that adjust for these characteristics. If there is a mismatch between the characteristics of the patient and those of the normative sample, this must be kept in mind when interpreting the patient's data, as described in Chapter 11.

In neuropsychological evaluation of older individuals, the availability of normative data for older age groups is obviously critical. Use of data from younger age groups may result in interpretation of an older individual's score as impaired when, in fact, it is within normal limits for his age group. The psychologist should be prepared to identify sets of normative data most appropriate for a given patient and consider updating the selection of normative data sets as newer, perhaps more appropriate, sets become available.

Several large sets of normative data for a variety of different tests have recently become available and include norms for older age ranges. One is the normative data from the WAIS-III and WMS-III, which include national standardization samples representing adults between ages 18 and 89 years from the United States (Wechsler, 1997a; Wechsler, 1997b). A strength of this data set is that it includes representative proportions of adults based on the 1995 U.S. Bureau of the Census report using the demographic variables of age, sex, race/ethnicity, educational level, and geographic region. A weakness of the data is that candidates for the standardization sample were screened mainly through use of a self-report questionnaire asking them about their medical and psychiatric history. Therefore, the standardization sample may include some individuals with subtle cognitive dysfunction. Some clinicians have expressed concern that, among older age groups, patients exhibiting very poor performance (e.g., no delayed memory recall) may still obtain standard scores that approach normal limits.

A second large data set is from the Mayo's Older Americans Normative Studies (MOANS). The normative sample of the MOANS included individuals who were normal according to self-report and whose medical history had been reviewed by professionals to exclude those with neurologic, psychiatric, or medical history that might compromise cognitive function at the time of testing. Age-based norms are provided for 3-year age intervals, from age 55 to 97. The MOANS provide norms for ages greater than 55 for the following tests: WAIS-R, Wechsler Memory Scale-Revised (WMS-R), Auditory Verbal Learning Test, Controlled Oral Word Association Test (letter fluency), category fluency, Boston Naming Test, Multilingual Aphasia Examination Token Test, Wide Range Achievement Test - Revised Reading subtest, American New Adult Reading Test, Stroop Test, Trail-Making Test, and Judgment of Line Orientation (Ivnik, Malec, Smith, Tangalos, & Peterson, 1996; Ivnik et al., 1992a; Ivnik et al., 1992b; Ivnik et al., 1992c; Lucas et al., 1998; Malec et al., 1992).

Several features of the MOANS normative sample must, however, be kept in mind when these data are used to interpret an individual's performance. First, the sample is not representative of the general population. It was recruited from a specific region (around Rochester, Minnesota) and is largely (99.6%) Caucasian. Minority groups are not well represented. In addition, the Wechsler Adult Intelligence Scale-Revised (WAIS-R) IQ scores of the MOANS sample were higher than those of same age groups (age 56–74) included in the population-based normative sample used by the developers of the WAIS-R. Thus, the general intellectual functioning of the MOANS sample is somewhat higher than that of the general population. This difference may reflect sample differences in demographics, solicitation procedures, and accrual rates. In addition, since the MOANS sample received more health screening than the WAIS-R samples, the higher IQ scores of the MOANS sample may also reflect better exclusion of individuals with mild cognitive dysfunction.

Therefore, the extent to which an individual patient's premorbid characteristics matches that of the MOANS sample must be carefully considered in interpreting patient data using these norms. The MOANS norms are most appropriately applied to the evaluation of healthy, Caucasian, middle-class individuals. For individuals with limited education or from different cultural groups, the MOANS norms may be less valid and must be applied more cautiously.

Normative data for specific tests are also available from a number of other sources. Erickson, Eimon, and Hebben (1994) have developed a bibliography of articles including normative data for a variety of specific tests, although some of these tests are not typically necessary to the neuropsychological evaluation of the older adult. Spreen and Strauss (1998) also include or provide references to normative data for a wide range of tests and age groups. In Chapters 4 and 5, the discussion of specific tests recommended for use in evaluating older adults includes references to appropriate normative data that are currently available.

SELECTING THE TEST BATTERY

Standard test batteries generally include both tests of general intellectual function and instruments that assess specific neuropsychological domains, such as memory or attention. Measures of general intellectual function have the advantages of psychometric reliability and comprehensiveness, tapping a range of specific abilities. During the initial neuropsychological evaluation, a measure of general function is helpful in determining if the patient has experienced a significant decline from the characteristic level of functioning (known as the *premorbid level*). During subsequent evaluation, administration of the same measure is useful for tracking the presence and rate of change in intellectual function.

However, tests of specific neuropsychological domains often have greater neuropsychological utility for developing hypotheses concerning specific areas of brain dysfunction and the etiology of such dysfunction. The domains that are often of greatest importance include attention, executive function, verbal abilities, visuospatial and visuoconstructive abilities, and memory. The neuropsychological evaluation also includes screening of affect, particularly anxiety and depression.

A test battery useful for addressing many common referral questions is outlined in Table 3.2. This test battery can be administered in less than 3 hours and does not exceed the level of energy and motivation of most patients. A major portion of the test battery consists of subtests from the WMS-III and the WAIS-III. The earlier versions of these scales (the WMS-R and WAIS-R) have recently been revised and include updated normative data derived from a population-based sample. The statistical properties of the test measures, including reliability and validity, are described in the technical manual for these tests, facilitating interpretation of test scores, particularly the inference of scores representing significant impairment or significant change.

The WAIS-III and WMS-III have a number of features that are attractive for the evaluation of older adults. Most importantly, they include population-based

TABLE 3.2   Test Battery for Neuropsychological Evaluation of Older Adults

American New Adult Reading Test (AMNART)
WMS-III Information and Orientation
WMS-III Mental Control
WMS-III Logical Memory I
WMS-III Visual Reproductions I
Trail-Making Test
Judgment of Line Orientation
WMS-III Logical Memory II
WMS-III Visual Reproductions II
Mattis Dementia Rating Scale
WMS-III Word Lists I
WMS-III Digit Span
Clock Drawing
WAIS-III Block Designs
WMS-III Word Lists II
Boston Naming Test
Letter and Category Fluency
WAIS-III Similarities
Geriatric Depression Scale or Beck Depression Inventory

Optional tests:
   Complete WAIS-III
   Wisconsin Card Sorting Test
   California Verbal Learning Test
   Motor tests: Finger Tapping, Grooved Pegboard

For movement-impaired patients:
   Replace WMS-III Visual Reproductions with WMS-III Faces
   Replace Trail-Making Test with WMS-III Letter–Number Sequencing
   Replace WAIS-III Block Design with WAIS-III Matrix Reasoning

---

norms for age groups between 16 and 89 years. Visually presented test materials have been enlarged and clarified, thus decreasing the potential that impaired visual acuity in older individuals will confound their performance. There is decreased reliance on mental speed, except in tests specifically designed to tap this variable.

Administration of either the complete WAIS-III or complete WMS-III to older adults has, however, several disadvantages, the most important of which is the time required to administer the scales. While the test manuals indicate that the WAIS-III primary tests can be administered in 60 to 90 minutes and the WMS-III primary tests in 30 to 35 minutes, these times are likely to be exceeded in evaluating older adults, who may respond more slowly and require more frequent rest breaks. Older patients often have limited patience and energy, and the inclusion of the full WAIS-III and WMS-III may limit their ability to complete other tests, particularly if they have become frustrated or fatigued by the time these tests are completed. Since the scales were designed for assessment of both younger and older age groups, more difficult test items are quite challenging, and inability to complete these items may frustrate older patients, even when they are informed beforehand that they are not expected to perform perfectly. Inclusion of the full WAIS-III and WMS-III is costly and may require additional justification of the hours billed for testing, and this may be problematic for both the patient and the psychologist. While some of the primary tests are revisions of instruments commonly used in neuropsychological evaluation of older adults (e.g., Logical Memory), the clinical correlates of other primary tests are currently less well understood. For example, the WMS-III Spatial Span and Letter–Number Sequencing have not been widely applied to the clinical evaluation of older adults, and the Family Pictures test is entirely new. Therefore, the implications of performance on these tests for differential diagnosis are currently less clear.

Therefore, it may be desirable to administer only selected tests from the WAIS-III and WMS-III, rather than all of the primary tests. While this approach violates the standardized procedure for administration of these scales, it may be more consistent with the goal of performing an efficient evaluation that is within the limits of the patient's energy and motivation. The recommended WAIS-III and WMS-III tests are indicated in Table 3-2. Descriptions of each of these tests are provided in Chapters 4, 5, and 10.

4

EVALUATION OF GENERAL INTELLECTUAL FUNCTION, ATTENTION, EXECUTIVE FUNCTION, VERBAL ABILITIES, AND VISUOSPATIAL AND VISUOCONSTRUCTIVE ABILITIES

This chapter describes tests useful for evaluating general intellectual function, attention, executive function, verbal abilities, and visuospatial and visuoconstructive abilities in older adults. For each test, the purpose and general procedures for administration and scoring are described, with references to documents providing additional details. For some instruments, suggestions for clinically useful extensions of the standard tests are provided. The interpretation of test findings is discussed, including those distinguishing different neurobehavioral disorders and the neuroanatomical basis for test performance.

ASSESSMENT OF GENERAL INTELLECTUAL FUNCTION

Wechsler Adult Intelligence Scale–III

One important decision is whether it is necessary to perform comprehensive evaluation of general intellectual function or whether a briefer measure will suffice. The WAIS-III can be used to obtain a comprehensive measure of general intellectual function (Wechsler, 1997a). In addition to producing measures of Full-Scale, Verbal, and Performance IQ (FSIQ, VIQ, PIQ), the WAIS-III generates index scores identified as reflecting Verbal Comprehension, Perceptual Organization, Working Memory, and Processing Speed.

A major advantage of the WAIS-III for the evaluation of older adults is the availability of population-based normative data. However, a major disadvantage is the time required to administer even the primary tests, typically between 60 and 90 minutes.

Therefore, the psychologist must carefully decide whether it is necessary to administer the entire WAIS-III or whether it is more appropriate to administer a briefer test of general intellectual function. Information gathered during the clinical interview and during the initial testing done by the psychologist can contribute to making this decision. The complete WAIS-III may be unnecessary if the patient exhibits significant deficits during the clinical interview. These might include dysnomia during conversational speech, difficulty formulating focused responses, inaccurate reporting of the current year or month, inability to remember recent visits to other clinicians, or impaired ability to complete simple mental control tasks, such as reciting the months of the year forward and backward.

However, it may be necessary to administer the full WAIS-III to patients in whom deficits are suspected to be subtle. This most commonly occurs with patients who are active and functioning independently and may still be employed. These patients often are self-referred because they have become concerned about changes in memory. In such cases, deficits may be very specific and subtle. Here, briefer tests may not be adequately sensitive for assessing and tracking mild decline in general intellectual function.

Administration of the complete WAIS-III is also advisable in cases where the psychologist suspects that the legal system may become involved, such as custody or guardianship cases. The WAIS-III is well validated, and professionals within the legal system, such as attorneys and judges, are more likely to be familiar with the WAIS-III than with other measures. Therefore, use of the WAIS-III may increase the psychologist's credibility and facilitate communication in legal settings.

Wechsler Abbreviated Scale of Intelligence

The Wechsler Abbreviated Scale of Intelligence (WASI) was designed to provide a reliable but less time-consuming measure of general intellectual functioning (WASI Manual, 1999). It consists of four tests (Similarities, Vocabulary, Block Design, and Matrix Reasoning), which are similar to their counterparts in the WAIS-III. However, the items comprising each test are different from those in the WAIS-III, and easier items have been inserted to facilitate use of the test with children.

When all four tests are administered (known as the WASI-4), estimates are obtained of VIQ, PIQ, and FSIQ. Administration of the Vocabulary and Matrix Reasoning alone (known as the WASI-2) allows estimation of the FSIQ. Tables are provided for estimating the range of the WAIS-III IQ scores based on WASI estimates and the magnitude of the difference between the WASI VIQ and PIQ required for statistical significance. The correlations between the WASI-4 IQ scores and WAIS-III IQ scores are high: .88, .84, and .92 for the VIQ, PIQ, and FSIQ, respectively. The correlation between the WASI-2 FSIQ and the WAIS-III FSIQ is .87. The test manual indicates that the WASI-4 takes about 30 minutes and the WASI-2 about 15 minutes to administer, although test time is typically increased for older adults. Normative data are available based on the performance of a large sample of English-speaking children and adults from the United States ranging in age from 6 to 89 years.

The WASI manual recommends administration of this instrument when limited testing time is available and there is a need for obtaining estimates of general intellectual functioning. It is not recommended that the WASI be used in isolation for diagnostic purposes or for cases involving the legal system. In the evaluation of older adults, the WASI can be particularly useful for detecting subtle change in relatively high functioning individuals without obvious deficits and when testing time is limited. The WASI may be used for tracking change in general intellectual function within the context of a more comprehensive battery including tests focusing on specific neuropsychological domains.

Dementia Rating Scale

When a less time-consuming and comprehensive measure is deemed appropriate for quantifying general intellectual function, one commonly-used instrument is the Mattis Dementia Rating Scale (DRS) (Mattis, 1988). The DRS was originally designed as a "brief measure of cognitive status in individuals with known cortical impairment, particularly of the degenerative type" (Mattis, 1988), and was intended for use in tracking the cognitive status of patients previously diagnosed with dementia. However, because it is brief and includes items examining a range of cognitive abilities, the DRS has been increasingly applied to screening patients for mild dementia.

The DRS has a maximum of 144 points and includes items examining five areas: attention, behavioral initiation and perseveration, construction, conceptualization, and memory. Within four of these (attention, behavioral initiation and perseveration, construction, conceptualization), the successful completion of more difficult items allows omission of less difficult items. The test can be administered within 20 to 30 minutes, and scoring takes an additional 5 minutes.

The psychometric properties of the DRS have been examined in a number of studies. The DRS total score is reliable in normal control subjects, dementia patients, and individuals with mild cognitive impairment (Coblentz *et al.*, 1973; Smith *et al.*, 1994). There is substantial support for the validity of the DRS total score for quantifying general intellectual function in both cognitively intact individuals and those with dementia. The total score correlates significantly with more comprehensive measures of general intellectual function (Coblentz *et al.*, 1973; Smith *et al.*, 1994). In patient groups having either Alzheimer's disease or dementias of varied etiologies, the DRS total score is related to other measures of behavioral functioning (Shay *et al.,* 1991; Vitaliano *et al.,* 1984).

Several studies have demonstrated that the DRS total score can be used to accurately classify healthy control subjects and patients diagnosed with Alzheimer's disease or other dementias (Green *et al.,* 1995; Monsch *et al.,* 1995; Vangel & Lichtenberg, 1995). However, a concern is that the criterion cutoff score for discriminating between demented and nondemented individuals has varied between studies, ranging from 120 (Vangel & Lichtenberg, 1995) to 133 (Green et al., 1995). The variability in criterion scores most likely reflects differences in the characteristics of the subject samples, particularly socioeconomic status and the extent to which the control subjects were screened for subtle cognitive and neuropsychological dysfunction. As the screening of control subjects for mild cognitive dysfunction becomes less extensive, the lower will be the criterion score for distinguishing these individuals from patients diagnosed with mild dementia.

The DRS has recently been applied to screening patients for mild cognitive impairment. It is important, however, that this application occur in a cautious and conservative manner. Even though the DRS score can be used to accurately discriminate between healthy control subjects and patients already diagnosed with dementia, the test will not necessarily have similar accuracy in discriminating between individuals with and without the mild cognitive impairment that may signal the early phases of Alzheimer's disease or another dementia.

A variety of factors complicate the use of the DRS for detecting mild cognitive dysfunction in apparently well-functioning individuals. A major concern is the availability of normative data for healthy older samples. The DRS manual includes normative data based on a relatively small sample of 85 community-dwelling individuals averaging 74 years of age (standard deviation [SD] 6.05, age range 65–81 years) (Mattis, 1988). Other characteristics of this sample (education, health status, methods used to screen for neuropsychological dysfunction) are not described in the manual. The mean total DRS score for this sample was 137.3 (SD 6.9). The manual recommends that scores below 123 (two standard deviations below the mean) be considered abnormal.

Normative data for the DRS are also available from a well-characterized larger sample (N=280) of somewhat older individuals (mean age 79.2 years, SD 8.0; mean education 12.8 years, SD 3.3), who were rigorously screened by medical, neurologic, and neuropsychological evaluation (Smith *et al.,* 1994). For this group, the total DRS score averaged 136.5, with a standard deviation of 6.2, values similar to those reported in the DRS manual. The convergence between these values suggests that DRS total scores below 123 may be considered abnormal.

This cutoff score of 123 for identifying a patient as impaired should, however, be applied with several considerations in mind, particularly the possible impact of patient age, education, cultural background, and previous screening for neurologic abnormality. The DRS total score significantly decreases with age and increases with years of education (Green *et al.*, 1995; Schmidt *et al.*, 1994; Smith *et al.*, 1994; Vangel & Lichtenberg, 1995). Thus, a DRS total score of 120 for a 90-year-old patient with a tenth grade education may not represent abnormality. Conversely, a DRS total score of 130 for a 60-year-old patient with a college education may raise significant concerns.

In addition, cultural variables may affect the DRS score. One study of an Austrian control sample reported a mean DRS total score of 141 (SD 2.4) for individuals between 70 and 80 years of age having 10 to 13 years of education (Schmidt *et al.*, 1994), which implies that a relatively higher criterion may be necessary for such individuals. In contrast, for an American urban inpatient sample, the majority of whom were African-American, a much lower criterion score of 120 was observed to discriminate well between cognitively intact individuals and those with impairment (Vangel & Lichtenberg, 1995). Thus, it is important that the criterion score applied to determine impairment be based on a sample having cultural characteristics similar to those of the patient being examined.

However, even when adequate normative data are available, use of the DRS score alone may result in misclassification of patients. For example, patients having focal deficits in recent memory and naming, possibly signaling the early phases of Alzheimer's disease, may have DRS scores exceeding 123 (see Case 1 in Appendix G). Scores can occasionally exceed 123 even for patients with significant dementia, particularly for individuals who have characteristically been very high functioning and for whom the DRS is not adequately challenging to detect mild cognitive change. On occasion, the DRS score may be well below the cutoff of 123, and yet detailed neuropsychological testing may not reveal a significant degree of dementia (see Case 11 in Appendix G). The DRS is also less useful for quantifying general intellectual function in patients experiencing significant movement disorder in their hands or arms, such as tremor or motor rigidity. Several of the DRS subscales (Initiation and Perseveration, Construction) are heavily dependent on motor abilities, and performance on these subscales may be lowered owing to motor impairment alone. Patients with movement disorders may thus have an abnormal DRS total score even when they do not exhibit significant cognitive dysfunction. Thus, the DRS total score cutoff of 123 must be applied very cautiously in screening patients for mild cognitive change, and patient characteristics affecting interpretation of the score must be carefully considered.

The DRS also includes subscale scores for each of the abilities that are examined, and it is not uncommon for psychologists to interpret these subscale scores to infer domain-specific deficits or even to resolve diagnostic issues (Paolo, Troster, Glatt, Hubble, & Koller, 1995; Rosser & Hodges, 1994; Salmon, Kwo-on-Yuen, Heindel, Butters, & Thal, 1989). There is some support for the validity of the subscales (Marson, Dymek, Duke, & Harrell, 1997), but their reliability is more questionable. Current data indicate that the subscale scores are adequately reliable for normal control groups. In one study of normal control subjects, each of the DRS subscales had acceptable test–retest reliability over an interval of 1.4 years, with the exception of the memory subscale, which showed a small but statistically significant decline of one-half point (Smith *et al.,* 1994). This suggests that, although the memory subscale may decline slightly, the other subscale scores of healthy older individuals can be expected to remain stable over the course of a year.

For patients having significant impairment, however, the reliability of the DRS subscale scores is less consistent, and reports of the reliability vary between studies (Coblentz *et al.,* 1973; Smith *et al.,* 1994; Woodard, Salthouse, Godsall, & Green, 1996b). The reliability of the Attention and the Initiation-Perseveration subscales is particularly suspect (Smith *et al.,* 1994). Therefore, it is not recommended that interpretations be based on DRS subscale scores, particularly the Attention and Initiation-Perseveration subscales.

How can the DRS be best applied within the context of neuropsychological evaluation? First, the test is useful for quantifying general intellectual function in patients receiving initial evaluations when there is other evidence, based on history or clinical interview, that deficits are significant rather than subtle. Second, the DRS can be performed within the context of detailed neuropsychological evaluation administered on a yearly basis to help determine whether there has been a change in neuropsychological status. One study observed that over an 18 month time interval, only 5% of normal older control subjects showed a decline in total score exceeding 10 points. In contrast, over the same time interval 61% of patients diagnosed with dementia showed a decline exceeding 10 points (Smith *et al.,* 1994). Thus, if an active, community-dwelling individual experiences a 10-point decline from the score obtained a year earlier, this supports the possibility that he may have experienced significant decline. In patients previously diagnosed with dementia, the presence of a greater than 10-point decline on yearly assessment is consistent with a progressive dementing disorder.

It is important to note, however, that some patients with dementia, even those with Alzheimer's disease, will have stable periods, sometimes lasting over a year, during which their DRS scores may not change. One study suggested that 39% of demented patients did not show a change exceeding 10 points over the course of 1.4 years (Smith *et al.,* 1994). Therefore, the absence of a decline in DRS total score over the period of a year does not rule out the presence of a progressive disease. In such cases, more challenging neuropsychological tests may be more sensitive for detecting subtle decline.

In addition, the total DRS score can be used cautiously to screen for abnormal cognitive function. For well-functioning individuals without complaints of cognitive dysfunction, it may be cost-effective to use the DRS alone to screen for possible mild dysfunction in conjunction with yearly medical evaluations. To reduce the possibility of failing to identify an individual with mild cognitive dysfunction, a more stringent criterion for identifying possible abnormality might be applied. For example, patients with total scores below 130 (about 1 SD below the mean) might be referred for more detailed neuropsychological and neurologic evaluation.

However, even for individuals with scores above 130, the DRS score alone cannot rule out the presence of neuropsychological dysfunction. If there is significant family or patient concern about decline in cognitive function, it is imperative to administer more challenging tests even when the DRS total score exceeds 130.

TESTS OF SPECIFIC ABILITIES

The following sections describe tests useful for assessing specific neuropsychological domains, including attention, executive function, verbal abilities, and visuospatial function. Assessment of memory and affect are described in Chapters 5 and 10, respectively. The tests described in these chapters have been selected because they are sensitive to major disorders affecting older adults, can be administered in an efficient manner, are well tolerated by most older adults, and have normative data for older age groups.

The review of the tests is organized in terms of the primary neuropsychological domain assessed by each. However, it is important to note that while neuropsychological tests are often described in terms of their utility for assessing a particular neuropsychological domain or brain region, most tests also contribute to the assessment of several interrelated domains and/or regions. It has been suggested that neuropsychological tests are "sensitive" but not "specific" to dysfunction (Costa, 1988). For example, although the Wechsler Logical Memory test is described as assessing "verbal memory," impaired performance could reflect deficits in attention, executive function, or verbal abilities that interfere with the acquisition of new information in memory. Thus, while each test is intended to assess a specific neuropsychological domain, that test also contributes to the evaluation of other domains and their associated brain regions.

Neuropsychological tests tap multiple neuropsychological domains because neuropsychological function depends on neural systems rather than focal brain regions. While a focal brain region may be critical to a specific ability, each ability is also dependent on other neural regions within a system interacting with the critical region. So, for example, executive function depends heavily on the functioning of the frontal lobes. However, the right and left frontal lobes interact heavily with each other and also with posterior cortical and subcortical regions (Alexander et al., 1986; Fuster, 1997; Stuss & Benson, 1986). Thus, a specific neuropsychological domain can be disrupted by a lesion in a brain region critical to that domain or in another regions participating in a neural network that includes the critical region. For example, tests of frontal lobe function are also sensitive to lesions in other brain regions (Anderson et al., 1991; Bigler, 1988).

Therefore, it is the overall pattern of test findings (rather than a particular test score) that is critical in interpreting the results of neuropsychological evaluation.

This overall pattern takes into account both the severity and qualitative characteristics of deficits on particular tests and the interrelationships between these. The pattern is identified by integrating individual test findings to identify an ability or a set of abilities that is consistently below expectation or impaired and then inferring the brain system and neurobehavioral disorder associated with this abnormality. The overall pattern of test findings is often most useful in diagnosing specific disorders and in suggesting compensatory strategies that may be implemented in rehabilitation therapy. An approach to discerning this overall pattern is detailed in Chapter 11.

Attention and Executive Function

Attentional behavior is complex and multidimensional, and different frameworks for conceptualizing attentional behavior have been proposed (Baddeley & Weiskrantz, 1993; Eysenck, 1982; Kahneman, 1973; Moray, 1970; Norman, 1968; Posner & Peterson, 1990; Schneider & Shiffrin, 1977; Zomeran, 1994). In general, attentional behavior refers to the distribution and control of limited-capacity mental resources in order to process information. This information may be internally generated, as during problem solving or remembering, or may be received from the external environment, as when comprehending the comments of another individual or trying to remember material that has just been read.

Because the magnitude of this information typically exceeds the capacity of available mental resources, attentional behavior determines which information is processed. From a clinical perspective, important aspects of attentional behavior include the ability to choose a task on which to attend (selective attention), to maintain mental resources focused on a specific task even in the presence of distraction (focused attention), to allocate mental resources between tasks that must be performed together (divided attention), and to sustain mental resources on a given task over longer periods of time (sustained attention).

Executive function refers to a diverse range of abilities that share the common feature of exerting higher-level control over behavior. One subset includes the abilities to establish and maintain behavior consistent with cues and task requirements (task sets) and to flexibly adjust behavior in response to changing task requirements. For example, when a patient is given test instructions, he must translate these instructions into behavior (establish a task set) and maintain that behavior until the test is complete (maintain a task set). When the task instructions change the patient must adjust his behavior to follow the new instructions (switch the task set).

A second major subset of executive abilities reflects higher-level reasoning. These include the development of task strategies, problem solving, conceptual inference, awareness of the quality of intellectual function, and recognition and display of socially appropriate behavior. For example, if a patient is attempting to remember a word list, the decision to cluster the words on the list based on similarity in meaning reflects use of both strategy and conceptual inference and, thus, executive function.

The clinical instruments useful for evaluating executive function, particularly abilities related to task sets, heavily overlap with those assessing attention. Executive function and attentional behavior also share the common feature of being heavily dependent on the integrity of areas within the frontal lobes (Stuss & Benson, 1986; Zomeran, 1994). The following sections describe instruments useful for evaluating attention and executive function in older adults.

WMS-III Mental Control

Purpose and Administration

This test from the WMS-III requires the performance of simple mental control tasks dependent on abilities to establish and maintain task sets and to focus attention over relatively short time intervals (Wechsler, 1997b). The test items are graded in difficulty, beginning with relatively simple items (e.g., counting from 1 to 20, reciting the alphabet) and progressing to more difficult items (e.g., reciting the months backward, alternating counting by sixes and reciting the days of the week).

Scoring and Interpretation

The score for each mental control item is based on both speed and accuracy of response, with a maximum of 5 points for each item. Analysis of the nature of the patient's errors can be very useful in suggesting difficulties related to task sets, to memory, and to inferential ability. The following examples describe common errors and possible interpretations of these.

• Errors on the later items include elements or reflect response sets from previous Items. For example, on Item 7, after being instructed to recite the months backward, the patient instead recites the months forward, as was done in Item 4. This type of error suggests a perseverative tendency that makes it difficult for the patient to flexibly switch between different task sets.

• The patient's response to an item is initially correct, but then he loses track of what he is doing and fails to complete the item. This suggests difficulty in maintaining the task set. When this occurs, it is often useful to extend the item by cuing the patient to continue. First, the patient can be asked if he remembers what instructions were given, providing an informal test of memory. If he remembers the instructions but is still unable to continue, this implies that the error is more closely related to impaired ability to establish and maintain the task set rather than to a memory deficit.

• The final mental control item requires the patient to alternate counting by sixes with reciting the days of the week. Some patients have difficulty understanding the instructions for this task, and persistent inability to understand the task even when instructions are repeated may reflect impairment in inferential ability.

WAIS/WMS-III Digit Span

Purpose and Administration

The WAIS-III and the WMS-III each include an identical Digit Span (Wechsler, 1997a; Wechsler, 1997b). The patient is instructed to recite digit sequences of increasing length either in the order presented (digits forward) or in reverse order (digits backward). There are two trials for each sequence length, and the standard administration requires that the test be discontinued when the patient makes errors on both trials of identical span length.

It is best to use the standard administration if it is important to minimize test time. However, when a patient without obvious attentional impairment or cognitive dysfunction suddenly misses two consecutive items of a relatively short span length, this suggests a transient lapse of attention, and it may be useful to continue the test beyond the scoring limit to test this hypothesis. If the patient correctly completes subsequent, more difficult trials, the testing can be continued until failure on two trials of identical span length occurs again.

The Digit Span requires comprehension and repetition of spoken digits and, thus, may be difficult for patients with receptive or expressive aphasia, even if they have relatively preserved attention. For aphasic patients, the WMS-III Spatial Span may be substituted for the Digit Span. The Spatial Span requires the patient to attend to a sequence of spatial locations that the examiner demonstrates by tapping with his hand. Then the patient is asked to replicate the tapping either in the order demonstrated by the examiner (forward visual span) or in the reverse order (backward span). Because the test requires visuospatial and motor skills, it is not useful for evaluating attention in aphasic patients with deficits in these skills.

Scoring and Interpretation

The total score is based on the sum of the points prior to failure on two trials of identical span length. Even if the testing is extended to examine the possibility of a transient lapse in attention, the total score is still computed according to standard procedure. Normative data are provided for the total score, combining points received on both forward and backward digit spans.

However, the forward and backward digit span reflect somewhat different abilities, and consideration of whether there is a difference between these spans is often helpful in distinguishing between neurobehavioral disorders (Black, 1986; Sullivan, Sagar, Gabrieli, Corkin, & Growdon, 1989). The forward digit span is a relatively unchallenging, structured test of attention, requiring the patient to attend to the digit list as it is presented and to maintain that list in short-term memory in order to repeat it back to the examiner. Accurate performance depends heavily on "freedom from distractibility" (Lezak, 1995), since the patient can perform well by simply attending to and mimicking the examiner, with little mental manipulation of stimulus material.

In contrast, the backward digit span places greater demands on attention. It requires not only that the patient hold the digit list in short-term memory, but also that the information be mentally manipulated so that it can be repeated in an order reverse to that of the initial presentation. The WAIS-III Administration and Scoring Manual provides separate norms for the longest digit forward span and the longest digit backward span.

Patients with mild neuropsychological dysfunction often show deficits on the backward digit span before these are present on the forward digit span. Even after age adjustments are applied, patients with neurodegenerative disease may exhibit an impaired backward span in the presence of a relatively preserved forward span (Loring & Largen, 1985). In contrast, if the forward span is shorter than the backward span, this suggests that the forward span was degraded by distractibility or inconsistent effort, a pattern often seen in individuals who are anxious or depressed. Distractability or inconsistent effort may also cause patients with affective disorder to exhibit variability over test trials, for example, missing relatively easy items and then completing more difficult items. Although the backward span requires comprehension of verbally presented material, the mental processes involved in reversing the digits may reflect the use of visual imagery and visuospatial abilities. Thus, patients with right brain lesions may have an impaired backward span (Costa, 1975; Rapport, Webster, & Dutra, 1994).

Trail-Making Test

Purpose and Administration

The Trail-Making Test was developed by the Army (1944) and is in the public domain. It has two parts, Trails A and Trails B. In Trails A, the patient is presented with a page on which randomly placed letters are enclosed in small circles. The patient is instructed to draw lines connecting the letters in alphabetical order. In Trails B, the page includes circled letters and also circled numbers. The patient is instructed to draw lines connecting the letters and numbers in an order that alternates between increasing numeric value and alphabetic order (1, A, 2, B, etc.). The instructions specify that the patient should work as quickly as possible, without lifting the pencil point off the page. If an error is made, this is pointed out to the patient, who then continues from the point at which the error occurred. The test score is the total time to complete the condition, including the time necessary to correct errors. If the patient fails to complete a condition within 5 minutes, it can be discontinued. Detailed instructions for the Trail-Making Test are provided elsewhere (Spreen & Strauss, 1998). An oral Trail-Making Test is available for evaluating attention and mental tracking in patients with known impairment in vision or motor abilities (Ricker, Axelrod, & Houtler, 1996).

Scoring and Interpretation

Separate measures are obtained for Trails A and Trails B, each representing the total time to complete the condition. The test score is age-sensitive (Ivnik *et al.*, 1996), with older adults requiring more time. In addition, the patient's education should be considered in interpreting test scores, particularly those having less than an eleventh grade education. Individuals having limited education may require more time to complete the test even in the absence of abnormality (Bornstein & Suga, 1988).

The Mayo's Older Americans Normative Studies (MOANS) provide norms for adults aged 56 to 97 years, although these are not education-adjusted and must be applied cautiously with individuals with limited education or with non-whites (Ivnik et al., 1996). Norms are also available as a function of age (range = 20 to 80 years), education (range = 6 to 18+ years) and sex (Heaton, Grant, & Matthews, 1991).

The Trail-Making Test places demands on a number of different abilities. Both Trails A and B require sustained attention, visual scanning and perception, and visuomotor ability. Because of its requirement to switch between numeric and alphabetic sets, Trails B places greater demands on divided attention and cognitive flexibility. Since the primary test score is the time to complete the test, overall mental speed affects performance.

The Trail-Making Test, particularly Part B, is highly sensitive to subtle brain dysfunction. The test was introduced as a measure of frontal lobe function (Halstead, 1947), and in healthy individuals, electrophysiological data suggest greater sensitivity of this test to the function of the anterior brain, including the frontal lobes, than to posterior brain function (Segalowitz, Unsal, & Dywan, 1992). However, test performance can also be impaired by lesions in posterior brain regions (Heilbronner, Henry, Buck, Adams, & Fogle, 1991; Reitan & Wolfson, 1995), most likely because such lesions disrupt a complex, interacting neural system including the frontal lobes. Thus, although impaired performance on Trails B does not necessarily imply a lesion within the frontal lobe, such performance can be interpreted as reflecting dysfunction with a brain system involving the frontal lobe.

The Trail-Making Test has the great advantage of being brief, sensitive to subtle brain dysfunction, and useful for tracking possible progression of neuropsychological dysfunction. Deficient performance on this test has been observed in the early phases of dementing illnesses such as Alzheimer's disease (Lafleche & Albert, 1995) and can contribute to the tracking of progressive decline (Greenlief, Margolis, & Erker, 1985; Storandt, Botwinick, & Danziger, 1986; Storandt, Botwinick, Danziger, Berg, & Hughes, 1984). Alzheimer's disease patients with parkinsonian features show greater deficits on Trails than do Alzheimer's patients without these features (Merello *et al.,* 1994). Patients with age-associated memory impairment, who are at increased risk for developing dementing illnesses, show deficits on tests of executive function, including the Trail-Making Test (Hanninen *et al.,* 1997). Trails B is also sensitive to subtle neuropsychological abnormalities associated with very mild cerebrovascular disease in apparently normal, nondemented older adults (Breteler *et al.,* 1994; Schmidt *et al.,* 1993), to hypoemia in chronic pulmonary obstructive disease (Grant *et al.,* 1987a), and to mild head injury (Leininger, Gramling, Farrell, Kreutzer, & Peck, 1990). Because of its sensitivity to dysfunction within frontal-subcortical systems, Trail-Making performance is often deficient in patients with movement disorders, including Huntington's or Parkinson's disease, although motor dyscontrol may make a major contribution to this impairment (Starkstein *et al.,* 1988; Taylor, Saint-Cyr, & Lang, 1986a). Alcoholics often show impaired performance on this test (Parsons & Leber, 1981).

Thus, while not specific to frontal lobe function, the Trail-Making Test is sensitive to dysfunction associated with a range of disorders affecting frontal lobe brain systems. Because of its brevity, its sensitivity to subtle neuropsychological dysfunction, and the availability of age-adjusted norms, Trails is one of the best tests to use in screening for neuropsychological function and in identifying individuals who require more detailed neuropsychological assessment and other diagnostic procedures. It also provides an efficient means for evaluating the presence and rate of neuropsychological change in disorders suspected to be progressive.

Wisconsin Card Sorting Test

Purpose and Administration

In the Wisconsin Card Sorting Test (WCST), the patient must infer and switch rules for card sorting based on feedback provided by the examiner (Berg, 1948; Grant & Berg, 1948; Heaton, Chelune, Talley, Kay, & Curtiss, 1993). The test requires the patient to integrate feedback received on each test trial to establish, maintain, and switch strategies for card sorting. The test also demands sustained attention in that it can take some time to complete and also involves analysis of visuospatial stimuli. Although some of the demands of the WCST are similar to those of the Trail-Making Test, the WCST is more difficult because of its greater reliance on the use of higher-level conceptualization, strategy, and integration of feedback.

The WCST has a number of other positive features. The full version of the test is well standardized and widely used. Normative data adjusted for age and education are available for age groups up to age 89 (Heaton *et al.,* 1993), although caution must be exerted when interpreting data for patients between ages 85 and 89 because of the small normative samples for this age group. The test provides a number of measures reflecting related but distinctive abilities, including facility in conceptualization, tendency toward perseverative responding, and the ability to maintain a task set. Among the most useful measures are the number of categories achieved (or a highly correlated measure, the total number of errors), the number of perseverative responses, and the number of response set losses. Because the test is challenging, it is sensitive to subtle neuropsychological dysfunction that may be present in high-functioning individuals who are developing dementia. Test scores do not depend heavily on mental speed.

However, the WCST has several significant disadvantages, the major one being that it is somewhat difficult and time-consuming to administer. Administration requires the examiner to record subject responses and determine feedback on each test trial, and administration and scoring errors are common (Flashman, Horner, & Freides, 1991; Paolo, Axelrod, & Ryan, 1994). Although a computer-administered version of the test is available (Heaton & PAR staff, 1999), the patient's lack of experience in using computers may compromise performance (Artiola i Fortuny & Heaton, 1996), thus making questionable the validity of the computer-based version in the assessment of older individuals with minimal computer experience. Standard administration may take only 20 minutes in relatively intact individuals but may take as long as 40 minutes in patients with significant dysfunction. Some patients become very frustrated by this test, and this may affect their motivation and cooperation during subsequent tests.

Several shortened versions of the WCST have been developed (Axelrod, Henry, & Woodard, 1992; Nelson, 1976; Robinson, Kester, Saykin, Kaplan, & Gur, 1991). The most attractive of these is the WCST-64, which requires administration of only one of the two card decks using otherwise standard administration procedures (Axelrod *et al.,* 1992; Axelrod, Jiron, & Henry, 1993). This form takes considerably less time to administer than the standard WCST and provides test scores that correlate well with those of the standard test (Axelrod *et al.,* 1992; Smith-Seemiller, Franzen, & Bowers, 1997). However, a major disadvantage of the WCST-64, as well as of the other alternative short forms, is the absence of age-adjusted normative data. Some normative data for older age groups are available for the WCST-64 (Axelrod *et al.,* 1993), but even these data are based on small sample sizes (N=20 per age group). The absence of adequate age-adjusted normative data is likely to produce a high rate of false positive errors, that is, identification of older individuals as impaired when, in fact, they are not (Smith-Seemiller *et al.,* 1997). Thus, the WCST-64 must be used cautiously until better age- and education-adjusted normative data become available.

Given these pros and cons, the decision to administer the WCST should be considered carefully. It may be most useful when evaluating individuals suspected to have relatively high premorbid function without obvious neuropsychological deficits during the clinical interview. If the patient becomes upset during administration of the WCST, it is recommended that only one deck be administered and that the age-adjusted norms for the WCST-64 (Axelrod *et al.,* 1993) be applied with caution.

Scoring and Interpretation

The WCST can be scored by the examiner, but this is complex and scoring errors are common (Flashman *et al.,* 1991; Paolo *et al.,* 1994). Fortunately, a computer-based scoring program is now available (Harris, 1999). In the long run, the use of computer-based scoring programs is cost-effective and increases the accuracy of scoring. The manual for the WCST suggests a classification system and guidelines for determining whether normative scores are within normal limits or, if not, the relative degree of impairment (Heaton *et al.,* 1993; Heaton *et al.,* 1991).

Since the WCST was originally developed to evaluate abstract reasoning and the ability to shift cognitive strategy in response to feedback (Berg, 1948; Grant & Berg, 1948), it has been considered a test of executive function. Neuropsychological interest in the test was stimulated by studies suggesting that dorsolateral frontal lesions resulted in pronounced deficits in performance (Drewe, 1974; Milner, 1963; Robinson, Heaton, Lehman, & Stilson, 1980), and the test has traditionally been used as a test of frontal lobe function. However, more recent structural imaging studies have observed that patients with non-dorsolateral frontal as well as nonfrontal lesions show impairment in WCST performance similar to that associated with dorsolateral lesions (Anderson *et al.,* 1991; Grafman, Jonas, & Salazar, 1990a).

This apparent contradiction between the earlier and more recent findings probably reflects the fact that performance of the WCST involves a complex neural network including the frontal lobes but other brain regions as well. In healthy individuals, performance of the WCST is associated with activation of the dorsolateral frontal lobe but also with activation of other more posterior brain regions, including the inferior parietal lobe, the visual association and inferotemporal cortices, and areas within the cerebellum (Berman *et al.,* 1995). It has been suggested that this network, particularly its frontal and parietal components, may be fundamental to working memory (Berman *et al.,* 1995), and since the WCST activates this network, the test is useful for assessing working memory. Thus, as with the Trail-Making Test, the WCST is sensitive but not specific to frontal lobe function. While the frontal lobe is important to performance of this test, this region is only one part of a neural network involving other, more posterior brain regions.

There has also been controversy as to whether impairment on the WCST implies asymmetry in frontal lobe dysfunction, that is, greater compromise of the left or right frontal lobe. Some studies have implied that the test has increased sensitivity to left frontal function (Grafman *et al.,* 1990a; Milner, 1963; Rezai *et al.,* 1993), some to right frontal function (Bornstein, 1986; Robinson *et al.,* 1980), and some have not observed asymmetry (Anderson *et al.,* 1991; Berman *et al.,* 1995). The absence of a reliable and pronounced asymmetry in WCST performance may, in fact, reflect the highly interconnected and interactive nature of the frontal lobes. It is not recommended that the WCST be used as a measure to determine asymmetry of brain dysfunction.

While not specific to dysfunction of the frontal lobes, the WCST is sensitive to impairment associated with a number of disorders compromising the function of these brain regions. High rates of perseverative responding are seen in both alcoholics (Jones & Parsons, 1971) and schizophrenics (Goldberg, Weinberger, Berman, Pliskin, & Podd, 1987; Van der Does & Van den Bosch, 1992). Impaired performance on the WCST is seen in Huntington's disease and other movement disorders compromising the function of frontal–subcortical neural systems (Pillon, Dubois, Lhermitte, & Agid, 1986). Cerebrovascular disease affecting the frontal lobes or neural regions closely interacting with the frontal lobes, particularly subcortical regions, may be reflected in impaired WCST performance (Anderson *et al.,* 1991; Robinson *et al.,* 1980). Patients with significant dementia generally perform poorly on the WCST, and the degree of impairment may reflect the relative involvement of frontal lobe systems in the dementia. For example, patients with Parkinson's disease with dementia may perform more poorly on the WCST than equivalently demented patients with Alzheimer's disease (Pillon *et al.*, 1986). In nondemented patients with Parkinson's disease, the WCST is sensitive to subtle deficits (Caltagirone, Carlesimo, Nocentini, & Vicari, 1989; Lees & Smith, 1983; Paolo, Axelrod, Troster, Blackwell, & Koller, 1996) and may be useful for tracking the progression and rate of neuropsychological change.

WAIS-III Similarities

Purpose and Administration

This test from the WAIS-III requires the use of higher-level conceptualization and reasoning abilities (Wechsler, 1997a). The examiner asks the patient to state the similarity between pairs of named items, for example, "In what way are a fork and a spoon alike?" Most of the items can be correctly answered in one or two words, although patients with intact reasoning but mild language dysfunction may have difficulty expressing themselves. The WAIS-III manual instructs examiners to use probe questions when the patient gives an unclear or ambiguous response, and use of such probes is particularly important when assessing older individuals who are suspected to have expressive speech impairment and who may require encouragement and extra time to express their knowledge.

For patients with severe expressive language difficulty (expressive aphasia), the examiner may chose to use the Similarities from the WAIS-R as a Neuropsychological Instrument (WAIS-R NI), which provides a multiple-choice format (Kaplan, Fein, Morris, & Delis, 1991). Patients are asked to choose the best response from multiple-choice alternative responses, which they can read or which can be read to them. The test may be particularly useful in rehabilitation settings involving assessment of preserved abilities in patients suffering from severe expressive aphasia. It is not uncommon for these patients to have relatively preserved language comprehension and reasoning abilities despite being unable to express themselves verbally.

Scoring and Interpretation

Test scoring is described in the WAIS-III Administration and Scoring Manual. Patients are given full credit (2 points) for higher-level, abstract responses and partial credit (1 point) for correct but more concrete responses.

The WAIS-III Similarities is a revision of the WAIS-R Similarities, and it is assumed that their neuropsychological correlates are similar. Education is an important variable affecting Similarities scores (Kaufman, McLean, & Reynolds, 1988; Kaufman, McLean, & Reynolds, 1991), so low test scores in poorly educated individuals may not represent a decline and must be interpreted cautiously. Several studies have observed that African-American patients also obtain lower scores (Kaufman *et al.*, 1991; Manly *et al.*, 1998), and a recent comprehensive study indicated that this difference did not reflect group variation in level of education or medical conditions such as hypertension or diabetes (Manly *et al.,* 1998).

Both metabolic studies of brain activation and lesion studies have related performance on the Similarities to the functioning of left temporal and frontal regions (Chase *et al.,* 1984; Newcombe, 1969). In patients with multiple sclerosis, lowered Similarities scores have been associated with bilateral frontal lesions (Rao, 1990). Decline in Similarities performance may be predictive of abnormal cognitive decline in middle-aged individuals (LaRue & Jarvik, 1987). In nondemented older adults, a relative weakness on the Similarities may be predictive of a later diagnosis of Alzheimer's disease (Jacobs *et al.,* 1995b; Manly *et al.,* 1998). Impaired performance is seen in patients with dementia (Whelihan & Lesher, 1985). However, in mildly demented patients, the deficit may be small or absent (Lafleche & Albert, 1995; Larrabee, Largen, & Levin, 1985), perhaps due to the test's relatively low dependence on concurrent manipulation of information in comparison with other tests of executive function (Lafleche & Albert, 1995).

Verbal Abilities

Speech Comprehension

Observation of the patient's behavior during the clinical interview and formal testing makes an important contribution to the evaluation of speech comprehension. Relatively preserved speech comprehension is suggested by the patient's ability to respond to questions about his concerns and history, to react appropriately to comments made by the examiner and accompanying family members, and to respond to instructions for simple tests.

Although difficulty in responding to questions or instructions raises the possibility of a deficit in speech comprehension (*receptive aphasia*), this may reflect impairment in other abilities. Patients may have difficulty responding to questions if they experience a lapse in attention or have difficulty remembering questions, expressing speech (*expressive aphasia*), or organizing behavior in response to commands (executive function). If the patient continues to exhibit confusion even when instructions or questions are repeated loudly and clearly, this reduces the possibility that a hearing deficit or an attentional lapse is critical in explaining the impairment. The contribution of deficits in memory, expressive speech, or executive function can be assessed within the context of other findings from formal testing.

In older patients, receptive aphasia is uncommon in patients with mild dementia, with the exception of those who have experienced strokes compromising the functioning of the posterior temporal lobe (Wernicke's area, see Chapter 7). In many cases, difficulty in responding questions is more closely related to deficits in other abilities rather than reflecting true receptive aphasia. However, if there is evidence of significant receptive aphasia, then more formal testing may be necessary, particularly for better specifying the nature of the aphasia in rehabilitation settings. This can be accomplished by using the Boston Diagnostic Aphasia Examination (Goodglass & Kaplan, 1983).

The presence of receptive aphasia may preclude administration of other tests involving comprehension of verbal language. In such cases, testing can focus on the evaluation of nonverbal abilities. Some patients with receptive aphasia may be able to understand written language better than spoken language, so it may be possible to evaluate other abilities by using written instructions. Although time-consuming, this may be particularly important where identification of preserved abilities is important, as in rehabilitation settings. Materials from the the WAIS-R NI may be useful in evaluating patients with receptive aphasia because they include written multiple-choice versions for the WAIS-R Similarities, Comprehension, Vocabulary, and Information (Kaplan *et al.,* 1991). Thus, with some flexibility and extra time, it is possible to assess patients with severe impairment in language comprehension.

Expressive Speech

Observation of the patient's behavior is also important to the evaluation of expressive speech. During the clinical interview, it is important to query the patient specifically about the presence of changes in expressive speech, particularly increased difficulty in word finding *(dysnomia).* If the patient is halting or slow in responding to questions, this suggests a deficit in word finding. Even if there is no evidence of dysnomia based on the patient's history or the clinical interview, formal testing of word finding should be conducted. The Boston Naming Test can be used for this purpose, as described in the following section.

The presence of significant dysnomia will compromise performance on other tests requiring production of verbal responses, and this should be considered in interpreting the findings from these tests. In cases of pronounced expressive aphasia, the multiple-choice tests from the WAIS-R NI may be administered.

Boston Naming Test

Purpose and Administration

The Boston Naming Test (BNT) is used in the evaluation of expressive speech, particularly the ability to recall (or find) the names of common objects. *Dysnomia* refers to difficulty in finding words; *anomia* is more severe and refers to the inability to find words.

In the BNT, the patient is presented with line drawings of 60 common objects (e.g., a house, a beaver), and is asked to name each item (Kaplan, Goodglass, & Weintraub, 1983). It is recommended that the following instructions be provided to patients (Lezak, 1995, p. 537): "I'm going to show you some pictures and your job is to tell me the common name for them. If you can't think of the name and it's something you know, you can tell me something you know about it."

Encouraging the patient to indicate recognition of each item, even if the specific name can't be retrieved, allows the examiner to better appreciate if the patient is accurately perceiving the items and facilitates the correct use of cues.

If the patient cannot correctly name the item within 20 seconds, a cue is provided. The nature of the cue depends on the nature of the patient's error. A *phonemic cue* is provided if the nature of the error indicates that the patient has correctly recognized the stimulus item but cannot retrieve the specific name. For example, the patient's response might be related in meaning to the correct response (e.g, naming a beaver as a rat or as an animal); this is labeled a *semantic error.* Another common type of error is a *circumlocutory error,* when the patient describes the item in several words (e.g., describing a beaver as "an animal that eats trees"). In cases of semantic or circumlocutory errors or when the examiner believes the patient has correctly perceived the stimulus item, the patient is provided with a phonemic cue, the initial phonemes (sound) of the correct response (e.g., for beaver, the phonemic cue is, "it begins with be...").

However, if the patient's response suggests that he has failed to recognize or has clearly misperceived the pictured item, a *semantic cue* is given. Difficulty perceiving the item is suggested if the patient makes a *stimulus* or *perceptual error* (e.g., names a beaver as a paddle) or fails to respond within 20 seconds of item presentation. Misperceptions sometimes reflect *inappropriate pull to stimulus detail*—the patient is perceiving the item with respect to one of its details rather than in terms of its gestalt. For example, naming a beaver as a paddle may represent inappropriate pull to stimulus detail in that the patient is naming the item in terms of one of its details (the beaver's tail) rather than in terms of its whole image. When perceptual impairment seems likely, the examiner provides a stimulus cue by describing the semantic class of the item (for example, "it's an animal"). If the patient still fails to correctly name the item, a phonemic cue is then given.

According to the instructions in the stimulus booklet, the testing is discontinued when the patient makes "six consecutive failures." It is recommended that this discontinuation rule be applied in a rigorous fashion by ending the test after the patient makes six naming errors. It is important to note that if the patient responds correctly following a semantic cue, that trial is not considered to reflect a naming error, since a perceptual deficit rather than a naming deficit may have accounted for the patient's initial difficulty. However, if a phonemic cue is followed by a correct response, this trial is counted as a naming error, since the patient's initial mistake is more likely to have reflected a naming deficit. If the patient receives frequent benefit from phonemic cues, this suggests that the naming deficit is not dense.

Although the BNT is relatively brief and easily administered, a number of "short forms" have been developed in which only a subset of the items from the standard BNT is administered (Mack, Freed, Williams, & Henderson, 1992; Williams, Mack, & Henderson, 1989). Use of a short form reduces testing time, but the absence of normative data for specific short forms increases the possibility that the patient may be misdiagnosed (Franzen, Haut, Rankin, & Keefover, 1995). However, if it is necessary to use a short form, it is recommended that one of the "odd-even" short forms be administered, in which only the odd or only the even-numbered items are presented to the patient. These 30-item versions better preserve the availability of the BNT's rich qualitative error data than is the case with even shorter versions. The scores on the odd and even versions correlate highly with each other (Mack *et al.*, 1992; Williams *et al.*, 1989), so they can be alternated in repeated testing to minimize practice effects. The total test score can be estimated by doubling the score obtained from performance on 30 items. This estimated total score correlates highly with the total test score obtained from standard test administration (Franzen et al., 1995; Williams *et al.*, 1989).

Scoring and Interpretation

The standard scoring for the BNT is described in the test booklet. The total raw score includes spontaneously correct responses plus responses correct after stimulus cues were provided. Crediting the patient for items that were initially misperceived but then named correctly after semantic cuing allows the total raw score to more accurately reflect the quality of naming alone independently of perceptual deficits.

Normative data are provided in the BNT booklet. These were based on a relatively small sample and apply only to age groups up to age 59. Age-related changes are not pronounced before 70 to 80 years, although between-individual variability and thus the standard deviation increase above age 60 (Ross, Lichtenberg, & Christensen, 1995; Van Gorp, Satz, Kiersch, & Henry, 1986; Welch, Doineau, Johnson, & King, 1996). The MOANS provides normative data for a large community-dwelling Caucasian sample between 56 and 97 years of age, the majority of whom are high school graduates. Age-stratified normative data are provided by Spreen and Strauss (1998, p. 436) based on the findings collected from several different centers and by Tombaugh and Hubley (1997) based on a large Canadian sample. Norms have also been published for older adults from middle Tennessee (Welch *et al.*, 1996), for urban elderly medical patients (Ross & Lichtenberg, 1998), for a Spanish-speaking sample (Allegri *et al.*, 1997), for native Americans (Ferraro & Bercier, 1996), and for older Australians (Worrall, Yiu, Hickson, & Barnett, 1995).

To avoid false positive errors, BNT scores must be interpreted cautiously for individuals having less than a high school education and for those with poor reading or verbal abilities or from minority groups. These individuals tend to obtain lower scores, particularly in comparison with relatively well-educated Caucasian individuals (Hawkins *et al.*, 1993; Ross *et al.*, 1995). Age-related changes may appear earlier in individuals with less than a high school education (Welch et al., 1996). African-American patients who are either community-dwelling or experiencing mild Alzheimer's disease may score lower than Caucasian patients even when matched for age and education (Fillenbaum, Huber, & Taussig, 1997; Welsh *et al.*, 1995a). It is recommended that regionally appropriate responses be scored as correct (e.g., in the southern United States, "tomwalkers" for stilts).

In addition to computing the patient's total score, the nature of errors and the benefits of cuing should be carefully analyzed. The examiner should summarize the kind of errors, particularly semantic, perceptual, and perseverative errors and those suggestive of pull to stimulus detail. In clinical practice, if a patient provides correct responses after phonemic cues on at least half of the semantic error trials, this may be interpreted as suggesting that the patient benefits from phonemic cues. For example, if the patient made 8 semantic errors but gave 6 correct responses after being provided with phonemic cues, this suggests that the patient benefits from phonemic cuing and that the naming deficit is not severely dense.

In community-dwelling individuals, relatively weak performance on the BNT raises the possibility that the patient is experiencing preclinical Alzheimer's disease (Jacobs et al., 1995b). The BNT is highly sensitive to mild Alzheimer's disease (Cahn *et al.,* 1995; LaBerge, Balota, Storandt, & Smith, 1992; Storandt *et al.,* 1984), and decline in performance is common as the disease progresses (Rebok, Brandt, & Folstein, 1990). In Alzheimer's disease patients, markedly impaired scores may be predictive of a more rapidly progressive disease course (Faber-Langendoen *et al.,* 1988). In these patients, semantic errors and circumlocutions have been associated with metabolic changes in the left mesial and lateral temporal lobe (Welsh *et al.,* 1995b), and performance on a 15-item short form of the BNT has been related to structural measures of the temporal lobe and hippocampus (Wilson *et al.,* 1996).

Patients having disorders other than Alzheimer's disease may also show impaired performance on the BNT, although the deficit may be small or absence in non-Alzheimer's disease patients with mild or no dementia. Patients experiencing diseases more strongly affecting subcortical structures often receive benefit from phonemic cues. The BNT may be useful in distinguishing between mild Alzheimer's disease and vascular dementia, with Alzheimer's disease patients performing more poorly (Barr, Benedict, Tune, & Brandt, 1992). In Parkinson's disease, the presence of naming deficits in nondemented, nondepressed patients is controversial. Some studies have failed to observe a naming deficit (Beatty, Stanton, Weir, Monson, & Whitaker 1989; Huber *et al.,* 1989a), but others have observed a mild decline in the naming scores of Parkinson's disease patients in comparison with community-dwelling control subjects (Goldman, Baty, Buckles, Sahrmann, & Morris, 1998; Matison, Mayeux, Rosen, & Fahn, 1982). In general, the naming deficit observed in Parkinson's disease patients without dementia is milder than that associated with Alzheimer's disease (Huber et al., 1989b), and phonemic cuing often facilitates naming in nondemented Parkinson's disease patients (Matison *et al.,* 1982). In Parkinson's patients, a rapid decline in naming may precede the development of dementia (Stern *et al.,* 1998). Patients with Huntington's disease may show impaired naming, but their errors are more likely to reflect visuoperceptual dysfunction rather than the semantic dysfunction associated with Alzheimer's disease (Hodges *et al.,* 1991).

In patients with depression, those with mild to moderate affective disorder often show normal performance (Boone *et al.,* 1995). The presence of impaired performance in depressed patients may be predictive of a poor prognosis (King, Caine, Conwell, & Cox, 1991b). Impaired naming in depressed patients may suggest an underlying nontreatable dementia rather than depression-related cognitive dysfunction (Hill *et al.,* 1992).

The presence of perceptual errors suggests a number of possibilities, including impairment in visual perception and inappropriate pull to stimulus detail. Visual perception is often deficient in individuals who have experienced right occipital or parietal brain strokes and in patients with neurodegenerative disorders, including Huntington's disease and Parkinson's disease. Although semantic errors are more common in Alzheimer's disease, some patients have pronounced visuoperceptual impairment, and subtypes of Alzheimer's disease have been described in which impairment in visual perception is more pronounced than impairment in language-related abilities such as naming (Becker, Hubb, Nebes, Holland, & Boller, 1988; Fisher *et al.,* 1996; Martin *et al.,* 1986; Weintraub & Mesulam, 1993; Weintraub & Mesulam, 1996). Perceptual errors raise the possibility of dysfunction in right hemisphere structures important for visual object recognition.

When patients make very rapid, impulsive responses resulting in perceptual errors, particularly inappropriate pull to stimulus detail, this may reflect dysfunction in frontal lobe–executive function systems important to controlling and monitoring the quality of behavior. Inappropriate pull to stimulus detail or fragmentation errors, in which parts of the stimulus are interpreted as the whole, may suggest right frontal lobe dysfunction.

Word Fluency

Purpose and Administration

Patients are instructed to generate as many different words as they can within a 1-minute time limit according to specified criteria. Two forms of this test are widely used in clinical practice, letter (phonemic) fluency and category (semantic) fluency.

In the letter fluency test, patients are cued to generate words beginning with a specified letter. Typically, patients are given three trials of 60 seconds each, with a different letter for each trial. A popular version of the letter fluency test employs the letters F, A, and S, and therefore is often referred to as FAS. Alternately, the Multilingual Aphasia Examination provides two equivalent letter sets (C,F,L and P,R,W) (Benton & Hamsher, 1989). Words beginning with FAS have a higher dictionary frequency than those beginning with CFL/PRW, which suggests that the FAS letter fluency test may be easier. Indeed, the equivalence of the two tests has been questioned (Ruff, Light, & Parker, 1996), although one study of hospital inpatients having varied diagnoses reported significant and high correlations between FAS and CFL test scores (Lacey *et al.,* 1996).

In general, it is recommended that norms be selected that are specific to the test version administered. Since norms for older age groups are more available for FAS than for CFL/PRW, the former test is often more useful in evaluating older adults. Instructions for administration of the FAS test are provided elsewhere (Spreen & Strauss, 1998). During test administration, it is important to record all of the patient's responses, including correct responses and errors, within each successive 15-second interval.

In the category fluency test, the patient is instructed to generate words representing specified categories, such as animals, supermarket items, fruits, and vegetables. One minute is allowed per category. In parallel with letter fluency tests, three category fluency trials are often administered, and there is evidence that performance based on three trials provides measures of greater utility than performance based on fewer trials. It is important to carefully select the category cues because test difficulty is greater for categories having fewer numbers of exemplars. It is recommended that the three categories of animals, fruits, and vegetables be used during evaluation of older adults because normative data for older age groups are available for these categories (Lucas *et al.*, 1998). In addition, category fluency is tested during administration of the Mattis Dementia Rating Scale using the category of supermarket items as the cue. As with the letter fluency test, it is important to record all of the patient's responses, including correct responses and errors, within each successive 15-second interval.

Scoring and Interpretation

For word fluency tests, the main quantitative score is the total number of words generated, and this is most critical for determining whether performance is within normal limits. Among demographic variables important in interpreting data, patient age is the most critical, particularly in interpreting category fluency performance. Age changes in letter fluency are minimal, but age-related decline is more pronounced for category fluency, and the extent of this decline varies as a function of the specific category cue (Bolla, Lindgren, Bonaccorsy, & Bleecker, 1990; Kozora & Cullum, 1995; Mittenberg, Seidenberg, O'Leary, & DiGiulio, 1989; Ruff *et al.*, 1996; Tomer & Levin, 1993). One study of healthy, relatively well-educated individuals averaging 14 years of schooling did not observe significant change in FAS performance between ages 50 and 89 (Kozora & Cullum, 1995). In this study, decline in performance occurred after age 69 for the categories of animal names and supermarket items but at age 50 for the category of first names (Kozora & Cullum, 1995). Therefore, in interpreting data it is important to apply normative data for the specific category cue used during testing.

Normative data for fluency tests are available for samples tested by specific groups of clinicians rather than based on a population sample. Such normative data must be applied cautiously, keeping in mind the exact cue used to elicit fluency and significant differences between characteristics of the patient being evaluated and the normative sample. The MOANS provides normative data for FAS letter fluency based on performance of a relatively well-educated, largely Caucasian sample between 55 and 97 years of age. Another set of normative data is available for FAS letter fluency for ages 16 to 95, including large older samples stratified by age (Spreen & Strauss, 1998). For CFL/PRW letter fluency, normative values are available for adults stratified by education and sex but not by age (Ruff *et al.*, 1996).

For category fluency, normative data for the categories of animals, fruits, and vegetables are available from the MOANS (Lucas *et al.*, 1998). Normative data are available for the category of animals alone for ages between 16 and 95 years stratified by years of education (Spreen & Strauss, 1998). Several experimental studies provide normative data for the combined categories of animals, fruits, and vegetables for middle-aged (mean age 50.8, standard deviation 17.2 years) and elderly (mean age 70.0, standard deviation 10.6 years), relatively well-educated (mean years of education = 14 years) control subjects (Monsch *et al.*, 1994; Monsch *et al.*, 1992).

Word fluency must be cautiously interpreted for individuals who are illiterate or poorly educated or those for whom English is not a first language. Reading ability has been significantly related to letter fluency performance (Crawford, Moore, & Cameron, 1992). Reports of sex differences have been inconsistent (Bolla et al., 1990; Kozora & Cullum, 1995).

Neuroanatomical studies implicate areas within the frontal, temporal, and parietal lobes, particularly within the left brain hemisphere, as being critical to word fluency performance. In healthy volunteers, performance of fluency tests is associated with increased activation in the frontal lobes. One study observed activation of bilateral frontal and temporal lobe regions during letter fluency performance (Parks *et al.*, 1988), while a later study observed prominent left dorsolateral prefrontal activation during letter and category fluency tasks, as well as less pronounced left parietal and bilateral anterior cingulate gyrus activation (Frith, Friston, Liddle, & Frackowiak, 1991).

Differences between the nature of the fluency tasks may help explain this variation in findings. A recent study of the impact of specific brain lesions on fluency performance observed that letter fluency was impaired by left dorsolateral, striatal, and parietal lesions or by superior (although not inferior) medial frontal lesions in the right or left hemisphere (Stuss *et al.*, 1998). Category fluency was impaired by lesions in similar sites and also those in right dorsolateral and inferior medial frontal regions.

Word fluency performance may contribute to both detection and tracking of neurobehavioral disorders. Impairment in fluency performance, particularly category fluency, may contribute to the detection of mild Alzheimer's disease (Cahn et al., 1995; Masur, Sliwinski, Lipton, Blau, & Crystal, 1994; Monsch *et al.*, 1992). Mildly impaired Alzheimer's disease patients may also have deficits in letter fluency (Lafleche & Albert, 1995). Deficits in letter and category performance in nondemented patients with Parkinson's disease may be predictive of the subsequent development of dementia (Jacobs *et al.*, 1995a). Impairment in letter fluency may be relatively more impaired in frontotemporal dementia than in Alzheimer's disease (Pachana, Boone, Miller, Cummings, & Berman, 1996). In patients with Alzheimer's disease, the progression of the disease may be indicated by a decline in category fluency (Barr & Brandt, 1996; Chan, Salmon, Butters, & Johnson, 1995; Welsh, Butters, Hughes, Mohs, & Heyman, 1992), and category fluency may also be sensitive to progression of vascular disease (Barr & Brandt, 1996). In contrast, in patients with Huntington's disease, changes in letter fluency may be more sensitive to disease progression (Barr & Brandt, 1996). In older patients with depression, changes in letter fluency may be subtle in mildly depressed patients, but the decline may be more pronounced in those experiencing more severe depression (Boone *et al.,* 1995). Thus, impairment in letter fluency performance may not be helpful in distinguishing between moderately depressed patients and those with mild dementia.

Comparison between the relative impairment in category fluency and letter fluency may be informative in differentiating between disorders. This comparison should be made between standardized test scores (see Chapter 11) rather than raw data scores. The use of letter and category fluency standard scores each based on the MOANS normative sample may be particularly useful. Alzheimer's disease patients may show disproportionate impairment in category fluency (Butters, Granholm, Salmon, Grant, & Wolfe, 1987; Martin & Fedio, 1983; Monsch *et al.,* 1992), while patients with more subcortically based disorders such as Huntington's disease often show deficits of similar magnitude on both fluency tests (Monsch et al., 1994). With disease progression, Alzheimer's disease patients may show an even greater deficit in category fluency as compared with letter fluency, while patients with subcortical disorders such as Huntington's disease may show the opposite pattern (Hodges, Salmon, & Butters, 1990). During tests of category fluency, patients with Huntington's disease or Parkinson's disease may benefit from cueing with subordinate categories (e.g., pets or farm animals for the category of animals), while Alzheimer's disease patients may not improve when cued (Randolph, Braun, Goldberg, & Chase, 1993).

The difference in fluency test performance between patients with Alzheimer's disease and those with more subcortically based disorders such as Parkinson's disease or Huntington's disease has been interpreted as reflecting disease-specific differences in the pattern of cognitive change. The disproportionate impairment of category fluency in Alzheimer's disease has been hypothesized as reflecting the breakdown and loss of semantic memory associated with this disorder (Hodges, Salmon, & Butters, 1992b; Monsch *et al.,* 1994). In contrast, the impairment of fluency performance in Huntington's disease and Parkinson's disease has been related to deficiencies in memory retrieval mechanisms (Monsch *et al.,* 1994; Randolph *et al.,* 1993).

Thus, tests of word fluency often make a major contribution to the early detection of dementia, to the tracking of the progression of dementia, and to specifying the etiology of the dementia. However, in interpreting test findings it is important to bear in mind a number of considerations. Because impaired fluency performance occurs in a number of different neurodegenerative disorders, fluency performance must be interpreted within the context of the overall test profile. There is some inconsistency in findings from different studies, and this is likely to reflect differences in the nature and difficulty of the fluency tests administered. Therefore, it is important to choose fluency tasks carefully and to interpret the findings in terms of the specific fluency cue that has been administered. In particular, the interpretation of category fluency findings depends on the number and nature of the category cues that are administered. The finding that Alzheimer's disease is associated with disproportionate impairment in category fluency seems dependent on inclusion of three categories of sufficient difficulty. The use of fewer categories, especially when those categories are very broad and include many exemplars (e.g., animal names), may not create adequately challenging conditions for detecting subtle dementia.

In addition to the total test score, the number and nature of errors made during word fluency performance can also be informative, particularly for distinguishing between different pathological etiologies. The presence of *perseverative errors* or *intrusion errors* may be of particular clinical utility. Word fluency instructions specifically tell the patient not to generate words representing variations on a previous generated word. Perseverative errors involve repetitions of words or variations of words previously generated during that trial. For example, for the letter F, if the patient generates the word "fly," and then subsequently says "fly" or "flying," either of these represents a perseverative error and is scored as incorrect.

It is useful to note whether a perseverative error is immediate or delayed, since this has implications for inferring the basis for the error. An immediate perseveration is a repetition or variation of a word that was just generated. For example, if the patient said "fly" and then the next word generated was "fly" or "flying," this represents an immediate perseveration. Immediate perseverations may reflect cognitive inflexibility, a tendency to be "stuck" to a particular response item, which is one aspect of executive dysfunction.

A delayed perseveration is a repetition of a word or a word variation that occurs after at least several intervening words have been generated. A delayed perseveration may also reflect cognitive inflexibility, particularly when the number of intervening words is few. However, when the number of intervening words is relatively large (more than 10), this type of error suggests a possible deficit in memory storage, that is, difficulty remembering that the word had already been mentioned.

Intrusion errors are said to occur when the patient begins a trial correctly but then generates one or several items that do not meet the criteria specified for that test trial. It is important to note the nature and extent of intrusion errors. For example, during the FAS test, the patient might complete the F trial, correctly begin the A trial with "and, act, apple," but then switch to "fear, frown" and continue to generate F words. This type of intrusion error suggests that the patient has had difficulty maintaining the response set appropriate for this trial and is perseverating on a response set appropriate to a previous trial, a sign of executive dysfunction. Patients who make only a few intrusion errors before switching back to the correct task set may be experiencing difficulty in switching task sets. If the intrusion errors are unrelated to previous task conditions and the patient never switches back to the correct condition, this suggests that the patient may have totally forgotten the task instructions, raising the possibility of a more severe memory deficit.

Writing

Purpose and Administration

Requiring the patient to perform some writing may be particularly useful for detecting behavioral changes associated with movement disorders and aphasic syndromes. A number of different writing tests have been described (Goodglass & Kaplan, 1983; Spreen & Benton, 1977).

A brief test of sentence writing, adapted from Spreen and Benton (1977), includes two conditions, writing to dictation and copying. First, the patient is told to write cursively a dictated sentence on a blank sheet of paper. Performance on two trials is obtained, first for the sentence "Today is a nice day" and then for the sentence "This brick building was built last year." In the copy condition, the patient is provided with printed versions of the same two sentences and is asked to copy each sentence.

Scoring and Interpretation

Qualitative features of the patient's writing are often most informative, particularly the presence of abnormal sizing, tremulousness, visuospatial problems, and executive function deficits.

Micrographia is writing that is abnormally small. Patients with micrographia often start writing in normal size, but then the writing becomes smaller and smaller. Writing that is wavy or shaky is described as *tremulous.* Both micrographia and tremulousness are observed in disorders affecting subcortical motor structures, such as Parkinson's disease or subcortical vascular disease.

Sometimes the patient will begin writing a sentence horizontally, but then the writing will slant notably upward or downward. This may suggest impairment in visuospatial function or visuomotor coordination necessary to maintain the horizontal orientation across the page. In the sentence copying condition, if the patient writes over the stimulus sentence, or if the patient's writing starts below the stimulus but then slants upward to converge with the stimulus, this suggests *stimulus boundedness.* Such behavior suggests that the patient's attention to the stimulus is guiding his behavior toward that stimulus and that there has been failure to monitor and control behavior so as to compensate for this attraction, which suggests impairment in executive function.

Visuospatial and Visuoconstructive Abilities

Visuospatial and visuoconstructive abilities are involved in the processing and manipulation of visual information from the environment. This information includes both the visual information that comprises written words and that which configures nonverbal stimuli such as faces, pictures, and other images of the external environment.

Neuropsychological assessment of visuospatial and visuoconstructive abilities typically focuses on the processing and manipulation of nonverbal information. These abilities may be conceptualized in a hierarchy ranging from relatively low level perceptual processes to more demanding higher-level skills. The lower-level abilities such as visual acuity, attention, scanning, and perception form a basis for higher-level abilities such as the appreciation of complex visual gestalts and the manipulation of visuospatial information during problem solving. The lower-level visual abilities are fundamental to the performance of the more complex visuospatial tasks. For example, if a patient is unable to deploy visual attention to effectively scan a visual stimulus or has difficulty accurately perceiving the stimulus, this will compromise the performance of higher-level visuospatial and visuoconstructive tasks requiring manipulation of information derived from visual stimuli, such as the configuration of block designs. In addition, deficits in these abilities may contribute to impairment on tests of verbal abilities. For example, impaired visual attention or perception could compromise the patient's ability to identify the stimulus items presented on the Boston Naming Test. The presence of perceptual errors during this test is consistent with this possibility.

Neuropsychological assessment includes tests that evaluate the integrity of different levels of visuospatial and visuoconstructive abilities. Appropriate tests for the evaluation of older adults are discussed in the following sections.

Visual Acuity

An initial step in evaluating visuospatial and visuoconstructive abilities is determining that the patient's visual acuity is adequate. During the clinical interview, it should be ascertained whether the patient wears corrective lenses and whether he feels that they are adequately corrective. The patient should be queried as to whether he ever experiences periods of double vision (*diplopia*) or blurred vision. The presence of these symptoms raises the possibility of a neurologic disorder in neural pathways underlying vision, which might require neurologic or neuro-ophthalmologic evaluation. In patients with Parkinson's disease, disturbances of visual acuity, particularly diplopia, are common.

At the beginning of formal testing, visual acuity can be screened by using a near-card acuity test. This test requires the patient to read letters and numbers from a card-sized version of an optometrist's wall chart which is held 14 in. in front of the patient. Acuity of at least 20/50 is typically adequate for formal testing. Errors not related to acuity may suggest other deficits. For example, skipping items that are within the limits of the patient's visual acuity may suggest a deficit in visual scanning or visual attention.

Screening Visual Attention, Scanning, and Perception

Purpose and Administration

Lower-level visual abilities can be screened by using portions of the DRS. Items AD and AE within the Attention subscale require the patient to scan a page to detect specified target letters. To increase the sensitivity of these items for detecting impaired processing of specific locations within the visual field, such as occurs in hemispatial inattention, the stimulus material should be placed centrally in front of the patient rather than skewed to one or the other side. Visual perception may be screened by using item AJ, which requires the patient to match four simple visual designs. Items L and Q in the DRS require the copying of a simple alternating design (referred to as *ramparts*) and a simple embedded design (a diamond within a square). These items may be used to screen for deficits in visuospatial and visuoconstructive ability.

Scoring and Interpretation

On DRS items AD and AE, normal individuals are highly accurate. If the patient makes more than two errors, this suggests impaired control of visual scanning or inattention to visual detail. The consistent failure to detect targets in one half of the visual field or in a specific visual quadrant raises the possibility of hemispatial inattention or a visual field defect (*hemianopsia*). Normal individuals are also highly accurate on DRS item AJ. Matching errors raise the possibility of deficits in lower-level visuoperceptual abilities.

Normal individuals are able to copy the DRS designs without error. In patients with significant disease, several types of ramparts errors are most common. First, patients may omit the small horizontal lines connecting the alternating figures. This "omission of detail" may suggest impairment in motor control or inattention to visual detail. Second, patients may have difficulty maintaining the alternation in the figures, often starting correctly but later copying one figure several times in succession rather than copying the two figures in alternation. This may reflect perseveration or mental inflexibility, both suggestive of deficits in executive (frontal lobe) function.

It must be emphasized that errors on these DRS items provide only a screening for deficits in visual scanning, perception and attention. The meaning of errors on these items must be interpreted in the light of other data gathered during the evaluation and from more extended testing of the suspected area of deficit. The tests recommended for evaluation of older adults (Table 3-2) include Judgment of Line Orientation, a test of visuospatial ability described later in this chapter. The Copy and Discrimination conditions from the WMS-III Visual Reproduction test may contribute to the evaluation of relatively low level visual abilities (see Chapter 5). Other tests that may be useful for assessing visual scanning and attention include tests of line bisection (Schenkenberg, Bradford, & Ajax, 1980) and verbal and nonverbal visual cancellation tests (Caplan, 1985; Mesulam, 1985). The Benton Visual Form Discrimination may be added as an additional test of visuospatial ability (Benton, Hamsher, Varney, & Spreen, 1983).

Judgment of Line Orientation

Purpose and Administration

Judgment of Line Orientation (JOLO) is a motor-free test of visuospatial ability (Benton *et al.*, 1983). On each item the patient is presented with two stimulus lines, each characterized by a specific spatial orientation and position, which must be compared with an array of lines varying in these features. The patient is asked to choose two lines from the array that match the stimuli in orientation and position. Specific instructions are provided elsewhere (Benton *et al.,* 1983). Two test forms are available, each consisting of the same 30 items presented in different but increasing orders of difficulty.

When time allows, it is preferable to administer the standard JOLO. However, when testing time is limited or when patients may become easily frustrated, a short form including only the odd or even-numbered items may be administered. The total raw score is estimated by doubling the raw score obtained on the short form. For most patients, this estimated total score is unlikely to differ significantly from the true total score (Woodard *et al.,* 1996a).

Scoring and Interpretation

Test scoring is straightforward, involving computation of the total number of correct responses (Benton *et al.,* 1983). Age and sex affect test performance, with older individuals and women performing more poorly (Benton *et al.,* 1983; Woodard *et al.,* 1996a). The MOANS provides age-adjusted norms for individuals above age 55 (Ivnik *et al.,* 1996). In addition, norms adjusted for sex and for ages up to 74 are also available (Benton *et al.,* 1983).

Impaired performance on this test suggests the presence of dysfunction in the right brain hemisphere. In one study of patients with unilateral brain disease, 92% of those with right brain disease showed defective to severely defective performance, in contrast to only 20% of those with left brain disease (Benton *et al.,* 1983). Lesions in right parietal regions often disrupt performance of the JOLO (Fontenot & Benton, 1970). In healthy volunteers, studies examining changes in regional cerebral blood flow have revealed bilateral temporo-occipital increases during performance of the JOLO, that were greater within the right hemisphere (Deutsch, Bourbon, Papanicolaou, & Eisenberg, 1988; Hannay *et al.,* 1987).

Patients with Alzheimer's disease often show impaired performance, and make errors distinct from those seen in control subjects (Ska, Poissant, & Joanette, 1990). While control subjects' errors often consist of the choice of a line just slightly shifted from the target line, Alzheimer's disease patients may also make other types of errors, for example, choosing a line from the wrong quadrant. Parkinson's disease patients also often do poorly on this test (Levin, Llabre, & Weiner, 1989). However, in patients with mild cognitive dysfunction or dementia, the presence of minor errors in identifying the orientation of the target line may reflect a more general impairment in frontal lobe-mediated executive function rather than a specific deficit in right hemisphere-mediated visuoperceptual ability (Bondi *et al.,* 1993). Age-related decline in JOLO performance may also reflect changes in frontal lobe, rather than right brain hemisphere, functioning (Mittenberg *et al.,* 1989).

Clock Drawing

Purpose and Administration

Clock drawing is a brief, easily administered test of visuospatial and visuoconstructive ability, which may also contribute to assessment of executive function and memory. There are several versions of clock drawing tests, which vary in the nature of instructions given to the patient, the amount of structure provided by stimulus material, and the scoring system (Freedman *et al.,* 1994; Goodglass & Kaplan, 1983; Sunderland *et al.,* 1989; Tuokko, Hadjistavropoulos, Miller, & Beattie, 1992; Tuokko, Hadjistavropoulos, Miller, Horton, & Beattie, 1995a; Wolf-Klein, Silverstone, Levy, & Brod, 1989). Several representative versions are the following.

Freedman *et al.,* (1994) have developed a clock drawing test that includes three conditions: free-drawn, pre-drawn, and examiner-drawn. In the free-drawn condition, the patients are provided with minimal external structure. They are given a blank sheet of paper and instructed to draw a clock and put the numbers on it. After completing this, they are told to set the hands at a quarter to seven. The pre-drawn and examiner-drawn conditions provide increasingly greater structure. In the pre-drawn condition, the patient is given a circle drawn on a sheet of paper and is instructed to number the clock face and set the time to five after six. In the examiner-drawn clock condition, the patient is provided with three sheets of paper each containing a numbered clock face and is asked to set the times to twenty after eight, ten after eleven, and three o'clock, respectively.

Tuokko *et al.,* (1992, 1995a) have developed another relatively structured version of clock drawing, The Clock Test. This test examines the ability to draw clocks within predrawn circles and and also includes tests of clock reading and hand setting. Prepared test materials and normative data from five Canadian age groups over age 65 are available. Test scores on this version of clock drawing have been reported to have high accuracy for distinguishing between patients diagnosed with Alzheimer's disease and healthy control subjects (Tuokko *et al.,* 1992).

Another briefer version of the clock drawing test, which can be useful in brief test batteries, originates from the Boston Parietal Lobe Battery and includes only "command" and "copy" conditions (Goodglass & Kaplan, 1983). First, in the command condition, the patient is given a blank sheet of paper and instructed (commanded) as follows: "I'd like you to draw a clock, put in all of the numbers, and set the hands for 10 after 11."

These basic instructions can be expanded slightly to obtain additional data. After drawing the circular clock face and attempting to number it, some patients indicate confusion about the time to be represented and ask for a reminder. The examiner can note this in the test protocol and respond, "Can you make a guess about the time I mentioned?" If the patient fails to recall the correct time, the examiner notes this memory failure and then reminds the patient of the correct time and instructs him to represent it.

After the patient has completed his drawing to command, if he did not require a reminder of the time but represented the wrong time, the examiner may ask, "What time did I ask you to draw?" The nature of the patient's response may indicate the reason for his error. For example, if he recalls the time incorrectly, then his misrepresentation of that time is likely to reflect memory impairment. However, if he recalls the time correctly, an error in representation is more likely to reflect visuoconstructive or executive dysfunction.

The command condition is followed by the copy condition, during which the patient is asked to copy a drawing of a clock. A drawing of a clock with the hands set to ten after eleven is placed centrally before the patient. If the patient had difficulty setting the clock hands in the previous command condition, he should be asked to interpret the time represented on the model. The patient is then instructed to copy the model on a blank page.

Scoring and Interpretation

The interpretation of clock drawing performance depends both on quantitative and qualitative data. For the clock drawing test developed by Freedman *et al.* (1994), a 33-point scoring system has been developed focusing on clock features that are drawn accurately by most normal individuals. Normative data are available for a large English-speaking Canadian sample between the ages of 20 and 90. Quantitative scoring guidelines are also provided for the test published by Tuokko *et al.* (1995a), as well as normative data starting at age 65. A 10-point scoring system for the command–copy clock drawing test and normative data for a population sample averaging age 71 are provided by Rouleau, Salmon, Butters, Kennedy, & McGuire (1992).

In addition to quantitative analysis of test scores, qualitative analysis of the nature and reason for errors is critical in interpreting clock drawing performance. With less structured versions of clock drawing, a richer source of qualitative data may be available because the patient has greater opportunity to make errors. For example, if the patient is informed of the time to be represented in the initial instructions (rather than after he has drawn the clock face and numbers), he must remember the time, and an error in representation may reveal a memory deficit. Errors in number positioning and hand setting may also reflect deficits in executive function. Detailed systems are available for describing errors as well as descriptions of the types of errors made by healthy individuals and by patients with Alzheimer's disease, Parkinson's disease, and Huntington's disease (Freedman *et al.*, 1994; Rouleau *et al.*, 1992).

The presence of a difference between the patient's ability to represent a specified time by drawing the clock hands and his ability to interpret the time from clock hands on the model may also be diagnostically useful. On the one hand, if the patient was unable to represent the time in the spontaneous drawing condition even though he remembered it but was able to accurately interpret the time from the model, this suggests a deficit in executive function rather than in visuospatial ability. On the other hand, if the patient had difficulty representing the time and also had difficulty interpreting it from the model, this increases the likelihood of impairment in visuospatial ability.

There is evidence that clock drawing performance declines with aging and may be weaker in individuals with limited education. Among community-dwelling individuals, those older than 70 years may show significantly worse performance than younger age groups, although after age 70 there may be little further decline (Cahn & Kaplan, 1997; Freedman *et al.*, 1994). Clock drawing performance may be significantly poorer in nondemented individuals with less than 9 to 10 years of education (Ainslie & Murden, 1993; Cahn & Kaplan, 1997). Thus, it is important to use age- and education-adjusted normative data when interpreting quantitative data and to cautiously interpret the scores of patients with limited education.

Clock drawing performance is likely to be impaired in patients with dementia. In one study of well-functioning older people residing in a senior citizen residence, clock drawing was significantly poorer for those classified as demented on the basis of DRS score of less than 123 (Freedman et al., 1994). A number of studies have observed that patients diagnosed with Alzheimer's disease perform worse than healthy control subjects (Pan, Stern, Sano, & Mayeux, 1989; Rouleau et al., 1992; Sunderland et al., 1989; Tuokko et al., 1992). Scores on The Clock Test developed by Tuokko and colleagues have been demonstrated to differentiate with high accuracy between patients diagnosed with Alzheimer's disease patients and control subjects (O'Rourke, Tuokko, Hayden, & Beattie, 1997; Tuokko et al., 1992). Other versions of clock drawing also have considerable, although lower, accuracy, particularly for correctly classifying healthy individuals (Cahn et al., 1995; Cahn et al., 1996; Lee, Swanwick, Coen, & Lawlor, 1996).

Clock drawing may be useful for tracking the progression of dementia. Performance declines as dementia becomes more severe, and significant correlations have been observed between clock drawing scores and measures of overall cognitive status such as the Mini-Mental State Examination or the DRS in both healthy controls and patients diagnosed with dementia, including Alzheimer's disease (Brodaty & Moore, 1997; Mendez, Ala, & Underwood, 1992b; Pan et al., 1989; Rouleau, Salmon, & Butters, 1996; Shulman, Gold, Cohen, & Zucchero, 1993; Sunderland et al., 1989).

Clock drawing performance may also contribute to the detection of mild cognitive decline in community-based individuals. In one study using command–copy conditions, groups of individuals identified either as at risk for Alzheimer's disease owing to mild cognitive deficit or as diagnosed with probable Alzheimer's disease were observed to have lower clock drawing scores than healthy control subjects (Cahn et al., 1995). In a prospective study of community-dwelling older men, those who produced an abnormal clock during an initial evaluation had an increased risk of decline in cognitive function within 4 years (Ferrucci et al., 1996). This study employed a relatively unstructured clock drawing task, in which a preprinted circle was provided with the instructions to "draw a clock" and abnormality was determined on the basis of 10 patterns of clock drawing that had previously been labeled as pathologic or nonpathologic (Cahn et al., 1996; Lee et al., 1996; Wolf-Klein et al., 1989).

These findings suggest that clock drawing may contribute to detection of mild cognitive dysfunction when included in a battery of neuropsychological tests. If clock drawing performance is abnormal and there is also other evidence of cognitive decline based on the patient's history or other test findings, this strongly suggests that future tracking of cognitive status is merited. However, in the absence of other evidence of cognitive change, the finding of an abnormal clock in an otherwise healthy individual should not raise undue alarm

It is important to note that although quantitative clock drawing scores may be sensitive to Alzheimer's disease, impaired performance is not specific to this disorder and may occur in a variety of neurodegenerative disorders, including Parkinson's disease, Huntington's disease, and cerebrovascular disease (Freedman *et al.,* 1994; Libon, Malamut, Swenson, Sands, & Cloud, 1996; Libon, Swenson, Barnoski, & Sands, 1993; Pan *et al.,* 1989; Rouleau *et al.,* 1992; Suhr, Grace, Allen, Nadler, & McKenna, 1998; Wolf-Klein *et al.,* 1989). However, comparison between performance in different conditions and the nature of qualitative errors may contribute to identification of the underlying dementia. When command–copy conditions are administered, patients with both vascular dementia and Alzheimer's disease may be impaired in the command condition, but in the copy condition the vascular dementia patients may be more impaired than the Alzheimer's patients and show a greater frequency of errors reflecting executive dysfunction (Libon *et al.,* 1996; Libon *et al.,* 1993). Qualitative errors may also be helpful in identifying patients with Alzheimer's disease and in distinguishing them from equally demented Huntington's patients. Although both groups may be impaired in command conditions, Alzheimer's but not Huntington's disease patients may show improvement in the copy condition (Rouleau *et al.,* 1992). In the command condition, Alzheimer's disease patients typically make conceptual and perseverative errors, as well as those reflecting inappropriate pull to stimulus detail, in contrast to the graphomotor and planning errors that are more characteristic of Huntington's disease patients (Rouleau *et al.,* 1992).

Patients with depression may also show impaired clock drawing (Lee & Lawlor, 1995). However, performance may improve once the depression is relieved (Lee & Lawlor, 1995). The presence of persistent impairment in clock drawing even when depression is relieved may suggest that an underlying neurodegenerative disease is compromising neuropsychological status.

WAIS-III Block Design

Purpose and Administration

In the WAIS-III Block Design, the patient is asked to use three-dimensional red and white blocks to configure a design identical to that appearing on a card placed before him. The instructions for administering the Block Design are detailed in the WAIS-III Administration and Scoring Manual (Wechsler, 1997a).

It is useful to track the patient's behavior during the attempt to complete each design because the quality of his strategy and errors may be informative. Information may be gathered concerning the location in which the patient begins the construction (left, right, top, bottom), the order of block placement, and the nature and location of errors. A system for tracking the patient's response and recording qualitative data is described in the manual for the WAIS-R NI (Kaplan *et al.,* 1991).

The WAIS-III manual indicates time limits for each test item. Although the scoring of each item must be based on the performance within the specified time limit, it may be useful to note what the patient has accomplished at the time limit and then allow him to continue until he is frustrated or no longer actively attempting to complete the design. This extra time may provide additional qualitative data and allow the patient the satisfaction of completing the item correctly.

However, this additional time has the practical disadvantage of extending the total evaluation time. For older patients, this extra work may cause them to become so fatigued or frustrated that they are unable to exert effort to complete other, equally important subsequent tests. Therefore, it may be most useful to allow additional time only if the patient appears to be approaching a solution, for example, if at least half of the blocks have been correctly placed when the time limit expires. In such cases, the examiner may choose to allow the patient to continue for 1 minute beyond the usual time limit. This approach will increase the availability of qualitative data without a lengthy extension of time.

Scoring and Interpretation

The standard technique for scoring and computing the total test score is described in the WAIS-III Administration and Scoring Manual (Wechsler, 1997a). Normative data for age groups between 16 and 89 are also available in this manual. Performance on the Block Design is highly age-sensitive, so it is critical to use age-based normative data.

Performance of this test is heavily dependent on higher-level visuospatial and visuoconstructive abilities, including mental and physical manipulation and problem solving based on information derived from visual stimuli. The test places major demands on *constructional praxis,* the ability to assemble or copy items in two- or three-dimensional space (Loring, 1999). Performance on the Block Design is significantly related to motor speed and dexterity (Schear & Sato, 1989), which is consistent with its requirement that patients manually manipulate the blocks. Thus, patients with movement disorders may exhibit lower performance even when higher-level visuospatial abilities are uncompromised. For such patients, it may be more appropriate to use the WAIS-III Matrix Reasoning to assess visuospatial analysis and reasoning. This test does not require motor performance but has the disadvantage that because it is a new Wechsler test, its neuropsychological and brain correlates are less well established.

Performance of the Block Design is heavily dependent on posterior brain regions, particularly in the right parietal lobe. In normal adults, Block Design performance has been associated with increased glucose metabolism in these regions (Chase *et al.,* 1984). In patients with brain lesions, performance may be lowered by lesions in a variety of different regions. However, deficits are more frequent and severe in patients with posterior lesions, particularly in the right brain hemisphere (Black & Strub, 1976; McFie, 1975; Newcombe, 1969; Warrington, James, & Maciejewski, 1986).

The total test score on the Block Design is sensitive to a number of disorders affecting older adults. Among the Wechsler intelligence tests, the Block Design is one on which patients with mild Alzheimer's disease often perform most poorly (Berg *et al.,* 1984; Fuld, 1984; Larrabee *et al.,* 1985; LaRue & Jarvik, 1987). Patients with mild Alzheimer's disease may understand the task requirements and successfully complete several of the easier designs but typically fail the more complex designs (Perez *et al.,* 1975). In these patients, relatively poor performance on the Block Design during an initial evaluation may be predictive of relatively rapid cognitive decline in the future (Rasmusson, Carson, Brookmeye, Kawas, & Brandt, 1996). Patients with Huntington's disease may show impaired performance independent of motor disability (Brouwers, Cox, Marin, Chase, & Fedio, 1984). In alcoholics, Block Design performance is often deficient, in part because of slowness, but without the configurational errors that are characteristic of parietal lesions (Akshoomoff, Delis, & Kiefner, 1989).

Kaplan and her colleagues have been instrumental in describing how qualitative analysis of block design performance may contribute to neuropsychological evaluation (Kaplan, 1988; Kaplan *et al.,* 1991; Milberg, Hebben, & Kaplan, 1986). If the patient's configuration reflects a gross distortion of the gestalt of the design, this suggests that the patient has failed to appreciate its overall configuration, a characteristic of patients with right hemisphere lesions (Ben-Yishay, Diller, Mandleberg, Gordon, & Gerstman, 1971; Kaplan *et al.,* 1991; Patterson & Zangwill, 1944). On the other hand, if the patient makes errors in individual block placement within a grossly correct gestalt, this suggests that the patient is having difficulty at the level of details, a characteristic of patients with left hemisphere lesions (Kaplan, 1983). Patients with focal lesions lateralized in one brain hemisphere tend to make more errors on the side of the design contralateral to their lesion. It has also been suggested that errors in the upper half of the visual field are more suggestive of temporal lobe lesions, whereas those in the lower half are more consistent with parietal lobe lesions (E. Kaplan, cited in Lezak, 1995).

Patients with frontal lobe lesions may also show distinctive types of errors on the Block Design. These patients may use an impulsive, disorganized approach to configuring the design, working on different parts of the design in an unsystematic fashion. Such behavior suggests a deficit in planning abilities associated with executive dysfunction. These patients may also exhibit perseverative responding and cognitive inflexibility, for example, repeating an error that does not advance construction of the design.

5

MEMORY EVALUATION
IN OLDER ADULTS

When older individuals are referred for neuropsychological evaluation, the most common concern is memory dysfunction. The patient may complain of losing items around the house, having difficulty finding words while speaking, or going into a room and forgetting what he intended to do. Family members may report that the patient repeats comments, becomes lost while driving, or has displayed paranoid behavior, for example, believing that someone has stolen his money or that his spouse is being unfaithful. Since Alzheimer's disease has been highly publicized in the media, these behaviors raise concern that the patient may be developing this disorder.

Determining the nature, extent, and possible basis for behavioral changes is not necessarily straightforward for several reasons. First of all, dysfunction of memory per se may not be the fundamental basis for the behavioral difficulty. Problematic behaviors are often attributed to memory impairment when, in fact, deficits in other cognitive areas constitute the primary difficulty. For example, a complaint that the patient "loses track" of what he intends to say during conversation may be more closely related to difficulty in sustaining attention rather than to a memory deficit. If the patient is relatively able to remember day to day information such as the date and appointments but loses track during conversation, this supports the hypothesis that he may be having difficulty sustaining attention.

Thus, even when memory dysfunction is the presenting complaint, neuropsychological evaluation must also include assessment of a range of other domains in order to determine the precise nature of the dysfunction.

To begin determining the severity of memory dysfunction relative to that in other domains, the psychologist obtains examples of the patient's difficulties during the clinical interview (see Chapter 3). The patient and family members can be asked to describe specific episodes during which the patient exhibited confusion. So, for example, if the patient initially says, "I've been having memory problems," the examiner can follow this up by asking, "Can you give me some examples of this?" The response to this query will begin to elucidate the nature of the patient's difficulty. The patient's ability to describe more specific details will indicate the degree and density of the memory problem, if there is one. For example, if a patient is able to remember detailed descriptions of episodes of "forgetfulness," this raises questions about whether memory dysfunction is the fundamental problem.

Another issue complicating the evaluation of memory is the fact that memory is complex and multidimensional. Recent research in experimental neuropsychology, cognitive psychology, and neuroscience has described multiple and separable memory systems in the brain as well as a number of specific processing activities fundamental to remembering. Understanding of current concepts of memory function and the changes that differentiate normal and pathological aging provides a framework for understanding and interpreting neurobehavioral data.

This chapter briefly reviews current models of memory systems within the brain and processing activities fundamental to remembering. This discussion will establish a conceptual framework for the clinical evaluation of memory, which is presented in the second section of the chapter.

MEMORY SYSTEMS: DECLARATIVE AND NONDECLARATIVE MEMORY

Research in neuroscience has revealed that remembering is not dependent on a single brain region or brain system but instead reflects the functioning of several neuroanatomically distinct and separable systems within the brain that modulate fundamentally different types of long-term memory (Schacter & Chiu, 1993; Squire, 1992; Squire, 1994; Zola-Morgan & Squire, 1993). From a cognitive perspective, the major components of these systems are illustrated in Figure 5-1. *Declarative memory* (or explicit memory) includes knowledge based on conscious experience and learning. *Nondeclarative memory* includes a heterogeneous variety of information, which shares the common feature of being accrued largely independently of the individual's awareness (Schacter & Chiu, 1993). It includes perceptual-motor skill learning, classical conditioning, and memory priming.

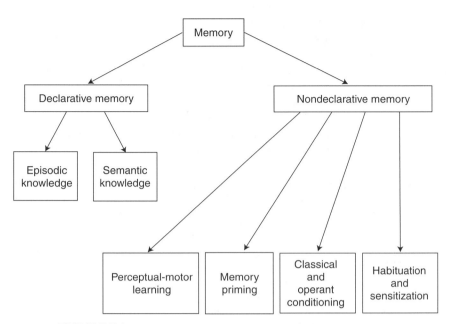

FIGURE 5-1 Memory systems of the brain (Adapted from Squire, 1992).

Within the declarative memory system, both semantic and episodic knowledge are stored (Tulving, 1972). *Semantic knowledge* consists of general concepts that have developed with experience and whose source can no longer be identified, such as knowledge of word meanings, the grammar of language, and abstract concepts. *Episodic knowledge* can more easily be associated with an experience occuring at a specific time or place (an "episode"). Examples of episodic memory include memory for the details of a news story you heard on the radio yesterday, for the name of a person you recently met, or for the location at which you left your keys or eyeglasses. When older individuals complain of memory problems, they are often describing difficulty with episodic memory, and this is becomes an important focus of neuropsychological evaluation.

Declarative memory is dependent on a neural system including three interrelated brain regions: the medial temporal lobe, proximal areas within the brain stem known as the diencephalon, and an areas just anterior to the diencephalon known as the basal forebrain (Damasio, Graff-Radford, Eslinger, & Damasio, 1985; Mair, Warrington, & Weiskrantz, 1979; Scoville & Milner, 1957; Zola-Morgan & Squire, 1993). These regions are illustrated in the drawings of basic brain neuroanatomy included in Appendix H. Lesions within this neural system are associated with *retrograde amnesia* (inability to remember information already stored in long-term memory) or *anterograde amnesia* (inability to store new information in long-term memory).

The medial temporal lobe and the structures proximal to it (the hippocampus, the perirhinal, parahippocampal, and entorhinal cortices, and the limbic regions, particularly the amygdala) play a crucial role in storing and consolidating new memories and in retrieving old memories. The amygdala is specifically involved in retaining the emotional associations of a memory, such as occurs with conditioned fears. The importance of the medial temporal lobe to anterograde memory was highlighted by the classic case of H.M. (Corkin, 1984; Scoville & Milner, 1957), who experienced severe anterograde amnesia after surgical removal of the hippocampus, amygdala, and adjacent medial cortex to relieve intractable epilepsy. H.M. remained intelligent with a preserved sense of humor and nondeclarative knowledge, but his ability to remember new information was severely impaired. The medial temporal lobe is also one of the brain regions earliest affected in Alzheimer's disease (DeLacoste & White, 1993; Hyman, Van Horsen, Damasio, & Barnes, 1984; Terry & Katzman, 1983), resulting in impaired ability to remember new information.

Lesions within the diencephalon, especially in the dorsomedial nucleus of the thalamus and the mamillary bodies, often result in amnesia and also in unusual behaviors suggestive of frontal lobe dysfunction. These behaviors may include interference between different episodes of memory, confabulation (false memories), and failure to appreciate the presence of memory dysfunction *(anosognosia)*. These lesions may disrupt a system involving the frontal lobe, medial thalamus, and medial temporal lobe that is important both for the formation of long-term memory and for retrieving and translating memories into action (Zola-Morgan & Squire, 1993). A striking example of dysfunction in the diencephalic-frontal system is seen in patients with *Korsakoff syndrome,* a consequence of thiamine deficiency associated with chronic alcoholism (Victor *et al.,* 1989). These patients suffer from anterograde and retrograde amnesia (Albert, Butters, & Brandt, 1980; Butters & Cermak, 1980; Salmon *et al.,* 1993; Squire, 1982). However, nondeclarative memory may be relatively unaffected. Neuropathological studies of the brains of Korsakoff syndrome patients indicate that they suffer bilateral damage to medial diencephalic structures, including the dorsomedial nucleus of the thalamus and the mamillary nuclei (Hata *et al.,* 1987a; Jernigan, Schafer, Butters, & Cermak, 1991a). Korsakoff syndrome and other alcohol-related disorders are further discussed in Chapter 9.

A third brain region important to declarative memory is the basal forebrain, the major source of innervation to the cerebral cortex by the cholinergic neurotransmitter system. Among the major neurotransmitter systems (cholinergic, serotonergic, dopaminergic, adrenergic), the cholinergic system is one of the most critical to memory. Dysfunction of cholinergic neurons is characteristic of Alzheimer's disease (Coyle, Price, & DeLong, 1983; Whitehouse *et al.,* 1982), and even in normal individuals, memory function can be degraded by administration of agents that interfere with the functioning of the cholinergic system, such as scopolamine (Drachman & Leavitt, 1974; Meador *et al.,* 1987). The major structures within the basal forebrain include the medial septal nucleus and the diagonal band of Broca, which project to the hippocampus, and the nucleus basalis of Meynert, which projects more widely to frontal, parietal, and temporal cortices (Mesulam, Mufson, Levey, & Wainer, 1983). It has been suggested that these structures may be involved in somewhat different functions, with the medial septal region being more important to long-term memory because of its direct projections to the hippocampus, and the nucleus basalis being more important in modulating attentional behavior (Olton, Wenk, Church, & Meck, 1988; Zola-Morgan & Squire, 1993).

Although the hippocampus, diencephalon, and basal forebrain are major anatomical regions involved in the consolidation and retrieval of new information in long-term memory, permanent memories may not be actually stored in these regions. This is suggested by the observation that although patients with diencephalon or medial temporal lobe lesions are unable to form new long-term memories, they often exhibit relatively preserved memory for information stored in long-term memory prior to when their lesions occurred. This suggests that the permanent long-term memory repository may be elsewhere, perhaps in associative regions in the neocortex (Squire, 1992).

There is also increasing evidence of the importance of the frontal lobes to declarative memory. Recent studies of dynamic brain function using positron emission tomography have demonstrated activation of the prefrontal cortex during episodic memory. The findings indicate that there is asymmetry in frontal activation during the initial acquisition of new information (memory encoding) and that this differs from the asymmetry when stored information is retrieved from episodic memory (Shallice *et al.,* 1994; Tulving, Kapur, Craik, Moscovitch, & Houle, 1994). The left prefrontal region is more involved than the right in episodic memory encoding, at least for verbal material. In contrast, the right prefrontal region may be more involved in retrieval of both verbal and visuospatial information from episodic memory. With respect to semantic memory, the left prefrontal region appears to be more activated than the right during retrieval, although asymmetry during acquisition has not been observed. Thus, it is clear that the frontal lobes play a major role in both the development and use of information in permanent memory.

The second major type of memory is nondeclarative (or implicit) memory, a heterogeneous variety of information with the common feature of being learned somewhat independently of the individual's awareness (Schacter & Chiu, 1993). Implicit memory was originally described as including perceptual–motor learning, several forms of memory priming, learning of procedural skills, and classical conditioning. More recently, another memory system, the perceptual representation system, has been described as underlying the phenomenon of memory priming (Tulving & Schacter, 1990).

The different types of implicit memory depend on brain systems that are distinct from those involved in declarative memory. For example, the learning of motor skills, such as those involved in controlling a car, are dependent on subcortical structures, including the caudate nucleus within the basal ganglia (Heindel,

Butters, & Salmon, 1988; Saint-Cyr, Taylor, & Lang, 1988). Priming of perceptual processing is dependent on posterior neocortical areas (Keane, Gabrieli, Fennema, Growden, & Corkin, 1991; Squire *et al.,* 1992), while lexical (word-based) priming depends on temporoparietal cortex (Keane, 1991). The cerebellum is critical to classical conditioning (Thompson, 1986).

Appreciation of the brain systems underlying different aspects of memory is important because some neurobehavioral disorders have relatively focal effects on specific brain systems, particularly early in the disease process. When brain dysfunction is relatively focal, some memory systems will be more impaired than others. For example, Alzheimer's disease compromises function of the medial temporal lobe and forebrain structures, and patients with this disorder show profound impairment of declarative memory and lexical priming. However, implicit memory is less affected in Alzheimer's patients, and they may exhibit relatively preserved motor skill learning and perceptual priming (Bondi & Kaszniak, 1991; Keane *et al.,* 1991). In contrast, patients with mild Huntington's disease, which compromises the function of the caudate nucleus within the basal ganglia, have impaired motor skill learning but preserved lexical priming (Heindel, Salmon, Shults, Walicke, & Butters, 1989). Patients with Parkinson's disease, which also compromises caudate function, have deficits in perceptual skill learning, while lexical priming is relatively intact (Bondi & Kaszniak, 1991). The presence of these characteristic patterns of memory dysfunction in different patient groups supports experimental research describing the existence of multiple memory systems.

A MODEL OF REMEMBERING NEW INFORMATION

Although disorders affecting the neuropsychological status of older adults may have distinctive effects on declarative as compared with nondeclarative memory, clinical evaluation typically focuses on the evaluation of declarative memory. Many common disorders have distinctive effects on this type of memory, and most of the clinical test instruments have been developed to focus on assessment of declarative memory. Although evaluation of nondeclarative memory could potentially be useful, many of the nondeclarative memory tasks, such as the priming tasks, were developed for research purposes and are impractical for clinical use because they produce only subtle effects and are time-consuming to administer.

A conceptual model of the phases and activities involved in developing new declarative memories provides a framework within which clinical data can be organized and interpreted. Cognitive psychology and neuroscience have provided a number of detailed models describing the stages and activities involved in remembering (Atkinson & Shiffrin, 1968; Atkinson & Shiffrin, 1971; Baddeley, 1986; Baddeley & Hitch, 1974). However, for clinical purposes, a relatively simple model is usually sufficient. This model includes three major components (memory acquisition, storage, and retrieval) and the concept of working memory, and is illustrated in Figure 5-2.

The first phase in remembering new information is the *initial acquisition* of that material. For information to be remembered, it must attended, perceived, and encoded in the memory system, and each of these activities contributes to the initial acquisition of that information in memory. Because the rich array of new information impinging on the senses at any given moment exceeds the processing capacity of the brain, attentional processes select information that will be perceived and will receive more intensive processing. However, even attended information is not necessarily well remembered because the quality of the memory depends on how the information is further processed, or encoded. *Encoding* is the processing of the information to be remembered into a form that identifies higher-level characteristics of that information and associates it with information already stored in memory. Attended information is often not remembered in its literal form, that is, in terms of its sensory or physical features, but rather is encoded into a form that facilitates remembering.

A variety of factors determine the precise nature of the encoding that occurs. The context in which the information occurs is one important variable, and information is more likely to be remembered if the cues available at the time of encoding match those available later when an attempt is made to retrieve that information (Tulving & Thomson, 1973). In addition, the kind of processing that to-be remembered information receives is an important determinant of how well that information will be remembered. Research in cognitive psychology has described different levels of processing, and there is evidence that memory is facilitated when encoding involves higher processing levels (Craik & Lockhart, 1972). Recognizing the physical features of a stimulus, such as its color, size or shape, represents a relatively low level of processing, whereas recognizing the conceptual attributes of a stimulus, such as its meaning, represents a deeper level of processing. For example, when a printed sentence is perceived in terms of the color of its

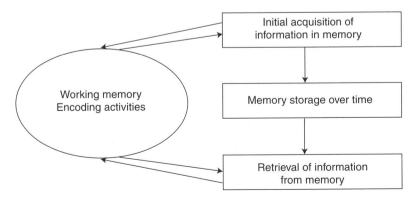

FIGURE 5-2 Critical components of remembering.

ink and font size, this represents a relatively low level of processing. Understanding of the meaning of the words in the sentence, the idea conveyed by the sentence, and its association with already stored knowledge represent deeper levels of processing and will facilitate memory for what has been read. When the face of a new person is perceived in terms of its specific physical features (for example, eye color, size, and shape), this reflects a relatively low level of processing, but appreciation of higher-level attributes, such as the person's affect (cheerful, sad), age (older, younger), or personality variables (friendly, reserved) represents a higher level of processing. Information that is encoded to a higher level is more likely to be remembered.

Information that is initially acquired enters long-term memory *storage*. Much of the huge wealth of information in long-term memory storage is not consciously perceived from moment to moment in daily life. However, this information can potentially be accessed and enter conscious awareness as remembered information.

When we consciously remember information, this reflects *retrieval* of that information from long-term memory. Often, we purposefully try to retrieve specific information, as when during a conversation we try to remember ideas from a book that we've read or the name of an acquaintance. Retrieval of information can also occur more automatically, as when cued by current information that we are processing or encoding. For example, when we are recalling a recent event (e.g., a recent birthday party) and suddenly remember a related past event (e.g., previous birthday parties), this reflects more automatic retrieval from long-term storage.

Retrieval and acquisition are heavily interdependent in that the efficiency of retrieval depends on the nature of the initial acquisition, and the quality of that acquisition depends, in part, on the nature of stored information that is activated by the information being acquired. Obviously, information that is not attended or perceived is less likely to be remembered. Deeper, more elaborate encoding during memory acquisition establishes retrieval cues and also associates new information with stored knowledge, thus facilitating later remembering of that information. Researchers generally agree that remembering is facilitated by the availability of specific cues that are highly similar to those established during initial encoding; this is known as *encoding specificity* (Tulving & Thomson, 1973). So, for example, if the name of a new person is associated with a visual image and with known information (e.g., the name Dr. Goldstein elicits an image of gold earrings and also the name of another person named Goldstein), this name is more likely to be remembered later, particularly if any of these encoding cues are available at the time of attempted retrieval. It has been hypothesized that decreased effectiveness in initial encoding, perhaps related to mental slowing or reduced attentional resources, is one factor contributing to the decline in memory associated with normal aging (Craik & Jennings, 1992).

The concept of *working memory* provides a powerful and neuropsychologically useful model for understanding processes facilitating the remembering of new information and the interactions between encoding, storage, and retrieval processes (Baddeley, 1986; Baddeley & Hitch, 1974; Gathercole, 1994). Working memory includes processes and structures that maintain a mental representation of information and manipulate and integrate that information with stored and other incoming information to facilitate remembering, decision making, and problem solving. The functioning of working memory helps determine how new information is encoded and the availability of cues during retrieval from memory storage.

Working memory has been described as including a *central executive* and two "slave" systems: a *phonological short-term store,* and a visual short-term store called the *visual sketchpad.* The phonological short-term store represents rapidly fading representations of verbal (word-based) information, which may be maintained in the short-term store by an articulatory subvocal rehearsal process. The left posterior temporoparietal junction has been identified as an anatomical locus of this store (Jonides *et al.,* 1993; Paulesu, Frith, & Frackowiak, 1993; Vallar & Baddeley, 1984a; Vallar & Baddeley, 1984b), and the left inferoposterior frontal lobe, critical to expressive speech (Broca's area), appears important to the rehearsal mechanism (Jonides *et al.,* 1993; Paulesu *et al.,* 1993). The visuospatial sketchpad represents rapidly fading representations of visual and spatial material. The anatomical locus of the visuospatial sketchpad has been more difficult to identify, although it may include temporal and right parietal areas (Ungerleider & Mishkin, 1982) as well as prefrontal cortex (Wilson, Scalaide, & Goldman-Rakic, 1993a).

From a clinical perspective, the central executive is the most conceptually useful feature of working memory because of its critical role in both memory acquisition and retrieval. The central executive is a flexible processor overseeing the coordination of mental activities and the deployment of limited-capacity attentional processing resources to mental activities involved in the rehearsal, manipulation, and organization of information in short-term memory as well as its retrieval from long-term memory. The frontal lobes have been hypothesized to be a major anatomical locus of both the central executive and working memory, specifically a system including the dorsolateral prefrontal cortex and the inferotemporal cortex (Wilson, Scalaidhe, & Goldman-Rakic, 1993). The dorsolateral prefrontal region may also be particularly important in coordinating the phonological store and the visuospatial sketchpad (Della Sala & Logie, 1993). As noted earlier, the frontal lobes are activated during both declarative memory encoding and retrieval (Shallice *et al.,* 1994; Tulving *et al.,* 1994), and this may reflect their participation in working memory.

DIMENSIONS FOR CLINICAL ASSESSMENT OF MEMORY

During formal testing, the patient's abilities to acquire, store, and retrieve information in memory are evaluated. In addition, the test battery also evaluates several other fundamental dimensions of memory function. The most important of these include:

- Recent as compared with remote long-term memory
- Immediate as compared with delayed recent memory
- Verbal as compared with visual recent memory
- Environmentally structured as compared with unstructured recent memory

The following discussion describes each of these dimensions.

The majority of clinical neuropsychological tests of memory assess *recent memory,* recently acquired memory of episodic information. Recent memory is typically evaluated by presenting the patient with new material to remember, such as stories (as in the WMS-III Logical Memory), word lists (as in the WMS-III Word Lists), or visual designs (as in the WMS-III Visual Reproduction). Memory for that material is assessed both immediately after presentation (immediate recent memory) and later, after a time delay of 20 to 30 minutes (delayed recent memory).

In contrast to recent memory, *remote memory* is memory for information accrued in the more distant past, typically at least several years earlier. Remote memory is often assessed by asking questions probing early personal history, distant historic events, or information learned in school. For example, remote memory is tapped when the patient is asked to recall places where he lived as a younger adult, the temperature at which water boils, or details of past job positions. Performance on tests of remote memory may reflect declarative memory but also semantic knowledge that cannot be tagged with a specific time or location of learning, such as general knowledge frequently learned during high school or college.

The pattern of strengths and weaknesses in immediate recent memory, delayed recent memory, and remote memory often makes an important contribution to diagnostic issues and planning of treatment. For example, patients with mild Alzheimer's disease often exhibit a significant deficit in delayed recent memory, although immediate recent memory and remote memory may be relatively stronger (Albert, 1996; Welsh, Butters, Hughes, Mohs, & Heyman, 1991). This pattern reflects the fact that mild Alzheimer's disease initially causes severe dysfunction in brain regions and systems underlying memory storage, including the medial temporal lobe (DeLacoste & White, 1993; Hyman *et al.,* 1984; Terry & Katzman, 1983) and the cholinergic neurotransmitter system (Coyle *et al.,* 1983; Whitehouse *et al.,* 1982). In contrast, patients with disorders affecting the frontal lobes, such as Parkinson's disease or subcortical vascular disease, may exhibit a relative weakness in immediate memory, reflecting dysfunction in memory acquisition, but are often able to retain most of their immediate memory over a time delay, particularly when retrieval is facilitated by cuing or other environmental structure (Heindel *et al.,* 1989). This pattern may reflect slowness during encoding as well as difficulty in self-organizing of both encoding and retrieval strategies (Huber, Shuttleworth, & Paulson, 1986a; Taylor *et al.,* 1990). Because they experience frontal lobe dysfunction, Parkinson's disease patients may also have difficulty spontaneously retrieving information from remote memory

(Freedman, Rivoira, Butters, Sax, & Feldman, 1984), particularly if they are developing dementia (Huber *et al.,* 1986a).

Verbal memory refers to memory for word-based information. Assessment of recent verbal memory typically involves asking the patient to remember stories or word lists, as is done during the WMS-III Logical Memory or Word Lists. *Visual memory* requires memory for visual images, and assessment of recent visual memory typically involves instructing the patient to remember abstract visual designs or pictures of faces, as during the WMS-III Visual Reproduction or Faces. Ideally, a visual memory test involves stimulus material that cannot easily be labeled with words, thus minimizing the involvement of verbal memory. For example, carefully selected abstract designs or faces are relatively difficult to remember in terms of words, and therefore are more dependent on visual than verbal memory. In contrast, pictures of common objects, such as of a table or of a house, can be easily labeled with words and therefore can be relatively easily stored in either visual or verbal memory or both. Thus, tests are more likely to assess visual memory to the extent that the stimulus material cannot be verbally labeled.

While recent verbal and visual memory both represent aspects of declarative memory, their neuroanatomical basis is different, and observation of a relative strength in verbal as compared with visual memory, or vice versa, is of clinical significance. Verbal memory is heavily dependent on left hemisphere brain systems, particularly in the medial left temporal lobe, whereas visual memory is more dependent on right hemisphere systems, particularly in the right medial temporal lobe (Milner, 1970). For example, patients with lesions in the medial left temporal lobe exhibit pronounced deficits in recent verbal memory, and those with lesions in the medial right temporal lobe lesions exhibit more pronounced visual memory deficits (Milner, 1968). Patients with right hemisphere lesions often exhibit impaired memory for visual information such as faces (Naugle, Chelune, Schuster, Luders, & Comair, 1994; Schweinberger, Buse, Freeman, Schonle, & Sommer, 1992).

Thus, the relative integrity of verbal as compared with visual memory performance suggests the relative integrity of left as compared with right hemisphere brain systems. The identification of relative strengths in verbal and visual memory may also contribute to the development of rehabilitation strategies for amnestic patients. For example, patients with pronounced verbal memory deficits might be able to compensate by increased reliance on visual memory.

Patients with mild Alzheimer's disease often exhibit bilateral deficits in both verbal and visual memory. However, if a patient exhibits an asymmetric deficit, in which verbal memory is considerably weaker than visual memory, or vice versa, this does not exclude the possibility that he may be experiencing this disorder. While the possibility of a unilateral focal lesion must be carefully considered, the presence of an asymmetric memory deficit may indicate that the patient has a subtype of Alzheimer's disease (see Chapter 6) in which either verbal or visuospatial deficits are initially more pronounced (Becker et al., 1988; Fisher *et al.,* 1996; Martin *et al.,* 1986)

The benefit of *environmental structure* in facilitating remembering is another important dimension in interpreting test data. Environmental structure can be provided either during memory acquisition, when information to be remembered is initially presented to the patient, or during retrieval, when stored information must be located in memory. For example, a relatively high level of environmental structure is provided during initial memory acquisition when the verbal information to be remembered is already organized into a story, as in the WMS-III Logical Memory. In contrast, the presentation of a randomly ordered list of words, as in the WMS-III Word Lists, represents an acquisition condition in which less structure is initially provided to the patient. The patient may impose structure to facilitate memory acquisition by use of a variety of *mnemonic aides*, strategies that facilitate remembering. These strategies include the clustering of words based on their meaning or the formation of a visual image integrating different words. For example, during the WMS-III Word Lists, the words "sunset, crocodile, ocean, giant" can be unified and more easily remembered as a "chunk" by forming a visual image of a giant crocodile watching a sunset over the ocean.

In word list learning tests of memory, the patient's ability to develop and apply strategies for structuring memory acquisition can be assessed by examining the order of recall. If the order is different for each recall trial, this suggests that the patient has not developed an effective strategy. However, if the order of recall is fairly consistent across trials, this might reflect rote memorization, or it could also suggest that the patient has applied a consistent strategy for remembering, even if that strategy is not obvious to the examiner. The consistent clustering of semantically or visually related words is particularly suggestive that the patient has self-imposed structure on memory acquisition.

The benefit of environmental structure provided at the time of memory retrieval can also be noted. Minimal structure for remembering is provided in conditions of *free recall,* in which the patient is asked simply to report material presented earlier. The patient must initiate the search of memory to locate the requested information, and cues are not provided for guiding this search. For example, in the WMS-III Logical Memory, after the patient has been read a story, he is instructed to recall the story that was just read to him. In the WMS-III Visual Reproduction, after the patient has been presented with a visual design, he is asked to draw the design from memory. In such conditions, relatively little environmental structure is provided to guide memory retrieval.

Memory retrieval is more environmentally structured when the patient is provided with external cues or when memory is tested in conditions of *recognition* rather than recall. In the WMS-III Logical Memory, the delayed free recall condition is followed by a more structured condition in which the patient is asked specific questions about the story. In the WMS-III Word Lists, the assessment of delayed memory includes a recognition test, in which the patient is asked to distinguish between previously presented words and distractor items. Both presentation of questions and conditions of recognition provide greater environmental structure than is present in conditions of free recall.

The extent to which environmental structure facilitates memory has clinical implications, particularly for the density of a memory deficit and the integrity of frontal lobe function. The frontal lobes provide a neuroanatomical basis for the working memory and executive functions that underlie the development of strategies for self-structuring both the encoding and the retrieval process. Patients with frontal lobe pathology often show pronounced memory deficits in unstructured conditions but perform significantly better in more environmentally structured conditions. For example, patients with focal frontal lobe lesions, as well as those with subcortical disorders compromising frontal lobe function such as Parkinson's or Huntington's disease, may show impaired memory retrieval in conditions of recall but perform significantly better in conditions of recognition (Butters, Wolfe, Granholm, & Martone, 1986; Heindel *et al.,* 1989; Jetter, Poser, Freeman, & Markowitsch, 1986; Moss, Albert, Butters, & Payne, 1986). Thus, if a patient exhibits impaired memory but benefits from environmentally provided structure and cuing during memory acquisition and retrieval, which are essentially externally provided frontal lobe functions, this raises the possibility that frontal lobe dysfunction may play an important role in the patient's memory deficit.

The following section describes test instruments that can be used to evaluate these different aspects of memory. Characteristic features of memory dysfunction associated with specific neurobehavioral disorders are detailed in Chapters 6 through 10.

TEST INSTRUMENTS FOR EVALUATION OF MEMORY

In order to assess each of the phases and dimensions of memory important to neuropsychological evaluation, the test battery must include several memory tests. The WMS-III, a recently revised and updated version of the Wechsler Memory Scale-Revised, consists of six primary tests (Logical Memory, Verbal Paired Associates, Letter-Number Sequencing, Faces, Family Pictures, Spatial Span) and five optional tests (Information and Orientation, Word Lists, Mental Control, Digit Span, and Visual Reproduction). Administration of the primary tests provides indices purported to be sensitive to what are labeled as immediate memory, auditory immediate memory, visual immediate memory, general memory (delayed), auditory delayed memory, visual delayed memory, auditory recognition delayed memory, and working memory.

The WMS-III has a number of features facilitating the evaluation of older adults. Most importantly, it includes population-based norms for ages between 16 and 89 years. Norms are presented for the index scores and for measures derived from both the primary and optional tests. In addition, the statistical properties of the index scores and tests are detailed in the technical manual, facilitating the interpretation of test scores.

There has also been significant improvement in the test materials. The administration instructions and test materials are included in two spiral-bound booklets, which stand upright between the patient and the examiner, allowing the tests to be administered in a standardized, efficient manner. Visually presented test materials are large and clear, which facilitates performance of older individuals whose visual acuity may be mildly compromised. The Logical Memory and Visual Reproduction have been modified and expanded, now examining both recall and recognition. The expansions of the Visual Reproduction allow closer examination of the contribution of motor and visuospatial variables to memory performance. The Faces test is a nonmotor test of visual memory, which may be particularly useful for evaluation of patients with significant motor impairment who are unable to draw. The optional Word Lists provides efficient evaluation of both environmentally structured and unstructured verbal memory.

Administration of the entire WMS-III to older adults has, however, several disadvantages. First, although the test manual indicates that the primary tests can be administered in 30 to 35 minutes, this time is likely to be exceeded in evaluating older adults, whose response rate is often slow. In addition, while some of the primary WMS-III tests are revisions of instruments commonly used in neuropsychological evaluation of older adults (e.g., Logical Memory), the clinical correlates of other primary tests are less well understood. For example, the Spatial Span and Letter-Number Sequencing have not been widely used in clinical evaluation of older adults, and the Family Pictures is entirely new. Some clinicians have expressed concern that older patients exhibiting very poor performance sometimes still obtain standard scores that approach the average range.

It may be desirable to administer only selected tests from the WMS-III, rather than all of the primary tests. While this approach violates the standardized procedure for test administration, it may be more consistent with the goal of performing an efficient evaluation that is within the limits of the patient's energy and motivation. As is indicated in Table 3.2, the following tests are often most useful: Information and Orientation, Mental Control, Digit Span, Logical Memory I and II, Visual Reproduction I and II, and Word Lists I and II.

Table 5.1 indicates measures derived from the WMS-III tests and their contribution to the evaluation of recent and remote declarative memory. Most of the tests contribute to the assessment of several different aspects of memory. As memory must be evaluated within the context of the functioning of other abilities, such as attention and verbal abilities, the findings from each memory test must be integrated with those derived from the others to infer an overall pattern of memory function.

The purpose, administration, scoring, and interpretation of each test are described in the next section. Detailed instructions for administration and scoring and normative data are provided in the WMS-III Administration and Scoring Manual.

TABLE 5.1   Aspects of Memory Evaluated by WMS-III Tests

WMS-III test	Aspects of memory evaluated
Information and Orientation	Recent memory
	Remote memory
Logical Memory	Immediate verbal memory
	Verbal acquisition (structured)
	Verbal storage
	Verbal retrieval (structured and unstructured)
Word Lists	Verbal acquisition (unstructured)
	Verbal learning
	Interference effects
	Verbal storage
	Verbal retrieval (structured and unstructured)
Visual Reproduction	Visual acquisition (structured)
	Visual storage
	Visual retrieval (structured and unstructured)
	Visuospatial ability
	Visuoconstructive ability

WMS-III Information and Orientation

Purpose and Administration

The Information and Orientation (I-O) test contributes to the evaluation of both recent and remote memory. The patient is asked to supply details concerning personal history dependent on remote memory (e.g., When were you born?) and details of orientation derived from recent memory (e.g., What year is this? What day of the month is this? Who is the president?) It is useful to administer this test at the beginning of evaluation because it is relatively nonthreatening and may motivate the patient to participate in additional testing. The test also provides initial data concerning the quality of the patient's memory that has implications for tailoring subsequent testing.

Scoring and Interpretation

The I-O provides an informal, preliminary impression of the patient's memory. Accurate performance on the I-O does not exclude the possibility that significant memory impairment may be revealed by more formal testing. Differences between the accuracy of details regarding personal history and details of orientation may suggest the relative impairment of remote and recent memory. Confusion about both suggests a significant memory problem, possibly affecting both remote and recent memory. In contrast, confusion about personal history only or orientation only suggests, respectively, a relative weakness in remote as compared with recent memory or in recent as compared with remote memory.

If the patient exhibits severe impairment on the I-O test, he is likely to have great difficulty with more formal tests of memory. Administration of these tests will be frustrating both to the patient and to the examiner. Therefore, if both performance on the I-O test and the findings from the clinical interview imply moderate to severe impairment of memory, it is often wise to limit subsequent memory assessment, perhaps including only one or two formal tests. The Logical Memory and Visual Reproduction may be sufficient in such cases.

WMS-III Logical Memory (LM)

Purpose and Administration

The Logical Memory (LM) test is used to examine both immediate and delayed recent verbal memory. The examiner reads the patient two stories, and the patient is asked for immediate recall after hearing each story. The second story is presented twice, with recall after each presentation, thus allowing the patient an additional opportunity to encode that story. After an interval of 25 to 30 minutes, preferably filled with nonverbal tests that minimize interference with verbal memory, the patient is asked to recall each story again. Then a structured recognition memory test is administered, during which the patient is asked specific questions about each story and must provide yes or no responses. The recognition test may be particularly useful for evaluation of patients having expressive aphasia.

Scoring and Interpretation

Test scores derived from LMI contribute to evaluation of immediate memory for structured verbal material, particularly the ability to initially acquire that information in memory. For the second LMI story, the difference between recall after the first and second presentation may suggest the density of the memory deficit, with improvement implying a milder deficit. The inclusion of scores reflecting both specific recall of story units (e.g., recall total scores) and more general recall of story themes (e.g., thematic total score) is also useful for evaluating the density of a memory deficit. If the patient's total score is impaired for both story units and story themes, this suggests that the memory deficit is dense.

Scores derived from LMII contribute to evaluation of delayed verbal memory. The LMII percent retention score reflects the difference between immediate and delayed memory, thus suggesting whether the patient has a deficit in storing new verbal material. The LM delayed memory evaluation includes a recall test and also a recognition test. Although normative data are not provided for the delayed recognition test, these data can be useful in assessing whether additional environmental structure benefits memory retrieval. A general rule is that if the patient's delayed recall scores are impaired but the accuracy of recognition exceeds 75%, this suggests that environmental structure is facilitatory and raises the possibility that the patient's memory dysfunction may primarily reflect a retrieval deficit.

WMS-III Word Lists

Purpose and Administration

Word Lists (WL) constitutes a test of verbal memory that complements LM. Unlike LM, which requires the patient to remember verbal material already structured in the form of stories, WL requires memory for unstructured verbal material. In addition to assessing immediate and delayed recent memory and structured as compared with unstructured memory retrieval, it also allows assessment of cumulative learning and of the extent of interference between different episodes of learning. The major phases of the test are as follows:

1. Learning of List A: The patient is instructed to remember List A, a 12-word list of unrelated items. The list is presented four times, with free recall after each presentation.
2. Presentation of List B: A different 12-word list is presented once, followed by immediate free recall of that list.
3. Short delay recall of List A: The patient is asked to recall List A. The patient is then instructed that memory for List A will be retested later during the evaluation.
4. Long-delay free recall of List A: After a delay of 25 to 30 minutes, the patient is asked to recall List A.
5. Long-delay recognition: The patient is presented with a list of 24 words, including the 12 items from List A and 12 distractor items. The patient is asked to indicate which words appeared in List A.

Scoring and interpretation

The measures derived from the test and their interpretation are as follows:

Word List I

Recall Total Score: This reflects cumulative learning over the four presentation trials and assesses immediate verbal memory acquisition of relatively unstructured material.

Learning Slope Calculation: This reflects improvement in memory with repeated presentation of material. If the recall total score is impaired and the learning slope score is impaired, this suggests a more profound deficit in memory acquisition, perhaps related to inability to self-structure material, or to interference between different episodes of learning. The latter is implied when learning is inconsistent, as when recall on the first two trials is stronger than on later trials.

Difference between Trial 1 Recall and List B Recall (Contrast 1): This is a measure of *proactive interference* (interference of previous learning with new learning). The presence of proactive interference is suggested if List B recall is less than Trial 1 recall, indicating that the learning of List A has interfered with ability to learn a new word list, List B.

Difference between Trial 4 and Short-Delay Recall (Contrast 2): This is a measure of *retroactive interference* (interference of new learning with previous learning). Retroactive interference may be present if short-delay recall of List A is less than Trail 4 recall of List A, suggesting that the presentation of List B caused some loss of memory for List A.

Word Lists II

Recall Total Score: This reflects relatively unstructured delayed verbal memory.

Percent Retention: This computation compares long-delay recall of List A with recall on Trial 4, thus reflecting the extent of memory loss between immediate and delayed remembering. An impaired score implies a defect in memory storage.

Recognition Total Score: This indicates the quality of delayed, more structured memory. If the recall total score is impaired but the recognition score is normal, this implies that the verbal memory deficit is not dense and raises the possibility of impairment in memory retrieval.

WMS-III Visual Reproduction

Purpose and Administration

The Visual Reproduction (VR) test contributes to the evaluation of immediate and delayed recent visual memory. The test requires memory for structured visual material (visual designs) and assesses memory retrieval in conditions of recall and recognition.

The examiner first presents the patient with five abstract visual designs, one at a time, each for 10 seconds. After the presentation of each design, it is removed and the patient draws the design from memory. After a 30-minute interval, preferably filled with verbal tests that minimize interference with visual memory, the patient is asked to reproduce each of the designs again. A recognition memory test is then administered, in which the patient views a series of 48 designs and is asked to distinguish between the designs that were presented earlier and distractor items.

Because VR requires drawing, patients with visuospatial or motor dysfunction may obtain impaired scores even in the absence of a deficit in visual memory. To evaluate the possible contribution of these factors, several additional items are administered after the delayed memory questions. Visuospatial abilities are evaluated by a visual discrimination test in which each design must be matched to one of five alternative designs. Visuomotor abilities are evaluated by a copying test in which each design is copied.

Scoring and Interpretation

In interpreting the findings from VR, the design copy and discrimination total scores are examined first because these may affect the interpretation of the other scores. If the discrimination score is impaired, this implies that visuospatial deficits may compromise visual memory. This hypothesis can be further tested by examination of performance on other tests of visuospatial function, such as Judgment of Line Orientation (see Chapter 4). If the discrimination score is unimpaired but the copy score is impaired, this implies that deficits in motor or visuomotor performance may compromise VR scores. This pattern is often observed in patients with movement disorders such as Parkinson's or Huntington's disease. These patients may have intact visual memory but may obtain impaired VR scores due to their motor deficits. In such cases the VRII recognition score, which does not depend on motor ability, should be more heavily weighed in evaluating visual memory.

If the patient exhibits unimpaired performance in the copy and discrimination conditions, then the other VR scores are more likely to reflect visual memory function. Scores on VRI contribute to assessment of immediate visual memory, whereas those on VRII contribute to assessment of delayed visual memory. Comparison of the VRI score with the VRII percent retention score reflects relative deficits in visual memory acquisition as compared with storage. If the percent retention score is higher than that on VRI, this suggests greater difficulty in initially acquiring new information than in storing this information over time. If the percent retention score is lower than that on VRI, this suggests dysfunction in visual memory storage. If percent retention score is very poor but delayed recognition is accurate, this suggests that the visual memory deficit is not dense, and that deficits in memory retrieval may be contributing to memory dysfunction.

Although performance on VR contributes to the evaluation of visual memory, inferences regarding the implications of test findings for the integrity of visual memory and right hemisphere function must be tempered by several considerations. Several of the VR stimuli can be verbally encoded, and, therefore test performance to some extent reflects the integrity of verbal memory as well as visual memory. This may be particularly true for patients with more highly developed verbal skills who may rely on verbal encoding even for visual material. Consistent with its sensitivity to both visual and verbal memory, the test is not reliably differentially sensitive to left as compared with right hemisphere lesions in patients with epilepsy (Chelune & Bornstein, 1988; Naugle, Chelune, Cheek, Luders, & Awad, 1993).

In cases in which memory dysfunction may be subtle or inconsistent, or when attentional dysfunction is suspected to be a contributing variable, the VR test may be particularly useful. Because the VR designs are presented for 10 seconds each, this allows the patient considerable time to attend to them and to apply encoding activities that facilitate their initial acquisition in memory. Some patients with attentional deficits may perform poorly during LM but perform relatively strongly in VR because they have more time to perceive and process the material to be remembered. When this occurs, however, the possibility of a relative strength in visual memory as compared with verbal memory must also be considered.

6

NEUROPSYCHOLOGICAL PROFILES OF COMMON DISORDERS AFFECTING OLDER ADULTS I

Alzheimer's Disease, Frontotemporal Lobar Degeneration

One major role of the neuropsychological evaluation is to determine whether a patient is experiencing cognitive dysfunction and to contribute to identification of the etiology of this dysfunction so that treatment can be offered. The major focus of Chapters 6 through 10 is to describe common disorders affecting the neuropsychological status of older adults and the neuropsychological profiles associated with these disorders. Chapter 6 begins by defining dementia and describing the distinction between cortical and subcortical syndromes. The neuropsychological profiles of two cortical dementing disorders, Alzheimer's disease and frontotemporal lobar degeneration, are then reviewed.

DEFINITION OF DEMENTIA

Dementia is a clinical syndrome characterized by deficits in memory and other cognitive domains that impair social or occupational functioning (American Psychiatric Association, 1994). Among individuals over the age of 65 worldwide, between 10 and 15% experience at least mild dementia and approximately 6% experience severe dementia (Cummings & Benson, 1992a). The prevalence of dementia doubles about every 5 years after age 65 (Jorm, Korten, & Henderson,

1987). Moderate to severe dementia occurs in approximately 2% of persons between the ages of 65 and 69, in 4% between the ages of 70 and 74, in 8% between the ages of 75 and 79, and in 16% above the age of 79 (Alzheimer's Disease and Related Dementias Guideline Panel, 1996).

Dementia can be caused by a number of different disorders. The most common cause of dementia in western European and North American countries is Alzheimer's disease (AD), accounting for 60% or more of all dementing illnesses (Alzheimer's Disease and Related Dementias Guideline Panel, 1996). Cerebrovascular disease is generally considered to be the next most frequent cause of dementia, accounting for perhaps 15 to 20% of cases (Katzman & Rowe, 1992; Mahendra, 1987). In some countries, including Japan, China, and Sweden, cerebrovascular disease may be more common than AD (Li, Shen, Chen, Zhao, & Li, 1989; Shibayama, Kasahara, & Kobayshi, 1986; Skoog, Nilsson, Palmertz, Andreasson, & Svanborg, 1993). Other disorders commonly causing cognitive dysfunction or dementia in older adults include frontotemporal lobar degeneration, dementia with Lewy bodies, Parkinson's disease and other parkinsonian syndromes, Huntington's disease, normal pressure hydrocephalus, traumatic brain injury, substance-related disorders, depression, and a variety of metabolic and toxic conditions.

The Diagnostic and Statistical Manual of Mental Disorders-IV (DSM-IV) provides criteria for diagnosing dementia caused by specific etiologies, as well as Dementia Not Otherwise Specified (American Psychiatric Association, 1994). Patients with milder cognitive dysfunction not meeting criteria for dementia may be diagnosed with Cognitive Disorder Not Otherwise Specified or, if there is focal memory dysfunction, with one of several amnestic disorders.

CORTICAL AND SUBCORTICAL DEMENTIA SYNDROMES

In neuropsychological assessment, a useful distinction has been made between *subcortical* and *cortical* dementing syndromes. The term *subcortical dementia* was initially proposed to describe a clinical syndrome associated with dysfunction in subcortical gray matter structures and their frontal lobe projections, including the basal ganglia, thalamus, subthalamus, and brain stem, as contrasted with cortical structures such as the frontal and temporal lobes. A distinctive pattern of neuropsychological and neurobehavioral findings was attributed to dysfunction in these subcortical structures, including mental slowness, forgetfulness related to mental slowness, impaired ability to manipulate acquired knowledge, and personality changes marked by apathy and failure of spontaneity (Albert, Feldman, & Willis, 1974; Cummings, 1990b; McHugh & Folstein, 1975). The prototypical disorders to which the term was initially applied were progressive supranuclear palsy (a parkinsonian syndrome) and Huntington's disease (see Chapter 8). It was proposed that subcortical dementias involved a relative absence of aphasia, amnesia, agnosia, and apraxia, which have been described as more characteristic of the *cortical dementias*. Alzheimer's disease was described as the prototypical representative of a cortical disease.

Since the distinction was initially proposed, there has been considerable debate concerning its validity, particularly with increasing recognition that both cortical and subcortical changes occur in most dementing disorders (Whitehouse, 1986). For example, it is well established that although AD involves major dysfunction in widespread cortical regions, including the frontal, temporal and parietal lobes, there is also early pathology in subcortical regions, notably the nucleus basalis of Meynert, which plays an important role in the cholinergic neurotransmitter system and deteriorates early in the course of AD (Whitehouse, Price, Clark, Coyle, & DeLong, 1981). Conversely, neuropathology in frontal cortical regions is often observed in subcortical disorders such as Huntington's and Parkinson's diseases (Boller, Mizutani, Roessmann, & Gambetti, 1980).

However, the syndrome of subcortical dementia continues to be useful for labeling disorders in which subcortical pathology is primary and cortical pathology is largely present in areas receiving subcortical neural projections (Cummings, 1990a; Cummings & Benson, 1984). In clinical practice, the subcortical–cortical distinction may be useful in initially describing profiles of neuropsychological dysfunction. While not specifying a particular disease, the labeling of a profile as more characteristic of subcortical or cortical disease directs the clinician toward hypotheses about groups of disorders that are more likely to be the cause of neuropsychological dysfunction and other clinical changes. For example, disorders of older adults that typically present with a subcortical neuropsychological profile include Parkinson's disease and parkinsonian syndromes, Huntington's disease, dementia with Lewy bodies, normal pressure hydrocephalus, and certain types of subcortical vascular disease. Disorders that typically present with a cortical dementia include AD and frontotemporal lobar degeneration. Within each of these groups, details of the neuropsychological profile allow the clinician to make a more specific diagnosis concerning the etiology of the patient's deficits.

Although brief mental status examinations may be unable to discriminate between subcortical and cortical syndromes, differences are often more apparent in formal neuropsychological test findings (Cummings, 1990a; Huber, Shuttleworth, Paulson, Bellchambers, & Clapp, 1986b; Mayeux, Stern, Rosen, & Benson, 1983). Classic features of subcortical and cortical dementia are summarized in Table 6.1. In subcortical disorders, patients often perform poorly on tests requiring speeded performance, and mental slowness may also contribute to dysfunction in memory and executive functions. Patients may have difficulty in developing and applying strategies to facilitate remembering and problem solving. For example, in memory tests involving word list learning, patients have difficulty in taking advantage of semantic and other relationships between words to facilitate encoding and retrieval. In problem-solving tests, they may have difficulty in maintaining attention and applying feedback to develop problem-solving strategies. Initial acquisition of new information in memory may be impaired,

TABLE 6.1   Major Neuropsychological Features of Mild to Moderate Subcortical and Cortical Dementing Syndromes

Characteristic	Subcortical dementia	Cortical dementia
Mental speed	Significantly slow	Relatively normal
Attention	Below expectation relative to other abilities	Relatively preserved
Memory	Deficient acquisition due to failure of organization; delayed recognition relatively preserved in comparison with recall	Impaired acquisition; impaired delayed recall and recognition
Executive	Disproportionately impaired relative to other abilities; deficient ability to self-initiate strategies and use feedback	Deficient in proportion to other abilities
Visuospatial	Variable	Variable
Language	Word fluency and naming may be below expectation but benefit from structure	Early impairment in naming and word fluency, with minimal benefit from structure
Motor	Motor abnormalities common	Motor abnormalities less common
Affect	Apathetic, inert, depressed mood	Relative lack of concern; defensive about deficits; impulsive; reduced interest in activities

with consequent impairment in delayed recall. However, delayed memory in structured conditions, particularly in conditions of delayed recognition, is often preserved. Patients may appear apathetic and uninterested in their usual activities. The frequency of clinical depression is higher in subcortical than in cortical illnesses. Abnormalities in movement and motor control are associated with subcortical disorders and may include tremor, chorea, impaired gait and balance, slowed movement, dysarthria, or masked facies.

In contrast, in the cortical dementias, dysfunction in memory, language, and visuospatial functioning is often most prominent. Patients have difficulty both with initial encoding of new information and with retaining that information over time. The provision of structure and cuing may not facilitate memory, and delayed memory is often poor in conditions both of recall and of recognition. Patients often exhibit dysnomia and show impairment on tests of word finding. Visuospatial dysfunction may be manifested by topographic confusion while driving. Patients may appear relatively unconcerned about neuropsychological change and are defensive in trying to rationalize episodes of forgetfulness described by their family members. They may show reduced interest in their usual activities, although the affect accompanying this is typically not depressed. Disinhibited and impulsive behaviors may occur.

Subtle differences are often important in determining whether deficient performance in a neuropsychological domain or on a particular test is more likely to reflect a subcortical or cortical syndrome. For example, memory may be affected by syndromes of both types, but the pattern of memory dysfunction is different, with subcortical disorders associated with less severe memory deficits, which that may be remediated by structure and cuing. Executive functions may be impaired in both syndromes, but in subcortical disorders this impairment is often pronounced in comparison with other test scores. Thus, to recognize that memory or executive function is impaired may not be diagnostically helpful; it is the nature of this dysfunction and its relationship to the overall neuropsychological profile that is most informative. It is also important to note that for patients with subcortical neuropsychological profiles, the term dementia may be a misnomer because their deficits may be subtle and not adequately severe to meet formal criteria for dementia (see Case 5 in Appendix G).

The designation of a neuropsychological profile as more characteristic of a subcortical than a cortical disorder has important implications in that it may suggest different options for patient management and treatment, even when the exact diagnosis is unclear. In general, a wider range of medical options is available for ameliorating and sometimes even reversing subcortical disorders. For example, in patients with a subcortical profile, behaviors such as disinterest and reduced activity are more likely to reflect a depressive syndrome, which may be treatable with antidepressant medication or psychotherapy. In contrast, these behaviors in patients with a cortical profile are less likely to reflect a depressive syndrome. Patients with a cortical profile are less likely to appreciate their neuropsychological deficits and may need to be strongly discouraged from continued involvement in behaviors that may endanger their well-being or that of others, such as cooking, driving, and financial management. In contrast, patients with a subcortical profile often appreciate their own decline in intellectual functioning and are able to make more appropriate decisions concerning the responsibilities for which they are competent.

ALZHEIMER'S DISEASE

Background

Alzheimer's disease is the most common dementing disorder in older individuals, accounting for 60% of all cases of dementia in western European and North American countries (Alzheimer's Disease and Related Dementias Guideline Panel, 1996). There are two closely related sets of criteria for diagnosing AD: those specified in the DSM-IV and those specified by A Work Group on the Diagnosis of Alzheimer's Disease, established by the National Institute of Neurologic and Communicative Disorders and Stroke (NINCDS) and the Alzheimer's Disease and Related Disorders Association (ADRDA)(McKhann *et al.,* 1984).

Both sets of criteria require that patients diagnosed with AD show gradually progressive deficits in at least two neuropsychological domains, including memory, that cannot be attributed to other psychiatric or medical conditions. The NINCDS-ADRDA criteria were developed to better define criteria for patients participating in research projects evaluating treatments for AD, and they distinguish between definite, probable, and possible AD. The definitive diagnosis of AD is made on the basis of a characteristic pattern of neuropathology identified in samples of brain tissue, most notably the presence of neuritic plaques and neurofibrillary tangles (Hyman, 1998; Mirra, Heyman, & McKeel, 1991). The NINCDS-ADRDA criteria are also more specific in describing behavioral, neurologic, and psychological features that are characteristic or unusual during the course of AD. When using the NINCDS-ADRDA criteria, experienced clinicians are able to diagnosis AD with high accuracy on the basis of clinical evaluation alone, with accuracy approaching 90% (Galasko *et al.*, 1994; Kawas, 1990).

Early in its course, the neuropathology of AD is often focused in medial temporal lobe structures, including the hippocampus and entorhinal cortex, with frontal, temporal, and parietal association cortices becoming more involved as the disease progresses (Hyman *et al.*, 1984). There is also loss of subcortical neurons in the nucleus basalis of Meynert, a major source of innervation within the cholinergic neurotransmitter system, and in the locus cereleus, a source of innervation within the noradrenergic neurotransmitter system (Bondareff, Mountjoy, & Roth, 1982; Whitehouse *et al.*, 1982). In mildly affected patients, temporoparietal metabolic abnormalities can often be detected through dynamic brain imaging, such as positron emission tomography (Haxby *et al.*, 1986; Haxby *et al.*, 1988). Such abnormalities may also be present in well-functioning middle-aged individuals at increased risk for developing AD (Reiman *et al.*, 1996). Structural brain imaging may reveal pronounced cortical atrophy, including enlarged ventricles and widened cortical sulci in more severely affected patients (Donaldson, 1979; Erkinjuntti *et al.*, 1984). However, mild atrophy may be present in both early AD and normal aging (Kemper, 1994).

There is increasing evidence that AD has a long, preclinical course and that it may be possible to detect changes in well-functioning individuals long before their symptoms achieve clinical significance (Snowdon *et al.*, 1996). Neuropsychological evaluation may contribute to early detection of AD, and neuropsychological changes have been observed in well-functioning, middle-aged persons at increased risk for developing AD (Hom, Turner, Risser, Bonte, & Tintner, 1994). Thus, it is important that middle-aged individuals who are complaining of memory decline receive neuropsychological evaluation, both for determining whether they are experiencing significant dysfunction in comparison with age peers and for obtaining baseline measures that can be used to track neuropsychological change. Such evaluation will be of increased importance as better treatment options become available, so that these can be offered before functional decline becomes pronounced.

There has been increasing interest in risk factors that may contribute to the development of AD. Late-onset AD, diagnosed in individuals after the age of 65, is more common than early-onset AD. Indeed, older age is a well-established risk factor for developing AD. After age 65, the overall prevalence of AD is between 5% and 10% increasing from 1% between the ages of 60 and 64 to 35 to 50% after age 85 (Evans et al., 1989).

In addition to age, a family history of AD increases an individual's risk of developing this disorder (Breitner et al., 1988; Huff, Auerbach, Chakravarti, & Boller, 1988; Mayeux et al., 1991). Although most AD cases are sporadic, occurring in individuals without a family history of AD, cases of familial AD have been observed in which multiple blood relatives from different generations are affected. One study reported that among patients diagnosed with AD, 33% had a first degree relative with dementia, in comparison with only 21% of non-AD dementia patients and 12% of normal older adults (Mendez et al., 1992a). In relatives of patients diagnosed with AD, as many as 50% may develop AD by their late eighties, even in patients unselected for their family history (Breitner et al., 1988; Huff et al., 1988). This is considerably greater than the lifetime risk in the general population of developing AD, which is about 10% (Rocca, Amaducci, & Schoenberg, 1986). Both the number of blood relatives and the number of first-degree relatives with AD increase the risk of developing this disorder (Amaducci et al., 1986).

In families with a strong history of AD, genetic inheritance may be an important variable. Mutations on chromosomes 1, 14 and 21 are known to transmit inheritance of AD in certain families with early onset disease, that is, onset before the age of 65 (Goate et al., 1991; Levy-Lahad et al., 1995; Sherrington et al., 1995; Sorbi et al., 1995). However, these mutations account for only a small percentage of the total number of AD patients, probably less than 5%.

The development of late-onset AD has been associated with the inheritance of the apolipoprotein-E (ApoE) $\varepsilon4$ genotype. This lipoprotein (fat-related protein) has been implicated in regulating levels of another brain protein, the amyloid B peptide, whose accumulation may be critical to the development of AD. Apolipoprotein-E has three common alleles, $\varepsilon2$, $\varepsilon3$, and $\varepsilon4$. The $\varepsilon3$ allele is most frequent, occurring in about 75% of the population, whereas the $\varepsilon4$ allele is least common, occurring in about 15 to 25% (Katzman & Kawas, 1994; Saunders et al., 1993). Each individual carries two alleles, and these may be either homozygous (e.g., $\varepsilon4/\varepsilon4$ or $\varepsilon2/\varepsilon2$) or heterozygous (e.g., $\varepsilon3/\varepsilon4$, $\varepsilon2/\varepsilon4$). The homozygous $\varepsilon4$ allele, which transmits the highest risk of developing AD, occurs rarely, in only about 2% of the population, while the $\varepsilon3/\varepsilon4$ genotype occurs in about 20% (Saunders et al., 1993).

It is well established that inheritance of an $\varepsilon4$ allele, located on chromosome 19, increases the risk of developing AD (Corder et al., 1993; Saunders et al., 1993; Strittmatter et al., 1993), particularly by the age of 70 (Blacker et al., 1997; Rebeck et al., 1994). An $\varepsilon4$ allele is present in 30 to 60% of AD patients, with the frequency generally being greater in patients with familial rather than sporadic AD (Katzman & Kawas, 1994; Saunders et al., 1993; Zubenko et al., 1994). The presence of the ε4 allele has been observed to increase the risk of developing AD in a dose-dependent fashion, such that the presence of two ε4 alleles increases the risk more than the presence of only one ε4 allele (Corder *et al.*, 1993; Saunders *et al.*, 1993; Strittmatter *et al.*, 1993). The relationship between the ε4 allele and the increased risk of developing AD may be stronger in Caucasians than in African-Americans or Hispanics (Mayeux *et al.*, 1993).

There is accumulating evidence that presence of the ε4 allele, particularly when homozygous, may also help determine certain characteristics of the disease, including the age at which clinical symptoms appear and features of the neuropsychological profile. In families with late-onset disease, the presence of the homozygous ε4 alleles has been associated with onset of disease earlier in the seventh decade (Blacker *et al.*, 1997; Corder *et al.*, 1993) and also with a faster rate of disease progression (Craft *et al.*, 1998), although the latter relationship has not always been consistently observed (Growdon, Locascio, Corkin, Gomez-Isla, & Hyman, 1996). Patients with homozygous ε4 alleles have been observed to have poorer verbal memory performance in comparison with other genotypes (Lehtovirta *et al.*, 1996), although this may not be true for patients carrying only a single ε4 allele (Tierney *et al.*, 1996). In nondemented older adults, episodic memory weaknesses have been observed in individuals carrying the ε4 allele (Bondi *et al.*, 1995).

It is important to note that the presence of the ε4 allele does not determine that an individual will develop the disease; its presence only confers a vulnerability to its development. Many AD patients do not carry the ε4 allele (Evans *et al.*, 1997; Welsh-Bohmer, Gearing, Saunders, Roses, & Mirra, 1997), and the ε4 allele may be present, even homozygous, in individuals who never develop the disorder (Farrer *et al.*, 1995; Henderson *et al.*, 1995). While the ε4 allele increases the risk of developing AD, it does not determine that an individual will develop the disease. It is currently hypothesized that a convergence of neuropathological and neurophysiological activities help determine whether an individual carrying the ε4 allele ultimately develops the clinical syndrome (Cummings, Vinters, Cole, & Khachaturian, 1998).

Therefore, the presence of the ε4 allele alone should not be used to diagnose individual patients. In fact, current research indicates that diagnosis is more likely to be accurate when based on clinical evaluation using NINCDS-ADRDA criteria than when based on ε4 genotype alone (Mayeux *et al.*, 1998). However, in individuals already meeting NINCDS-ADRDA criteria for probable AD, the presence of the ε4 allele increases the likelihood that the diagnosis is correct, that is, that the neuropathological hallmarks of the disease will be present in brain tissue (Mayeux *et al.*, 1998; Welsh-Bohmer *et al.*, 1997). In addition, the presence of the ε4 allele in individuals with mild cognitive impairment of unknown etiology has been observed to be predictive of the development of AD (Peterson *et al.*, 1995).

A previous history of traumatic brain injury is another variable that may increase the risk of developing AD, although this relationship is somewhat controversial. One study indicated that individuals having suffered a single traumatic brain injury sufficient to cause loss of consciousness or hospitalization had twice the risk of developing AD as individuals without this history (Mortimer *et al.,* 1991). There is some suggestion that this increased risk may be present for individuals without a genetic vulnerability for AD (Mortimer *et al.,* 1991; Rasmussen, Brandt, Martin, & Folstein, 1995). This conclusion is, however, questioned by other evidence indicating that the relationship between traumatic brain injury and increased risk of AD may be moderated by the presence of the ε4 genotype. One recent study observed that although individuals who had experienced a traumatic brain injury and also carried the ε4 allele had an elevated (tenfold) risk of developing AD, the risk was not increased in head injury victims who did not carry the ε4 allele (Mayeux *et al.,* 1995). Thus, while traumatic brain injury appears to increase the risk of developing AD, future research is needed to clarify whether other variables modulate this risk.

Female sex may slightly elevate the risk of AD, although this may largely reflect the fact that women tend to live longer than men (Jorm, 1990; Rocca *et al.,* 1986). Use of estrogen therapy after menopause has been associated with decreased risk of developing AD among women (Henderson, Paganini-Hill, Emanuel, Dunn, & Buckwalter, 1994; Kawas *et al.,* 1997). However, it is not well understood whether or how the concurrent use of progesterone may moderate this effect.

There is also evidence that lower education increases the risk of developing AD, while higher education or greater intellectual ability may be protective. The prevalence of AD is greater in groups with less education, particularly in those with less than 12 years of education (Katzman, 1993). It has been hypothesized that variables such as higher education may confer a "brain reserve," which raises the threshold for disease expression and delays the time at which clinical symptoms are manifested (Satz, 1993). It has been proposed that education may increase synaptic density in neocortical association cortex (Katzman, 1993), allowing synaptic function to become more degraded before clinical symptoms emerge. Education may be protective, in part, because better-educated individuals may follow better medical and nutritional practices and regularly engage in more cognitively stimulating activities.

As is consistent with a protective effect of education in delaying the appearance of clinical symptoms, patients diagnosed with AD who had greater education or more complex occupations have been observed to have more severe brain metabolic abnormalities than those with comparable dementia severity but less education (Alexander *et al.,* 1997; Stern, Alexander, Prohovnik, & Mayeux, 1992). Well-educated patients often have a later age of disease onset and a shorter survival time after becoming symptomatic (Stern *et al.,* 1994b; Stern, Tange, Denaro, & Mayeux, 1995), which also suggests that their brains have sustained greater damage before they become clinically symptomatic.

Neuropsychological Characteristics of Alzheimer's Disease

Neuropsychological assessment plays a critical role in the diagnosis of AD. Both the DSM-IV and the NINCDS-ADRDA criteria specify that findings of deficits in memory and other neuropsychological domains are necessary for diagnosing the disease.

The neuropsychological symptoms of AD can be heterogenous, but certain findings are frequently observed, particularly in late-onset disease (after the age of 65), the most common presentation. The following pattern of findings is highly characteristic of the initial symptoms of late-onset AD.

1. *Dysfunction in recent memory.* The patient has difficulty in remembering new information, as evidenced by clinical history as well as findings from formal testing. Immediate memory for new information (as during the WMS-III Logical Memory I) may be below expectation or impaired, and delayed memory dysfunction (as in Logical Memory II) is often even more pronounced. These findings suggest impairment in the initial acquisition of new information in memory as well as in memory storage. A deficit in memory storage, as indicated by marked memory loss after a short time delay, has been described as one of the most sensitive and specific findings observed early in the course of AD (Welsh *et al.,* 1991; Welsh *et al.,* 1992).

Recent memory is typically not facilitated by the provision of external structure. That is, memory is deficient in both conditions of recall and recognition. In contrast, remote memory may appear relatively preserved. During the early phase of the disease, the impairment in recent memory may occur in the absence of other deficits, qualifying the patient for a DSM-IV diagnosis of an Amnestic Disorder Not Otherwise Specified.

2. *Impaired naming.* The patient and the family may report that the patient seems to struggle "to find words," even when he knows what he wants to say. Even in the absence of this observation, a word-finding deficit is often observed in formal tests of naming such as the Boston Naming Test, on which the patient obtains a score that indicates impairment or is below expectation. Although the patient may not be able to retrieve the exact name of a pictured object, he is often able to recognize and describe the object, resulting in semantic paraphasic or circumlocutory errors. Perceptual errors are less common except in patients experiencing a visual subtype of AD. External structure such as phonemic cuing typically does not facilitate naming.

3. *Dysfunction in attention and executive function.* These deficits are often less pronounced than impairment in memory but may be revealed in tests requiring concurrent manipulation of information (Lafleche & Albert, 1995). Patients may make errors or be unable to perform the more demanding items on the WMS-III Mental Control, such as item 8, which requires alternation between counting by sixes and reciting the days of the week. Patients may exhibit a relative weakness on the backward digit span, although the forward span may be relatively preserved (Lafleche & Albert, 1995). A common pattern is for the backward digit span to be below expectation or impaired, although the forward digit span is within the expected range. Deficits may be present on the Trail-Making Test or on tests of word fluency. When standardized scores are compared,

category fluency may be weaker than letter fluency (Cahn *et al.,* 1995; Masur *et al.,* 1994; Monsch *et al.,* 1992), reflecting the breakdown of semantic memory associated with AD (Hodges *et al.,* 1992b; Monsch *et al.,* 1994).

Decline in executive function may also be revealed by *unawareness of deficit.* Patients may report that they are aware of only mild or no change in memory and may become defensive in trying to explain memory deficits exhibited during formal testing. Decline in planning and concreteness thinking may lower test scores in general, particularly on tests requiring self-structuring of behavior, such as Clock Drawing or WAIS Block Design. As discussed in Chapter 4, typical clock drawing errors made by patients with mild AD include mispositioning of numbers on the clock face related to impaired planning and inability to remember the time that must be represented. Even when reminded, patients may represent the time incorrectly, often pointing both hands toward the number 10 and making other errors suggestive of inappropriate pull to stimulus detail or concrete thought.

Alzheimer's Disease Subtypes

Although the previously described features are often characteristic of the neuropsychological profile of early AD, the disease presentation can be quite heterogeneous. Some patients exhibit a profile that overlaps with the characteristic profile but also has some highly distinctive features. Observation of variability in the neuropsychological profiles of AD patients has led to descriptions of disease subtypes.

Understanding of possible AD subtypes is important for a number of reasons. First, such understanding increases appreciation for the fact that atypical neuropsychological characteristics or profiles, particularly in the absence of other etiologies for cognitive dysfunction, do not exclude the possibility that AD may be the underlying disorder. Second, recognition of an AD subtype may be helpful in predicting the possible course of the patient's disease because some subtypes have been associated with a distinctive clinical course. Third, some subtypes may be associated with distinctive patterns of pathophysiology (Kanne, Balota, Storandt, McKeel, & Morris, 1998), raising the possibility that medication treatments that may eventually be subtype-specific. If this occurs, identification of the patient's subtype has the potential for contributing to identification of an optimal treatment for that patient.

Subtypes of AD are usually most prominent early in the course of the disease and have been classified along several dimensions. One set of subtypes distinguishes between patients having predominantly verbal, predominantly visuospatial, or global (both verbal and visuospatial) neuropsychological deficits (Becker et al., 1988; Fisher et al., 1996; Martin et al., 1986). The *verbal subtype* shows focal or more pronounced impairment in verbal abilities (as assessed by tests such as the Boston Naming Test and Word Fluency) and may have unimpaired or less impaired visuospatial abilities (as assessed by tests such as the WAIS-III Block Design or Judgment of Line Orientation). In patients with pronounced or isolated verbal deficits, it is important to consider the possibility of a progressive nonfluent aphasia or semantic dementia, both of which are rare forms of frontotemporal lobar degeneration described later in this chapter.

The *visuospatial subtype* has a neuropsychological profile that is the reverse of the verbal subtype, with pronounced impairment in visuospatial abilities, including visual memory, and relative preservation of verbal skills. In some cases, visuospatial impairments in the absence of verbal deficits may be present for as long as 2 years (Weintraub & Mesulam, 1993; Weintraub & Mesulam, 1996). The *global subtype* shows relatively equivalent impairment in both verbal and visuospatial abilities. The global presentation is most common, occurring in 50 to 60% of patients, with the verbal and visuospatial subtypes each equally represented in the remaining patients.

Metabolic studies have revealed patterns of brain dysfunction corresponding to these subtypes. The global subtype shows bilateral hypometabolism of temporal and parietal brain structures, the verbal subtype shows greater left temporal hypometabolism relative to other regions, and the visuospatial subtype shows relatively greater right temporal and parietal hypometabolism (Haxby, Juara, Grady, Cutler, & Rapoport, 1985; Martin *et al.*, 1986). Moreover, initial subgroup membership may be predictive of the pattern of subsequent deterioration, with patients in the verbal subgroup showing more pronounced deterioration of verbal abilities and those in the visuospatial subgroup having more pronounced deterioration of visuospatial abilities (Haxby *et al.*, 1990; Martin *et al.*, 1986).

There has been some examination of the other clinical correlates of the verbal, visuospatial, and global subtypes. The subtypes do not appear to differ in age of disease onset or rate of disease progression. Right hemisphere lesions have been associated with unawareness of deficit, and there is some evidence that AD patients with more pronounced visuospatial as compared with verbal dysfunction are more likely to experience unawareness of deficit (Auchus, Goldstein, Green, & Green, 1994; Starkstein *et al.*, 1995). Left hemisphere lesions have been associated with an elevated rate of depression (Robinson & Szetela, 1981), and it might be hypothesized that the verbal subtype of AD is more vulnerable to depression.

A second classification of subtypes distinguishes between a late-onset "temporal lobe" subgroup in whom dysfunction in recent memory and language are most pronounced (with other neuropsychological domains being mildly or unaffected) as compared with comparably aged patients with more widespread impairments including attention/executive function and recent memory (Butters, Lopez, & Becker, 1996). In the *temporal lobe subtype,* impairment is pronounced on tests such as the WMS-III Logical Memory, Visual Reproduction, Word Lists, Boston Naming Test, and Word Fluency, suggesting pronounced temporal lobe dysfunction, but visuospatial function is relatively spared. In the *attention/executive dysfunction subtype,* impairment is more pronounced on part B of the Trail-

Making Test or the Wisconsin Card Sorting Test, suggesting deterioration of frontal lobe function. The temporal lobe subgroup has been observed to exhibit a slower rate of neuropsychological and functional decline than other patients (Butters *et al.*, 1996).

A third classification of AD subtypes distinguishes between patients who experience *early-onset AD* (with clinical symptoms appearing before the age of 65) as opposed to *late-onset* disease. Early onset patients have been described as having more pronounced deficits in attention/executive function than late-onset patients, even when the overall severity of dementia is similar (Jacobs *et al.*, 1994; Koss *et al.*, 1996; Loring & Largn, 1985). In addition, early-onset patients often experience more rapid deterioration (Jacobs *et al.*, 1994; Koss *et al.*, 1996). Consistent with this rapid deterioration, studies of the structural and neurochemical changes associated with early-onset disease have observed more severe and widespread degeneration than that associated with late-onset disease (Prohovnik, Smith, Sackeim, Mayeux, & Stern, 1989). An unanswered question is whether the early-onset subtype is related to the more rapidly progressive late-onset subtype in which deficits in attention/executive function are also pronounced.

It has been suggested that early- and late-onset patients differ in their language functioning, although this is controversial. Initial studies suggested that the early-onset patients showed specific deficits on language tests more dependent on syntactic abilities (rather than semantic access), such as language comprehension and writing (Becker *et al.*, 1988; Filley, Kelly, & Heaton, 1986). One study indicated that informants describing early-onset patients more frequently noted impairment in language as an initial symptom than was the case for late-onset patients (Jacobs *et al.*, 1994). However, several more recent reports have described greater language deficits in late-onset patients. Confrontation naming has been observed to be more impaired in late- as compared with early-onset patients (Jacobs *et al.*, 1994; Koss *et al.*, 1996), and late-onset disease was also associated with greater impairment on a composite language measure including naming, reading, auditory comprehension, and writing to dictation (Bayles, 1991). One possible explanation for this inconsistency is that the early-onset patients may experience greater dysfunction in higher-level language abilities that are not assessed in existing studies. For example, it is possible that increased dysfunction in executive abilities in early-onset patients may degrade the organization of more complex verbal expression.

A fourth classification of AD subtypes distinguishes between patients with and without *extrapyramidal motor symptoms* (EPS) (Chui, Teng, Henderson, & Moy, 1985; Mayeux, Stern, & Spanton, 1985; Merello *et al.*, 1994). These symptoms are characteristic of Parkinson's disease and include features such as motor rigidity, tremor, motor slowness (bradykinesia) and impaired gait. Estimates of the prevalence of EPS in patients with mild AD have ranged between 20 and 50% (Chui *et al.*, 1985; Mayeux *et al.*, 1985; Merello *et al.*, 1994), varying as a function of the classification criteria. Subtle forms of EPS are also common in nondemented community-dwelling older individuals, with estimates ranging from 32 to 57% (Merello et al., 1994; Richards, Stern, & Mayeux, 1993d), and have been associated with subtle cognitive dysfunction as well as with increased risk for developing AD (Richards, Stern, Marder, Cote, & Mayeux, 1993c; Richards et al., 1993d).

The neuropsychological profile of AD patients with EPS differs from that of AD patients without EPS. When groups with and without EPS are matched on critical variables such as age or disease duration, AD patients with EPS may exhibit more severe neuropsychological impairment, particularly in recent memory, naming, word fluency, and visuospatial construction, although not in long-term memory, language comprehension, or abstract reasoning (Richards et al., 1993a). The neuropsychological profile of AD patients with EPS is often similar to that observed in Parkinson's patients having significant cognitive dysfunction, with the exception that the AD patients may show poorer naming ability (Richards et al., 1993a; Soininen et al., 1992).

Alzheimer's disease patients with EPS also exhibit greater dysfunction in executive abilities. When patient groups with and without EPS were matched for overall intellectual function, AD patients with EPS exhibited more severe deficits on tests such as the Wisconsin Card Sorting Test, Trail-Making Test and letter fluency, with the severity of these deficits being greatest for patients having the greatest number of EPS (Merello et al., 1994). In contrast, patients with and without EPS did not differ on tests of verbal or visual memory.

Alzheimer's disease patients with EPS show more rapid disease progression (Chui et al., 1994; Mortimer, Ebbitt, Jun, & Finch, 1992). For patients initially without motor symptoms, the emergence of clinically detectable EPS may be predictive of disease acceleration or deterioration (Stern et al., 1996). Also, AD patients with EPS are more likely to show psychotic features such as hallucinations, delusions, or depression and behavioral problems such as agitation (Mayeux et al., 1985; Merello et al., 1994).

It has been suggested that the appearance of EPS in AD patients reflects the presence of another disease overlapping with AD. Some patients may have medication-induced EPS, and it is important to evaluate this possibility in patients who have been treated for psychiatric disorder with neuroleptic medications known to induce EPS, such as haloperidol. Some AD patients with EPS may also have Parkinson's disease, and indeed, neuropathologic studies have suggested that some patients experience these two disorders concurrently (Ditter & Mirra, 1987; Leverenz & Sumi, 1986). However, some AD patients with EPS do not show the responsiveness to dopaminergic medication that is characteristic of Parkinson's disease patients, which suggests that the motor symptoms may have a different pathophysiology (Merello et al., 1994). The presence of EPS together with a relatively rapid course of deterioration accompanied by visual hallucinations raises the possibility that the patient may be experiencing dementia with Lewy bodies (McKeith et al., 1996), either alone or overlapping with AD (see Chapter 7).

Neuropsychiatric Symptoms in Alzheimer's Disease

It is not uncommon for AD patients to exhibit neuropsychiatric symptoms (Cummings & Victoroff, 1990). Early in the disease, family members often report that the patient has lost interest in his usual hobbies and activities and spends considerable time being inactive or uncharacteristically watching television. The patient may exhibit paranoid or delusional thought, for example, believing that others are stealing his belongings or intending to harm him. In some cases, the patient becomes suspicious of his spouse, for example, believing that she is having an affair.

In a study using the Neuropsychiatric Inventory (NPI), 44 (88%) of 50 consecutive outpatients with AD were observed to exhibit behaviors suggestive of psychopathology (Mega, Cummings, Fiorello, & Gornbein, 1996). In patients with mild AD, the most frequent symptoms were apathy and agitation, occurring in 47% of the patients. Irritability and disinhibited behaviors were also common, each occurring in 35% of the patients. In patients with moderate or severe disease, apathy was the most frequent symptom. In contrast, few patients met clinical criteria for depression, and even dysphoria was uncommon in mildly affected patients (12%), although dysphoria increased with disease severity. Although the level of overall psychiatric disorder for the entire patient group increased as neuropsychological status declined, the neuropsychiatric symptoms of individual patients were variable over time and not necessarily linked with changes in overall mental status. Some patients showed a pattern of psychiatric symptoms early in the course of the disease that was different from that observed later in the disease.

One advantage of the Neuropsychiatric Inventory for evaluating psychiatric symptoms in AD is that it has been validated specifically for use in this population and attempts to distinguish symptoms reflecting depression from those more closely related to apathy (Cummings *et al.,* 1994). This is an important distinction, with significant implications for treatment. There is evidence that caregivers of patients with AD tend to overreport the occurrence of depression in patients (Mackenzie, Robiner, & Knopman, 1989), and it is not uncommon for family members to infer that the loss of interest in usual activities or other apathetic behaviors suggest that the patient is depressed. In fact, such behaviors, particularly in the absence of other symptoms of depression such as tearfulness, insomnia, or appetite disturbance, may reflect apathy rather than depression. The most common treatment for depression in older adults is administration of antidepressant medication. However, these medications may have undesirable side effects, and treatment of patients who are actually exhibiting apathetic behavior more intrinsic to AD rather than depression may unnecessarily expose them to these side effects.

While some studies have reported a relatively high prevalence of depression among AD patients, this may in part reflect failure to distinguish between depression and apathy. The reported prevalence rates for depression are usually below

50%, and symptoms of mild depression are more common than major depression, with most estimates ranging between 10 and 30% (Lyketsos, Tune, Pearlson, & Steele, 1996; Reifler, Larson, Teri, & Poulsen, 1986; Rovner, Broadbent, Spencer, Carson, & Folstein, 1989; Teri & Wagner, 1992; Wragg & Jeste, 1989). Depressive symptoms are often in response to episodic events (such as frustration about difficulty in performing a formerly easy activity) rather than being continuous. The risk of depression in patients with AD has been observed to be higher in those having a personal or family history of depression (Zubenko, Rifai, Mulsant, Swett, & Pasternak, 1996).

A number of studies have examined whether the neuropsychological performance of AD patients with clinical depression is different from that of AD patients without depression. The findings suggest that depression does not superimpose greater cognitive dysfunction and in fact, that depressed patients may be less cognitively impaired than those who are not depressed (Lopez, Boller, Becker, Miller, & Reynolds, 1990; Pearson, Teri, Reifler, & Raskind, 1989). This may reflect the fact that depression is more likely to be present in patients with mild to moderate cognitive impairment than in those with more severe dementia (Rabins, Merchant, & Nestadt, 1984; Reifler, Larson, & Hanley, 1982). Treatment of depression in AD patients may not significantly improve neuropsychological performance (Reifler *et al.,* 1986; Reifler et al., 1989), with the exception of possible subtle improvement in patients from relatively high socioeconomic and educational backgrounds (Raskin, 1986). However, the diagnosis and treatment of depression in AD patients is important in that it may improve the patient's mood and functional status (Pearson *et al.,* 1989; Reifler *et al.,* 1986; Reifler *et al.,* 1989).

Identification of psychiatric symptoms in patients with AD has both treatment and prognostic implications. Neuropsychiatric symptoms can often be relieved with medication, allowing the patient to become more functional and easier for the family or spouse to care for. However, in patients who are experiencing delusions and hallucinations, rapid intellectual decline is more likely (Lopez *et al.,* 1991; Stern *et al.,* 1994a).

FRONTOTEMPORAL LOBAR DEGENERATION

Background

Frontotemporal lobar degeneration (FTLD) comprises a group of progressive dementing disorders associated with distinctive neuropathology of the frontal and temporal lobes of the brain and sharing a number of clinical features (Brun *et al.,* 1994; Neary *et al.,* 1998). Disorders in this group have several common features. First, early in its course, each disorder is characterized by distinctive deficits in neuropsychological abilities mediated by the frontal and/or temporal lobes. Second, symptoms of FTLD often appear before age 65. Third, neuropathological findings are distinct from those of AD and other common dementing disorders.

Two major types of neuropathological change are seen in the frontal and tempo-ral lobes: the *frontal lobe degeneration type,* consisting of loss of large cortical cells with nonspecific microvacuolar or spongiform change; and the *Pick type,* consisting of loss of large cortical cells with severe astrocytosis, with or without intranuclear inclusion bodies and swollen neurons (Brun et al., 1994; Neary & Snowden, 1996).

Frontotemporal lobar degeneration commonly presents as one of three clini-cal syndromes: frontotemporal dementia, progressive nonfluent aphasia, or semantic dementia. Each of these is described below.

Frontotemporal Dementia

The most common form of FTLD is frontotemporal dementia (FTD), which includes what has been called Pick's disease (Pick, 1977), frontal lobe degenera-tion (Brun, 1987; Miller *et al.,* 1991), dementia of the frontal lobe type (Neary, Snowden, Northen, & Goulding, 1988), dementia lacking distinctive histological features (Knopman, Mastri, Frey, Sung, & Rustan, 1990), and disinhibition-dementia-parkinsonism-amyotrophic syndrome (Lynch et al., 1994). Because this disorder is distinguished by insidious and progressive behavioral changes in personality and mood, it has also been called progressive comportmental dys-function (Weintraub & Mesulam, 1993).

The behavioral change associated with FTD usually begins between ages 45 and 65, with several studies reporting a mean age of onset of about 55 years (Gre-gory & Hodges, 1996; Gustafson, 1987; Neary *et al.,* 1988). Reports of the preva-lence of FTD among cases of dementia are variable, with most estimates ranging between 10 and 20% (Brun, 1987; Cole, 1992; Neary *et al.,* 1988; Stevens *et al.,* 1998). Among patients with symptoms appearing before age 65, FTD may be more common than AD (Brun et al., 1994). Genetic inheritance appears to play an important role, with between 40 and 60% of FTD cases having a positive fam-ily history (Gustafson, 1993; Lynch et al., 1994; Neary et al., 1987; Stevens et al., 1998). In rare cases, the early personality change associated with FTD is fol-lowed by the development of rapidly progressive motor changes such as motor weakness and dysarthria, reflecting motor neuron disease similar to that associ-ated with amyotrophic lateral sclerosis (Lou Gehrig's disease) (Lynch *et al.,* 1994; Neary *et al.,* 1990). The mean duration of the nonmotor forms of FTD is 8 years, although some patients have survived as long as 15 years. Patients with the motor neuron form have a shorter survival, often dying within 3 years of disease onset.

Brain imaging of FTD patients often reveals distinctive findings. Patients may have pronounced bilateral, asymmetric atrophy of the frontal and temporal lobes with relative preservation of posterior structures (Kitagaki *et al.,* 1998). The striatum of the basal ganglia may also be atrophic, producing parkinsonian motor dysfunction later in the course of the disease. In FTD motor neuron dis-ease, atrophy may be restricted to the orbitomedial frontal and anterior temporal lobes. Metabolic and blood flow studies reveal dysfunction in the anterior frontal lobes (Miller *et al.,* 1991; Neary *et al.,* 1987; Starkstein *et al.,* 1994). Electroencephalographic activity is often normal.

Neuropsychological changes, reflected in personality and mood abnormalities, are among the earliest symptoms of FTD. These changes may initially be dominated by one of several patterns of personality change: overactive, disinhibited, impulsive behavior, which has been associated with more severe pathology in the orbitomedial frontal lobe; inert, apathetic behavior, which has been associated with dorsolateral prefrontal dysfunction; or repetitive, stereotypic behavior, which has been associated with more severe atrophy of the striatum of the basal ganglia and the temporal lobe and is often accompanied by parkinsonian motor symptoms (Neary & Snowden, 1996). Overactive, disinhibited personality changes are more common in patients with FTD motor neuron disease, which is consistent with the pronounced orbitomedial frontal atrophy often observed in these patients. In general, patients who are initially overactive and disinhibited often later become apathetic and inert as the disease progresses.

Mood disorders are common, including depression, emotional lability, manic behavior, and irritability. Patients may exhibit symptoms of Kluver-Bucy syndrome, such as hypersexuality, hyperorality, and compulsive attention to detail (Cummings & Duchen, 1981). Awareness of change may be limited and judgment compromised. Because of the prominent changes in personality and mood, patients with FTD are often initially diagnosed as having a primary psychiatric illness such as schizoaffective disorder, depression, or bipolar disorder (Gregory & Hodges, 1996).

Although patients with FTD may perform within normal limits on mental status screening tests (Gregory & Hodges, 1996), they typically exhibit deficits on formal neuropsychological instruments, particularly on less structured tests and those sensitive to frontal lobe function (Miller *et al.,* 1991; Neary & Snowden, 1996). Patients may exhibit cognitive inflexibility, perseverative behavior, difficulty in planning performance of novel tasks, and inability to recognize and correct errors. Behaviors reflecting stimulus-boundedness and environmental dependence (L'Hermitte, 1986) are common, such as *echolia* and *echopraxia* (repeating the speech and action of others) and *utilization behavior* (spontaneous handling of objects despite instructions to the contrary). Expressive speech is often impaired by a *dynamic aphasia* (Costello & Warrington, 1989), in which speech may be fluent, but the content is repetitive, stereotyped, and echolalic of others. Mutism may occur later in the disease. Early in the course of the disease, memory may be relatively preserved or deficits on memory tests may largely reflect lack of effort or concern rather than a fundamental deficit in memory storage or retrieval. Confabulation, the recall of information that was not presented, is common. Visuospatial skills and praxis are often relatively preserved, particularly early in the course of the disease.

Progressive Nonfluent Aphasia

Progressive nonfluent aphasia (also called primary progressive aphasia) is a relatively rare, progressive language disorder in which the most prominent early symptom is a gradually progressive expressive aphasia (Mesulam & Weintraub, 1992). Patients often present with difficulty in word finding and make phonemic paraphasic errors in spontaneous speech and during tests of naming. Speech output is characterized by hesitancy, abnormal articulation and prosody, phonological errors, and agrammatic sentence structure. Knowledge of word meaning may be relatively intact, although comprehension of more complex language constructions may become progressively more compromised. Visuospatial skills, recent and remote memory, reasoning, and personality are initially preserved, although behavioral changes more characteristic of FTD may appear later in the course of progressive nonfluent aphasia. Brain imaging indicates that this disorder is often associated with asymmetric involvement of the left frontal and perisylvian cortex (Chawluk et al., 1986; Tyrrell, Warrington, Frackowiak, & Rossor, 1990).

Semantic Dementia

Semantic dementia is a rare disorder characterized by early speech deficits suggesting a marked deterioration in semantic knowledge, particularly that underlying language (Hodges, Patterson, Oxbury, & Funnell, 1992a). This clinical syndrome has been described as a fluent form of progressive aphasia (Weintraub & Mesulam, 1996). Although conversational speech appears effortless, with normal articulation, prosody, and syntax, speech content is notable for being relatively empty and conveying little information. Patients often use vague, imprecise, or idiosyncratic terms, such as referring to objects as "things" or making semantic paraphasic errors. The semantic paraphasic errors often consist of equal-level rather than superordinate terms, for example, "rat" or "squirrel" instead of "beaver," but not the superordinate word "animal." Patients exhibit a severe deficit in comprehending single words or in naming objects that they see or touch. Patients may have difficulty in remembering not only the identity of objects but also their use. There is pronounced impairment in the ability to generate exemplars of semantic categories (e.g., to generate animal names) as well as reduced knowledge of category and word meanings (Hodges & Patterson, 1996; Hodges et al., 1992a; Snowdon, Goulding, & Neary, 1989). In some cases, patients are unable to recognize familiar faces because they cannot recall the contextual cues in which they were initially seen. Memory for new information may be compromised because of the deterioration in semantic knowledge. Patients with semantic dementia may exhibit behavioral changes, including reduced concern about others and a restricted range of interests, sometimes neglecting routine everyday activities. Some patients have been described as having an abnormal preoccupation with their financial affairs.

Early in the disease, patients with semantic dementia are often able to match visuospatial stimuli and copy simple line drawings. They may initially be able to read, write, and repeat short phrases and sentences, although they may not fully comprehend them, particularly as the disease progresses. It has been suggested that semantic dementia begins with focal dysfunction of the left inferolateral temporal lobe (Hodges et al., 1999).

Distinguishing Frontotemporal Lobar Degeneration from Alzheimer's Disease

Some of the characteristics of FTLD overlap with those of AD, but differences in the overall pattern of behavioral and neuropsychological findings can be helpful in distinguishing between these disorders. Prominent early changes in personality or language before the age of 65 together with relatively preserved recent memory strongly raise the possibility of FTLD rather than AD.

Behavioral abnormalities and neuropsychiatric dysfunction are more frequent among patients with FTLD than among those with AD. During the clinical interview, patients with FTLD may be more inclined to imitate behaviors of the examiner, even when instructed not to do so (Kitagaki et al., 1998). Loss of personal awareness, hyperorality, stereotyped and perseverative behavior, progressive reduction in speech output, and preserved spatial orientation may be more strongly suggestive of FTLD than of AD (Miller et al., 1997). Using the Neuropsychiatric Inventory, one study observed that FTLD patients were rated as having higher disinhibition and apathy with relatively lower levels of depression in comparison with AD patients (Levy, Miller, Cummings, Fairbanks, & Craig, 1997). The presence of psychotic behavior such as delusional thought or hallucinations is more characteristic of AD than FTLD (Lopez et al., 1996).

A number of studies have directly compared the neuropsychological performance of patients with FTLD and AD. In several studies focusing on patients with FTD and AD, both groups showed impaired performance in comparison with healthy control subjects on multiple tests, including naming, memory, word fluency, and verbal inference (Mendez et al., 1996; Pachana et al., 1996). However, one study indicated that the overall pattern of deficits may be different, with FTD patients having greater executive than memory dysfunction and AD patients showing the opposite pattern (Pachana et al., 1996). Patients with FTD may show stronger and relatively better preserved visuospatial skills than patients with AD (Mendez et al., 1996).

A study comparing groups of healthy control subjects and patients diagnosed with AD, FTD, or semantic dementia also observed a pattern of neuropsychological strengths and weaknesses that may be helpful in distinguishing between these groups (Hodges et al., 1999). On single-word reading, the semantic dementia group performed significantly more poorly than the other three groups, who did not differ from each other. On tests of immediate and delayed verbal recall, the performance of the semantic dementia and AD groups was notably worse than that of the FTD group, although even this group was impaired relative to the control group. However, on a test of visual memory, the AD group stood out, being worse than the other three groups, who were similar to each other. On a test of category fluency, the semantic dementia group was again the poorest, with the AD and FTD groups being significantly better, although worse than the control group. On letter fluency, the semantic dementia and FTD groups were both worse than the AD group, which was impaired relative to the control group. Comparing category and letter fluency performance, both the control and the FTD groups showed stronger category than letter fluency, while the semantic dementia group showed the opposite pattern. On a test of picture naming, the semantic dementia group was worse than the other three groups, who did not differ from each other. The performance of all the groups was similar on tests of attention and visuospatial ability.

7

NEUROPSYCHOLOGICAL PROFILES II

Cerebrovascular Disease, Dementia with Lewy Bodies

CEREBROVASCULAR DISEASE AND VASCULAR DEMENTIA

Background

Cerebrovascular disease compromises the blood supply to the brain and is one of the most common life-threatening illnesses, ranking third as a cause of death behind heart disease and cancer. The rate of cerebrovascular disease increases with age, affecting about 6% of those over age 75 (Wolf, Kannel, & Verter, 1984). Hypertension is the most important variable placing individuals at increased risk for this disorder, and other contributory factors include diabetes mellitus, hyperlipidemia (elevated levels of fat in the blood), heart disease, atherosclerosis (buildup of plaque in the blood vessels), cigarette smoking, alcohol consumption, and family history (Hachinski & Norris, 1985; Meyer, McClintic, Rogers, Sims, & Mortel, 1988).

Understanding of the organization of the brain and the cerebrovascular system is critical for understanding the neuropsychological sequelae of cerebrovascular disease. Detailed description and representation of this system can be found in the books by Lezak (1995) and Netter (1989). Major structures and blood vessels associated with cerebrovascular disease are represented in Appendix H. The anterior cerebral arteries (ACAs) and the middle cerebral arteries (MCAs) emerge at the end of the internal carotid arteries. The ACAs and their smaller branches supply the medial and polar surfaces of the frontal and parietal lobes, the corpus callosum, and the basal ganglia. The right and left ACAs are connected by the anterior communicating artery (ACoA). The MCAs and their subsidiaries supply the lateral frontal, temporal, and parietal lobes, the basal ganglia, the thalamus, and the internal capsule. The posterior cerebral arteries (PCA) emerge from the basilar artery and supply the inferior medial and polar regions of the temporal lobe, occipital lobe, and posterior corpus callosum (splenium). The posterior communicating artery (PCoA) connects the juncture of the ACA and MCA with the PCA. The circular network formed by a branch of the ACA, the ACoA, the PCoA, and the end of the basilar artery is known as the *circle of Willis*. Each of the major vessels has smaller branches (arteries and arterioles), which penetrate below the cerebral cortex to supply subcortical structures. The term *watershed* refers to regions supplied by networks of tiny vessels at the terminations of the distributions of the major vessels.

The blood supply of the cerebrovascular system nourishes the brain with oxygen and nutrients and removes heat and by-products of metabolic activity. Reduction in this supply can result in tissue death (*infarcts*) and *lesions* (areas of dead brain tissue). The most common etiologies of cerebrovascular disease are *ischemia*, reduction in the blood supply, and *hemorrhage*, which is abnormal bleeding into surrounding tissue. The neurologic and neurobehavioral abnormalities associated with these events are commonly referred to as *strokes*.

Ischemic strokes account for about 80% of strokes and are more common than hemorrhagic strokes. Ischemic strokes occur when there is a reduction or blockage of the blood supply, resulting in oxygen deprivation to proximal tissue. Ischemia is most frequently subsequent to atherosclerotic *thrombosis,* a buildup of plaque in the large or medium-sized vessels that initially reduces and may eventually occlude the blood supply. Blood flow may also be restricted by an *embolus,* a fragment of thrombotic material that has broken away from a vessel upstream from the area of blockage. Heart disease is often related to atherosclerosis and thus increases the risk of embolic stroke. Emboli are sometimes released following medical procedures used to treat heart disease, such as coronary artery bypass surgery (CABG) or carotid endarterectomy.

Transient ischemic attacks (TIAs) involve a temporary vascular blockage that is sufficient to alter brain function but without significant tissue death. Patients display transient symptoms lasting only several minutes, for example, temporary dysarthria or hemiparesis. Patients experiencing multiple TIAs are at increased risk for a major ischemic event.

Ischemia may also occur subsequent to other medical conditions that reduce the brain's oxygen supply, such as cardiopulmonary arrest (heart attack), cardiac arrhythmia (irregular heart rate), recurrent hypotension with syncope (low blood pressure with faintness), severe anemia, or restriction or spasm of blood vessels caused by a cerebral aneurysm (an abnormal, balloon-shaped dilatation of a blood vessel).

Hemorrhagic strokes occur when blood vessels rupture, and typically present as a gradually increasing neurobehavioral abnormality, with symptoms worsening over 5 to 30 minutes, usually with disrupted alertness and severe headache. Blows to the head incurred during a fall or automobile accident may result in a *subarachnoid hemorrhage,* a bleed into the subarachnoid space between the brain and the skull due to rupture of vessels on the brain's surface. Pockets of blood may exert pressure on and cause damage to underlying brain tissue. Older individuals who frequently fall, such as patients with Parkinson's disease, are at increased risk for subarachnoid hemorrhage (Bornstein, Weir, Petruk, & Disney, 1987). Intracranial hemorrhages in deeper brain tissue may occur following the rupture of a cerebral aneurysm or of an *arteriovenous malformation* (AVM) a relatively rare, congenital abnormal tangle of the blood vessels connecting the arterial and venous circulation. In some cases, aneurysms may be surgically removed before they rupture.

Neuropsychology of Cerebrovascular Disease

The nature and severity of neuropsychological sequelae of cerebrovascular disease reflect the location and quantity of the affected brain tissue. However, because most brain regions participate in distributed neural systems, it is rare that a lesion will result in a single neuropsychological deficit. More typically, pronounced impairment in a particular neuropsychological ability or domain is accompanied by less severe deficits in other abilities modulated by the affected neural network.

Major types of cerebrovascular disease include cortical infarctions, strategically located small infarcts, and small-vessel disease (lacunar disease and leukoaraiosis). *Cortical infarctions* involve blockages of the large vessels (the ACAs, PCAs, or MCAs) supplying cortical gray matter (the frontal, temporal, parietal, and occipital lobes). These blockages often have an acute onset, resulting in prominent impairment in specific abilities or neuropsychological domains, accompanied by less pronounced deficits in other areas. Cortical infarctions are often responsible for the abnormalities referred to as strokes.

Table 7.1 indicates some of the neuropsychological sequelae associated with lesions in specific brain regions. Comprehensive reviews of these sequelae can be found in Lezak (1995) and Heilman and Valenstein (1993).

Frontal lobe lesions are associated with changes in executive function, attention, personality, affect, and motor behavior that are somewhat specific to the areas affected within the frontal lobe (Stuss & Benson, 1986). Medial frontal lobe lesions are associated with apathy, poor motivation, and reduced spontaneity of behavior. Dorsolateral prefrontal lesions are associated with reduced verbal fluency, impairment of motor control, and cognitive inflexibility. Orbitofrontal lesions are associated with personality change, including disinhibited behavior, failure to follow social custom, emotional lability, and childlike behavior.

Strokes involving the anterior and medial temporal lobe are associated with severe amnestic syndromes, particularly *anterograde amnesia,* that is, difficulty in

TABLE 7.1   Major Neuropsychological Sequelae Associated with Strokes in Specific Brain Regions

Lesion site	Vessels involved	Neuropsychological sequelae
Frontal lobe	ACA, MCA	
Medial		Apathy, poor motivation, reduced behavioral spontaneity
Dorsolateral prefrontal		Reduced verbal fluency, cognitive inflexibility, contralateral motor deficits
Orbitofrontal		Disinhibition, impaired social judgment, emotional lability, childlike behavior
Temporal lobe	MCA, PCA	Amnesia, aphasia, apraxia
Left angular gyrus (posterior)	MCA branch	Acalculia, right–left disorientation, dysgraphia, finger agnosia
Parietal lobe	ACA, MCA	Visuospatial and visuoconstructive deficits, anosognosia, hemispatial neglect, especially following right hemisphere lesions
Occipital lobe	PCA	Visual deficits (visual agnosias, anopsias)
Anterior corpus callosum	ACA	Disconnection syndromes
Caudate nucleus	ACA or MCA branch	Deficit in memory retrieval, fluency, attention, cognitive flexibility, motor programming
Globus pallidus	MCA branch	Deficit in memory retrieval, cognitive flexibility
Thalamus	PCA branch	Amnesia, deficits in fluency, attention, cognitive flexibility, motor programming

ACA, anterior cerebral artery, MCA, middle cerebral artery; PCA, posterior cerebral artery.

remembering new information. The laterality of a temporal lobe stroke often determines its relative impact on verbal as compared with visual memory. Left temporal lobe strokes are associated with more pronounced deficits in verbal memory, whereas right temporal lobe strokes produce more severe visual memory deficits. Naming may be impaired, particularly following left temporal lesions. Posterior left hemisphere lesions may produce *acalculia* (impairment in mathematical calculation), *apraxia* (impairment in symbolic movement), *alexia* (impairment in reading) and *agraphia* (impairment in writing). Lesions of the angular gyrus, at the juncture of the temporal and parietal lobes, may produce a cluster of deficits known as *Gerstmann's syndrome,* which includes acalculia, right-left disorientation, agraphia, and finger agnosia (Benton, 1992; Strub & Geschwind, 1983). As described below, specific aphasic syndromes are associated with left temporal lobe lesions.

Strokes involving the parietal lobe, particularly the right parietal lobe, often impair visuospatial and visuoconstructive abilities (Benton & Tranel, 1993; Egelko *et al.,* 1988). Patients experiencing right hemisphere lesions may fail to appreciate the overall organization, or gestalt, of visual stimuli, resulting in a segmented and disorganized approach to performance of visuospatial and visuoconstructive tasks. In contrast, left hemisphere lesions may impair appreciation of detail, resulting in simplification of drawing and absence of detail. *Hemispatial neglect* (or *inattention*), impaired awareness of stimuli contralateral to the side of the lesion, is frequently associated with right parietal lesions, although lesions in frontal and subcortical regions may also produce this syndrome (Caplan *et al.,* 1990; Heilman, Watson, & Valenstein, 1993b). *Anosognosia* (defective awareness of poststroke deficits, such as hemiplegia or amnesia) has been associated with right hemisphere lesions involving the parietal and temporal lobes, thalamus, and basal ganglia (Starkstein, Fedoroff, Price, Leiguarda, & Robinson, 1992a). Anosognosia is often accompanied by a relative weakness on neuropsychological tests of frontal lobe function.

Lesions of the occipital lobes may affect visual perception (Benton & Tranel, 1993). Occipital lesions may produce *anopsias,* or visual field "cuts," in which quadrants *(upper quandrant anopsia)* or halves *(hemianopsia)* of the visual field cannot be perceived. Occipital lesions also may produce one or several *visual agnosias,* impairments in specific aspects of visual perception. Patients with *simultanagnosia (Balint's syndrome)* are unable to perceive simultaneous visual stimuli. Patients with *cortical blindness* are able to perceive light and dark but cannot distinguish forms or patterns. Some patients with bilateral occipital lesions experience *Anton's syndrome,* in which they fail to appreciate that they have cortical blindness. *Prosopagnosia,* the inability to recognize faces, is associated with bilateral, inferior occipitotemporal lesions.

In individuals with left hemisphere dominance for language, aphasic syndromes are associated with infarctions in specific regions within the left frontal, temporal, and parietal lobes. Over 95% of right-handers and at least two-thirds of left-handers have left hemisphere speech dominance (Bradshaw & Nettleton, 1983). Aphasic syndromes differ in the relative severity with which they impair aspects of expressive and receptive speech, such as speech fluency, comprehension, repetition, and naming. Features of the major aphasic syndromes are indicated in Table 7.2, and detailed descriptions can be found in Goodglass and Kaplan (1983) and Heilman and Valenstein (1993).

One characteristic that distinguishes aphasic syndromes is the quality of speech fluency, the ability to produce a stream of language. In the fluent aphasias, patients are able to produce a stream of language, although the organization and content of this language stream may be deficient. *Broca's aphasia* is the prototypical *expressive aphasia,* involving severely impaired speech fluency, with relatively preserved speech comprehension. In contrast, *Wernicke's aphasia* is the prototypical *receptive aphasia,* involving devastation of speech comprehension. Persons with Wernicke's aphasia have fluent speech, although the content of their speech is often jargonistic, and they may be unaware of this deficit. In patients with expressive or receptive aphasia, particularly in the absence of other symptoms of stroke, the possibility of a frontotemporal lobar degeneration should be considered (see Chapter 6).

TABLE 7-2   The Relationship between Aphasic Syndromes and Left Hemisphere Lesion Sites

Syndrome	Lesion location	Fluency	Comprehension	Repetition	Naming
Broca's	Inferior frontal gyrus	Weak	Strong	Weak	Weak
Transcortical motor	Middle frontal gyrus	Weak	Strong	Strong	Weak
Wernicke's	Posterior superior temporal gyrus; inferior parietal gyrus	Strong	Weak	Weak	Weak
Anomic	Temporal-parietal juncture	Strong	Strong	Strong	Weak
Conduction	Arcuate fasciculus (connecting inferior frontal and temporal gyrus)	Strong	Strong	Weak	Weak
Trancortical sensory	Inferior parietal gyrus	Strong	Weak	Strong	Weak

Patients with *conduction aphasia* are unique in having a severe deficit in the ability to repeat language spoken by others. Patients with *transcortical sensory aphasia* have preserved fluency and repetition, but the content of their speech is deficient and has been described as "empty" and filled with jargon. Naming is the most pronounced deficit in patients with *anomia,* resulting in the use of circumlocution during expressive speech.

Strategically located small infarcts may also have significant neuropsychological sequelae. Lesions of the anterior corpus callosum may produce a disconnection syndrome, disrupting behaviors requiring communication between the brain hemispheres. For example, such patients are unable to name unseen objects held in the left hand because the right hemisphere's perception of the stimulus is unavailable to the left hemisphere, the repository of stimulus names (Bogen, 1993). Basal ganglia infarcts, particularly within the caudate nucleus, may affect the functioning of a circuit also involving the dorsolateral frontal lobe, producing deficits in memory retrieval, attention, word fluency, cognitive flexibility, motivation, mental speed, behavioral control, and executive function (Caplan *et al.,* 1990). Lesions of the thalamus, particularly the dorsomedial nucleus, have been associated with severe deficits in episodic and retrograde memory, although other brain regions are often involved when the amnesia is severe (Katz, Alexander, & Mandell, 1987; Markowitsch, 1982; Sala, Spinnler, & Venneri, 1997). In some cases, small infarcts in critical locations, such as the thalamus, genu of the internal capsule, caudate nucleus, and angular gyrus may be sufficient to cause dementia (Benson & Cummings, 1982; Bokura & Robinson, 1997; Graff-Radford, Eslinger, Damasio, & Yamada, 1984; Katz *et al.,* 1987; Mendez, Adams, & Leewandowksi, 1989; Wallesch, Kornhuber, Kunz, & Brunner, 1983).

Small-vessel disease (*lacunes* and *leukoaraiosis*) produces small lesions, usually of ischemic origin, in the small vessels (arterioles) nourishing deep white or gray matter structures. Lacunes are small infarcts most frequently occurring within the basal ganglia, thalamus, internal capsule, cerebellum, and brain stem. *Lacunar infarcts* are often "silent," occurring without dramatic behavioral or neurologic change and may be detected only by brain imaging. Nondemented patients with multiple subcortical lacunes may exhibit a mild frontal lobe syndrome with impairment on tests dependent on cognitive flexibility and self-structuring, such as letter fluency, WMS-III Words, and the Wisconsin Card Sorting Test (Wolfe, Linn, Babikian, Knoefel, & Albert, 1990). Because the subcortical regions vulnerable to lacunes are important to the modulation of motor behavior, patients with lacunar infarcts may present with parkinsonian symptoms such as dysarthria, gait abnormalities, mood disturbance, and reduced behavioral initiative (Ishii, Nishihara, & Imamura, 1986; Van Zagten, Lodder, & Kessels, 1998).

Lacunar states are often accompanied by *leukoaraiosis* (Hachinski, Potter, & Merskey, 1987), ischemic disease in the capillaries and other tiny vessels supplying tissue around the brain ventricles, resulting in multiple microinfarcts of the cerebral white matter. Leukoaraiosis represents another type of vascular disease that is often silent. This condition is often undiagnosed because its presence, particularly when mild, may be associated with little or no neuropsychological or neurologic change. In older individuals with leukoaraiosis, some studies have not detected neuropsychological change (Hunt *et al.,* 1989; Rao, Mittenberg, Bernardin, Haughton, & Leo, 1989), whereas others have reported decline in memory retrieval, mental speed, attention, and executive function (Junque *et al.,* 1990; Libon, Scanlon, Swenson, & Coslet, 1990; Steingart *et al.,* 1986; Ylikoski *et al.,* 1993), producing what has been described as a mild frontal lobe syndrome (Boone *et al.,* 1992). From a clinical perspective, among individuals showing evidence of leukoaraiosis based on brain imaging, there is considerable variability in neuropsychological findings, and the observation of leukoaraiosis does not necessarily imply the presence of deficits. Although individuals with mild small-vessel disease may function well without obvious neuropsychological sequelae, the presence of this condition places an individual at increased risk for developing neuropsychological deficits and dementia (Loeb, Gandolfo, Croce, & Conti, 1992). One explanation for the variability in neuropsychological findings as well as the increased risk of dementia is that neuropsychological deficits may become significant only when a threshold amount of brain tissue has been lesioned (Boone *et al.,* 1992).

More severe leukoaraiosis is associated with dementia, a condition that has been referred to as *senile dementia of the Binswanger type* or *subcortical ischemic leukoencephalopathy* (Babikian & Ropper, 1987; Roman, 1987). This is a progressive disorder, often accompanied by lacunes and by neurologic abnormalities that include lateralized motor signs, parkinsonian features such as disturbance in gait, and urinary urgency or incontinence. The progression of symptoms may be gradual or abrupt, even in the absence of stroke. Brain images of these patients display patchy symmetrical abnormalities in areas around the lateral ventricles, often accompanied by lacunar infarcts.

Neurobehavioral and neuropsychological changes are prominent in Binswanger's dementia. Early changes often include mental slowing, memory deficits, emotional dyscontrol, apathy, and loss of motivation (Babikian & Ropper, 1987). Memory deficits may be characterized by slow learning, failure to structure material during learning, and poor delayed recall but with facilitation of delayed memory by cuing (Gupta *et al.,* 1988). Spontaneous speech and cued word finding may be relatively preserved.

Neuropsychological deficits have been associated with both the rupture and removal of aneurysms, with AVM, and with hemorrhage of the ACoA. A variety of deficits have been associated with aneurysms in specific sites (Barbarotto *et al.,* 1989; DeLuca, 1992; Richardson, 1991). Anterior communicating artery aneurysm has been associated with anterograde amnesia and executive dysfunction (DeLuca, 1992). With respect to AVM, the nature of the neuropsychological deficits may reflect the laterality of the AVM (Brown, Spicer, Robertson, Baird, & Malik, 1989; Mahalik, Ruff, & U, 1991; Waltimo & Putkonen, 1974), with left hemisphere AVM being associated with greater deficits in neuropsychological function modulated by the left hemisphere, and the opposite being true for right hemisphere AVM.

Neuropsychological changes have also been associated with CADASIL (cerebral autosomal dominant arteriopathy with subcortical infarcts and leukoencephalopathy), a recently identified inherited disorder affecting the cerebral arterioles (Joutel *et al.,* 1997). The disorder typically appears in midlife, with early abnormalities including mood disturbance and progressive cognitive decline. In nondemented patients, neuropsychological deficits may be most pronounced on frontal lobe tests, including the Wisconsin Card Sorting Test and the Trail-Making Test (Taillia *et al.,* 1998).

The diagnosis of cerebrovascular disease is facilitated by findings from brain imaging by magnetic resonance imaging (MRI) or computed tomography (CT) (Brown & Bornstein, 1991). The CT scan has the advantages of being less costly, less uncomfortable for many patients, and better at detecting acute intracerebral hemorrhage than MRI. However, MRI is generally considered to be more sensitive for detecting ischemic abnormalities, particularly small regions of subcortical infarction such as lacunar infarcts, intermediate stages of stroke, TIAs, and leukoaraiosis. It is also more sensitive to small aneurysms and AVM.

Vascular Dementia

Vascular disease has been described as the second leading cause of dementia in older age groups, accounting for 15 to 25% of cases of cognitive decline (Roman, 1991; Tomlinson, Blessed, & Roth, 1970). It is diagnosed when neuropsychological deficits meet criteria for dementia and the major etiology of this change is determined to be cerebrovascular disease. The risk of vascular dementia (VaD) is increased by variables similar to those that increase the risk of cerebrovascular disease without dementia, including hypertension, older age, cardiac disease, and previous history of TIAs or stroke.

Several sets of criteria for diagnosing VaD are available. The DSM-IV provides criteria that define subcodes for identifying the neuropsychiatric correlates of the dementia (American Psychiatric Association, 1994). The criteria require the presence of multiple cognitive deficits, including memory impairment, that cause significant impairment in social or occupational functioning. The patient must have focal neurologic signs and symptoms that are judged to be etiologically related to the cognitive disturbance. Separate diagnostic codes are provided for VaD with and without correlates such as delirium, delusions, or depressed mood.

Another set of criteria has been developed by the National Institute of Neurological Disorders and Stroke (NINDS) in conjunction with the Association Internationale pour la Recherche et l'Enseignement en Neurosciences (AIREN) (Roman et al., 1993). The NINDS-AIREN criteria parallel the NINCDS-ADRDA criteria for AD in defining characteristics of definite, probable, and possible VaD. Like the criteria for definite AD, criteria for definite VaD require neuropathological confirmation of cerebrovascular disease. The NINDS-AIREN criteria are more specific than the DSM-IV criteria in listing a range of vascular disorders that may cause dementia, including that associated with large cortical ischemic infarcts (formerly referred to as multi-infarct dementia), strategically located small strokes, small-vessel disease (lacunes, leukoaraiosis), ischemic-hypoxic lesions such as those associated with cardiac arrest or severe hypotension, and hemorrhagic lesions. The NINDS-AIREN criteria also provide criteria for diagnosing "AD with cerebrovascular disease." It is recommended that this diagnosis be given to patients who meet the diagnostic criteria for AD and who also have clinical or brain imaging findings consistent with cerebrovascular disease.

Differentiating between Vascular Dementia and Alzheimer's Disease

Because the treatments and prognosis for VaD and AD are different, a frequent diagnostic issue is whether a patient's dementia is related to vascular disease alone, to AD alone, or to a combination of the two disorders. There is considerable overlap between the dementias caused by vascular and Alzheimer's disease, and significant vascular disease is present in 15 to 20% of patients diagnosed with AD (Gearing et al., 1995; Victoroff, Mack, Lyness, & Chui, 1995). Even in their pure forms, it may be difficult to distinguish between VaD and AD. A recent neuropathological study reported that over 20% of patients with AD were misdiagnosed with VaD (Fischer, Jellinger, Gatterbi, & Danielcyzk, 1991).

Several approaches may be useful in differing between VaD, AD, and an overlap syndrome. Medical records can be examined to determine the presence of relevant neurologic and brain imaging findings as required by the DSM-IV and NINDS-AIREN criteria for diagnosing VaD. During the clinical interview, questions based on items from the Hachinski Ischemic Scale (Table 7-3) may be

TABLE 7-3   The Hachinski Ischemic Score

Feature	Score
Abrupt onset	2
Stepwise deterioration	1
Fluctuating course	2
Nocturnal confusion	1
Relative preservation of personality	1
Depression	1
Somatic complaints	1
Emotional incontinence	1
History of hypertension	1
History of strokes	2
Evidence of associated atherosclerosis	1
Focal neurological symptoms	2
Focal neurological signs	2

useful in determining the likelihood of cerebrovascular disease (Hachinski et al., 1975). Total scores of 7 or greater are associated with VaD, and those of 4 or lower are more common in patients with pure AD. Scores of 5 or 6 suggest a mixed etiology. The Hachinski scale has high sensitivity for distinguishing pure multi-infarct dementia and pure AD but is insensitive for distinguishing between pure multi-infarct dementia and an AD-VaD overlap (Chui et al., 1992; Rosen, Terry, Fuld, Katzman, & Peck, 1980).

In addition, neuropsychological and neuropsychiatric features may be useful in distinguishing between pure VaD and pure AD. When matched for overall severity of dementia, both immediate and delayed memory are often less impaired in VaD than in AD (Gainotti, Parloato, Monteleone, & Carlomagno, 1989). The presence of consistent impairment in memory, even in structured or cued conditions, is more strongly suggestive of AD than VaD. Although VaD patients may actually perform more poorly than AD patients in unstructured conditions (Mendez & Ashla-Mendez, 1991), they often show greater facilitation when structure is provided. On tests of delayed memory, VaD patients may perform considerably better on tests of recognition as compared with recall, while AD patients often show impairment in both of these conditions. Patients with VaD may be relatively more impaired on tests dependent on frontal lobe function, such as those involving planning, sequencing, or verbal fluency, whereas AD patients may show greater deficits in memory (Kertesz & Clydesdale, 1994; Starkstein *et al.*, 1996). Emotional lability and affective disorder may be more common in patients with VaD (Starkstein *et al.*, 1996)

The presence of cerebrovascular disease alters the neuropsychological profile of AD. Patients with mild AD and leukoaraiosis may have a greater rate of disease progression, with more severe dementia during the mild phases of the disease and at death (Diaz *et al.,* 1991; Heyman *et al.,* 1998; Steingart *et al.,* 1987). Patients with mixed etiology also may exhibit greater apathy and have a higher frequency of parkinsonian motor signs (Starkstein *et al.,* 1997).

Neuropsychiatry of Cerebrovascular Disease

Psychiatric complications are common after stroke (Starkstein & Robinson, 1994). Most common is affective disorder, with 20 to 50% of poststroke patients meeting criteria for major depression or dysthymia (Robinson, Starr, Kubos, & Price, 1983). Depression is most likely following anterior left hemisphere lesions, particular those involving the left frontal dorsolateral cortex and head of the caudate (Robinson, Kubos, Starr, Rao, & Price, 1984). In patients with right hemisphere lesions, depression is more frequently associated with frontal or parietal damage (Starkstein *et al.,* 1989b). In depressed poststroke patients, more pervasive neuropsychological deficits are more common in those with left hemisphere lesions than in those with right hemisphere lesions (Bolla-Wilson, Robinson, Starkstein, Boston, & Price, 1989).

Anxiety is also common following stroke, occurring in about 20% of patients and often coexisting with depression. Anxiety without depression is more frequent following right hemisphere lesions, whereas left hemisphere lesions often produce a mixed anxiety-depression syndrome (Castillo, Starkstein, Fedoroff, Price, & Robinson, 1993). Among patients with right hemisphere lesions, anxiety is often associated with posterior (parietal) lesions (Castillo *et al.,* 1993).

Less common neuropsychiatric disorders following stroke include apathy, psychosis, catastrophic reactions, and emotional lability. Apathy has been associated with subcortical lesions such as in the posterior limb of the internal capsule (Starkstein, Fedoroff, Price, Leiguarda, & Robinson, 1993a). Poststroke psychosis (e.g., hallucinations, delusions, agitated delirium) is rare, but has been associated with right hemisphere lesions accompanied by subcortical atrophy or the occurrence of poststroke seizures (Levin & Finklestein, 1982; Rabins, Starkstein, & Robinson, 1991). Catastrophic reactions are characterized by inability to cope with physical or cognitive deficits, as expressed by severe anxiety, tearfulness, agitation, and poor cooperation (Goldstein, 1939). Catastrophic reactions occur in about 20% of stroke patients and are more likely in patients with previous personal or family history of psychiatric disorder, particularly depression, and in aphasic or depressed patients. These reactions have been associated with basal ganglia lesions (Starkstein, Fedoroff, Price, Leiguarda, & Robinson, 1993b). Stroke patients sometimes experience emotional lability, mood variability, and *pseudobulbar affect*, which is sudden outbursts of strong emotion such as crying or laughing often in response to appropriate stimuli but sometimes occurring without obvious provocation. Such emotional dysregulation has been associated with lesions affecting the frontal lobe and their pathways to subcortical brain structures (Heilman *et al.,* 1993a).

DEMENTIA WITH LEWY BODIES

Background

Dementia with Lewy bodies (DLB) is a dementing illness with neuropsychological, neuropsychiatric, and motor features that are associated with neuropathological findings of diffuse and numerous Lewy bodies in the neocortex, diencephalon, brain stem, and basal ganglia. Lewy bodies are specific, neuropathological abnormalities (eosinophilic inclusions in neuronal bodies), which are present in a number of different disorders, including Parkinson's and Alzheimer's disease. However, the neuropathological distribution and frequency of Lewy bodies as well as the neurobehavioral profile are distinctive in DLB.

Clinical criteria for diagnosing DLB have been defined (McKeith *et al.,* 1996). A central feature of these criteria is progressive cognitive decline that interferes with normal social or occupational functioning. Early in the disease, deficits on tests of attention, executive function, and visuospatial abilities are prominent. Memory impairment may not be pronounced early in the disease but usually occurs with its progression. To be diagnosed with probable DLB, patients must have two of the following: fluctuations in cognition, with variation in attention and alertness; visual hallucinations, which are often well formed and detailed; and extrapyramidal motor features similar to those associated with Parkinson's disease. The diagnosis of possible DLB requires only one of these features.

Recent studies have suggested that DLB may be responsible for 15 to 30% of all cases of dementia (Hansen et al., 1990; McKeith *et al.,* 1996), perhaps making this neuropathologic subgroup the second largest after AD. Progression is often rapid, with the patient becoming severely demented and parkinsonian within 1 to 5 years. As with AD, the apolipoprotein E ε4 genotype increases an individual's risk of developing DLB (Galasko et al., 1995).

There has been controversy concerning whether DLB is a distinct disorder or represents a variant of other disorders, although the extensiveness and range of the neuroanatomical structures affected by Lewy bodies seems unique to DLB. A distinction has been made between common DLB, in which there are widespread Lewy bodies plus neuropathology sufficient to meet criteria for AD, and pure DLB, in which there is little or no Alzheimer's pathology (Cercy & Bylsma, 1997; Kosaka, 1990). One recent meta-analysis attempting to outline the clinical differences between these subtypes suggested that common DLB typically presents late in the seventh decade, with early dementia and delusions, while pure DLB typically appears somewhat earlier, in the first half of the seventh decade, with pronounced extrapyramidal motor features, less pronounced cognitive dysfunction, a fluctuating course, and a higher frequency of depression (Cercy & Bylsma, 1997). In many medical centers, clinicians follow guidelines for the clinical and pathologic diagnosis of DLB specified by the Consortium on Lewy Body Dementia (McKeith *et al.,* 1996), which allow the disease to be diagnosed in the presence of diffuse Lewy bodies plus Alzheimer's pathology.

Patients with DLB have a number of unique features. Difficulty in maintaining alertness during the day is common, and episodes of brief unresponsiveness or inattentiveness are characteristic. Visual hallucinations of people or animals in the home are common, recurrent, and well detailed. The patient often realizes that these perceptions are unreal and may find them disturbing but not frightening.

Patients with DLB often exhibit the motor abnormalities associated with Parkinson's disease, including rigidity, bradykinesia, hypophonia, masked facies, and impaired gait. These patients are often hypersensitive to the neuroleptic medications used to treat the psychiatric disorder and experience increased parkinsonism when these are administered. The diagnostic criteria for DLB suggest that cognitive dysfunction should appear within 12 months of the onset of the extrapyramidal motor symptoms, that is, temporally proximal to the appearance of the motor abnormality. It is recommended that patients with Parkinson's disease who develop dementia at least 12 months after the onset of motor symptoms are more appropriately diagnosed as having Parkinson's disease with dementia.

Neuropsychological Characteristics of Dementia with Lewy Bodies

Although the neuropathology of DLB affects both cortical and subcortical structures, the neuropsychological profile of this disorder most closely resembles that of a subcortical dementia. Dementia with Lewy bodies is characterized by pronounced impairment in executive functions as assessed by the Wisconsin Card Sorting Test, the Trail-Making Test, or word fluency. Patients exhibit deficits on tests of visuospatial abilities, such as Block Design or Clock Drawing. When memory is impaired, it may be facilitated by the provision of external structure, as in conditions of recognition (Salmon & Galasko, 1996; Salmon *et al.,* 1996).

In comparison with AD patients, DLB patients may exhibit greater executive and visuospatial dysfunction, milder impairment in memory, and more frequent hallucinations and delusions (Galasko, Katzman, Salmon, & Hansen, 1997; Hansen *et al.,* 1990; Shimomura *et al.,* 1998b). The presence of pronounced and rapidly progressive cognitive dysfunction, which is temporally proximal to the onset of motor symptoms and accompanied by fluctuation in cognitive confusion and frequent visual hallucinations, is highly characteristic of DLB and less characteristic of Parkinson's disease or other parkinsonian syndromes.

8

NEUROPSYCHOLOGICAL PROFILES III

Parkinsonian Disorders, Corticobasal
Degeneration, Huntington's Disease

PARKINSON'S DISEASE

Diagnosis and Clinical Characteristics

Parkinson's disease (PD) is a progressive neurodegenerative disorder with prominent motor symptoms first described by James Parkinson in 1817 (Parkinson, 1817). Although its major symptoms are motor abnormalities, as is detailed later, it is now well established that patients may also experience neuropsychological and psychiatric dysfunction. Although the fundamental causes of PD are not well understood, symptoms emerge after substantial deterioration of neurons within the substantia nigra, a structure in the midbrain section of the brain stem. The substantia nigra is a major source of the neurotransmitter dopamine in the extrapyramidal motor system, which also includes the basal ganglia (the caudate nucleus, putamen, and globus pallidus), the thalamus, the subthalamic nucleus, and the interconnections between these structures (illustrated in Appendix H). The deterioration within the substantia nigra occurs slowly over many years, and 60 to 80 % of nigral cells are lost before the symptoms of PD appear (Snow & Calne, 1992; Stacy & Jankovic, 1992). The dopamine depletion has a profound impact on the functioning of the neural pathways between the substantia nigra and the major input structures to the basal ganglia, known as the striatum, including the caudate nucleus and the putamen.

Dysfunction within the basal ganglia and interconnected structures is responsible for the cardinal extrapyramidal motor signs of idiopathic PD: a low-frequency resting–postural tremor (typically 3 to 5 Hz), muscular rigidity (stiffness), and bradykinesia (slowed execution of movement) (Paulson & Stern, 1997). Most clinicians diagnose PD based on the presence of at least two of the three cardinal motor signs, accompanied by relief of these symptoms by dopamine replacement therapy, typically using levodopa (L-dopa) (Paulson & Stern, 1997).

Other motor symptoms of PD may include *masked facies* (restricted facial expression, also called *hypomimia*), impairment in gait (e.g, slowed or very rapid, propulsive gait with short steps), freezing of movement, postural instability, poor balance, sudden falls, *akinesia* (difficulty initiating movement), *hypophonia* (reduced speech volume), *dysarthria* (slurred speech), *micrographia* (decreased size of writing), and *monotonia* (restricted range of speech inflection) (Stacy & Jankovic, 1992). Ocular dysfunction is common, including impaired eye movement (slow saccades, jerky ocular pursuits), blurred vision related to poor convergence, and limited eye blinks (Paulson & Stern, 1997). The severity of motor symptoms is often rated using the Hoehn and Yahr Scale (Hoehn & Yahr, 1967), which assesses patients on a scale from 1 to 5, where 5 represents the most advanced disease. A more detailed scale is the Unified Parkinson's Disease Rating Scale (UPDRS), on which a maximum of 144 points represents the most advanced disease (Fahn, Elton, & Corporation, 1987).

Parkinson's disease is an age-related disorder, affecting less than 0.001% of persons below age 50 but increasing to 1% of those over age 60 and 2.5% of those over age 85 (Hoehn & Yahr, 1967; Rajput, Offord, Beard, & Durland, 1984). Clinical symptoms usually appear in patients between 50 and 60 years of age, with slow progression over the next 10 to 20 years (Hoehn & Yahr, 1967; Rajput *et al.,* 1984). However, some PD patients (5 to 10%) develop "young onset" PD, with symptoms appearing before the age of 40 (Golbe, 1991; Quinn, Critchley, & Marsden, 1987).

There is increasing evidence that genetic inheritance confers a susceptibility to developing PD (Tanner *et al.,* 1997). Several large pedigrees have been described in which multiple family members from several generations are affected (Golbe, Di Iorio, Bonavita, Miller, & Duvoisin, 1990). However, most cases of PD occur randomly. For random cases, the risk of developing PD is greater for individuals having an affected parent or sibling (Martin, Young, & Anderson, 1973), and 10 to 15% of PD patients have affected relatives (Duvoisin, 1986). It is currently hypothesized that individuals may inherit a susceptibility for developing PD, perhaps related to a reduced ability to metabolize or inactivate environmental or internally generated neurotoxins (Johnson, 1991).

Parkinson's disease is slightly more common in men than in women (Mayeux *et al.,* 1992; Shoenberg, Anderson, & Haerer, 1985). Caucasians may be at greater risk than Africans or Asians, although the research findings are somewhat inconsistent. Increased risk of PD has been associated with rural living, farming, and exposure to pesticides, herbicides, and well water (Gorell, Johnson, Rybicki, Peterson, & Richardson, 1998; Koller *et al.*, 1990; Lewin, 1985), possibly because of increased exposure to environmental neurotoxins.

It is well established that, in addition to motor abnormalities, some patients with PD experience neuropsychological and psychiatric dysfunction. This dysfunction has been attributed in part to deterioration within several of the five parallel, segregated circuits that link the basal ganglia, thalamus, and frontal cortex (Alexander *et al.*, 1986; Alexander, Crutcher, & DeLong, 1990). Three of these circuits (the associative, the orbitofrontal and the limbic) are believed to modulate neuropsychological and psychiatric function. Dysfunction within the associative circuit is believed to be particularly important in compromising neuropsychological function because this circuit communicates between the basal ganglia and the dorsolateral prefrontal cortex, a region implicated in executive function and working memory.

Changes in other neural regions and neurotransmitter systems also play an important role in the neuropsychological and psychiatric dysfunction sometimes associated with PD. The functioning of the prefrontal cortex is particularly dependent on dopamine supplied by the ventral tegmentum, a midbrain region within the brain stem, that deteriorates in PD (Scatton, Javoy-Agid, Rouquier, Dubois, & Agid, 1983). The frontal lobe is modulated by nondopaminergic neurotransmitter systems that also become depleted over the course of the disease, most notably the cholinergic system, which is essential to memory, and the serotonergic system, which modulates affect (Brown, Crane, & Goldman, 1979; Dubois, Ruberg, Javoy-Agid, Ploska, & Agid, 1983; Scatton *et al.*, 1983; Scatton, Rouquier, Javoy-Agid, & Agid, 1982).

After death, neuropathological findings in PD patients include neuronal loss in the substantia nigra and the ventral tegmentum (sources of dopamine) and also in subcortical brain nuclei modulating nondopaminergic neurotransmitter systems, including the locus coeruleus (the noradrenergic system), the raphe nucleus (the serotonergic system), and the nucleus basalis of Meynert (the cholinergic system). These changes result in widespread dysfunction in brain systems modulating neuropsychological, affective, and autonomic function (Brown *et al.*, 1979; Dubois *et al.*, 1983; Scatton *et al.*, 1983; Scatton *et al.*, 1982). Another characteristic and abnormal neuropathological finding is the presence of diffuse Lewy bodies, signifying neuronal degeneration, within the cytoplasm of neurons in the substantia nigra, ventral tegmentum, and locus cereleus (Gibb & Lees, 1988). Although Lewy bodies are present in other disorders (e.g., Alzheimer's disease, dementia with Lewy bodies) and thus are not specific to PD, their distribution and frequency in PD is distinctive and can reliably be distinguished from that associated with other disorders (Cornford, Chang, & Miller, 1995).

It is important to note that while idiopathic PD is the most common cause of parkinsonism, other disorders can also produce parkinsonian symptoms.

Idiopathic PD typically (although not always) includes tremor, is responsive to dopaminergic therapy, and occurs in the absence of identifiable etiologies. There are a wide variety of other parkinsonian syndromes in which motor symptoms similar to those observed in idiopathic PD are predominant, although these disorders are generally less responsive to dopaminergic therapy and may include unusual motor features. Non-PD parkinsonian syndromes have been associated with vascular disease, neurotoxin exposure, metabolic disorders, brain trauma, encephalitis, and normal pressure hydrocephalus (Cummings & Benson, 1992a; Watts & Koller, 1997). A group of disorders known as the Parkinson's plus syndromes, discussed later in this chapter, also produce parkinsonian symptoms (Watts & Koller, 1997). Long-term use of medications that either deplete dopamine or block dopamine receptors, such as antipsychotics and antiemetics, may produce parkinsonism, which may be treatable when the medications are adjusted.

Special Issues in Evaluation of Patients with Parkinson's Disease

In patients with PD, it is particularly important to consider how disease-related impairments in motor behavior, speech, eye movements, and other behaviors may compromise test performance. The motor symptoms of the disease often interfere with performance of tests requiring verbal responses, drawing, writing, or manual manipulation of test materials. For example, a patient with a pronounced tremor, rigidity, or bradykinesia may show impaired performance on the WAIS-III Block Design that is more closely related to motor impairment than to a deficit in higher-level visuospatial construction. Speech disturbances such as hypophonia or dysarthria may compromise verbal expression, for example, on the WAIS-III Vocabulary. Impaired eye movement may compromise visuospatial scanning, for example, on the Trail-Making Test.

The test battery and the interpretation of findings can be adjusted to reduce the impact of confounding factors. For example, in patients with milder tremor or rigidity that may affect but not prohibit drawing, the findings from the WMS-III Visual Reproduction or Clock Drawing can be reviewed to determine the extent to which minor errors (e.g., minor distortions) may reflect motor symptoms rather than a deficit in visual memory. For patients with more severe symptoms, it may be necessary to exclude tests dependent on motor abilities, substituting other nonmotor tests when possible. For example, the Visual Reproduction from the WMS-III might be replaced with the Faces test and the WAIS-III Block Design with the Matrix Reasoning test.

Neuropsychological function in PD patients may be affected by antiparkinsonian medications. Some of these medications have anticholinergic properties (e.g., artane, cogentin, amantadine), which may degrade memory or frontal lobe function, particularly in older patients or those with dementia (Cooper et al., 1992; Dubois, Pillon, Lhermitte, & Agid, 1990a; Glatt & Koller, 1992). If patients taking these medications exhibit memory impairment, it may be advisable to reevaluate patients after these medications have been temporarily discontinued.

Although dopaminergic therapy relieves motor symptoms, its effect on neuropsychological function is inconsistent, which suggests that neuropsychological change in PD is to a significant extent dependent on nondopaminergic changes (Cooper et al., 1992; Pillon et al., 1989). During the first several years of the disease, dopamine replacement therapy may ameliorate or have little impact on mild cognitive dysfunction (Cooper et al., 1992; Growdon, Kieburtz, McDermott, Panisset, & Friedman, 1998). However, in patients with more advanced disease, the effect of dopaminergic therapy is more variable, improving performance on some neuropsychological measures while impairing performance on others (Gotham, Brown, & Marsden, 1988).

Patients with advanced disease are also more likely to experience fluctuation in the effectiveness of their medications for relieving motor symptoms. This fluctuation may produce periods when the patients are "on" and relatively asymptomatic and periods when they are "off," with more disabling symptoms. On–off fluctuations may cause mild variability in neuropsychological performance (Delis & Massman, 1992; Kulisevsky et al., 1996). If patients are tested when they are off, they may be experiencing increased levels of frustration, anxiety, or depression, which may compromise their performance.

Neuropsychological Function in Parkinson's Disease

Neuropsychological change is often subtle and not clinically detectable early in the course of the disease, particularly in younger patients. However, in patients with later onset or more advanced disease, neuropsychological dysfunction may be pronounced. Reports of the prevalence of cognitive impairment without dementia have ranged between 17 and 53% (Lieberman, 1998), and the rate of subclinical dysfunction may be even higher.

Dysfunction in processing activities mediated by the frontal lobes is believed to be fundamental to the deficits observed on conventional neuropsychological tests (Bondi et al., 1993; Taylor & Saint-Cyr, 1992; Taylor et al., 1986a; Taylor et al., 1990). These include decline in self-directed planning, which affects attention, memory, and problem solving; difficulty in remembering temporal order (Sagar, Sullivan, Gabrieli, Corkin, & Growdon, 1988); reduced capacity for cognitive processes requiring mental effort or central attentional resources (Brown & Marsden, 1991; Cooper & Sagar, 1993b); and compromise of working memory (Gabrieli, Singh, Stebbins, & Goetz, 1996; Postle, Jonides, Smith, Corkin, & Growdon, 1997). Many of these deficits may be overlapping. It has been proposed that slowing in psychomotor speed reduces frontal lobe–mediated working memory capacity, which may be fundamental to many other deficits (Gabrieli et al., 1996).

Neuropsychological change may not be clinically detectable early in the course of PD by using standard test instruments. However, experimental studies have demonstrated that even recently diagnosed PD patients show subtle but significant deficits in abilities, including attentional set shifting (Cooper, Sagar, Jordan, Harvey, & Sullivan, 1991), information processing speed during encoding of new information in memory (Cooper & Sagar, 1993a), speed of choice response decision making (Cooper, Sagar, Tidswell, & Jordan, 1994), and spatial working memory (Postle *et al.,* 1997).

Where deficits are clinically detectable, the following features are among the earliest noted on standard neuropsychological instruments in PD patients without dementia.

1. *Executive dysfunction:* Impairment is often, although not always, present during performance of the Wisconsin Card Sorting Test (Canavan *et al.,* 1989; Lees & Smith, 1983; Sagar, Sullivan, Cooper, & Jordan, 1991; Taylor *et al.,* 1986a). Common deficits include difficulty in achieving the first correct sort and in switching between sorting rules, often accompanied by perseverative use of a previously applied rule that is no longer appropriate. These deficits seem to reflect a failure in self-directed problem solving, including difficulty in integrating feedback with present performance to develop new hypotheses concerning rules for correct response. However, PD patients who were characteristically high functioning may not display deficits on this test (Mohr *et al.,* 1990), raising the possibility that such individuals may have a protective cognitive reserve (Satz, 1993).

On digit span tests, PD patients often have an impaired backward span, particularly in comparison with the forward digit span, which is often normal (Huber *et al.,* 1986a). These patients are often acutely aware of their deficits and do not typically exhibit the anosagnosia that is more characteristic of other disorders, such as Alzheimer's disease (Green *et al.,* 1993; McGlynn & Kaszniak, 1991).

2. *Memory:* On unstructured verbal memory tests involving repeated presentation and recall of a word list, PD patients often show a deficient learning curve (Buytenhuijs *et al.,* 1994; Taylor *et al.,* 1990). Recall after the first list presentation may be particularly weak, and even after several repetitions final recall may be below expectation or even impaired. However, immediate word list memory is often within normal limits in more structured retrieval conditions, including recognition or cuing (Breen, 1993; Buytenhuijs *et al.,* 1994). On memory tests involving material that is externally structured, such as the WMS-III Logical Memory or Visual Reproduction, immediate memory may be somewhat stronger than that observed for unstructured material, although often remaining deficient even in structured conditions (Mohr *et al.,* 1990; Taylor *et al.,* 1986a).

On tests of delayed memory, PD patients often do not show pronounced memory loss over a time interval when immediate memory is compared with delayed memory. Although the absolute level of delayed recall may be deficient, measures of delayed memory savings that take into account the level of immediate memory are often within normal limits (Taylor *et al.,* 1986a). Thus, delayed recall of a word list or of more structured verbal material, such as stories, may be equivalent to immediate recall, although each of these may be below expectation or impaired. As with immediate memory, PD patients typically show little if any impairment in delayed recognition conditions.

This pattern of deficient initial acquisition of new information (as tested by learning or immediate recall), relatively preserved recognition, and minimal memory loss over a time interval is characteristic of the memory performance of nondemented PD patients. It has been suggested that these features reflect deficiency in abilities to self-impose structure and strategy during memory acquisition, which compromises both the encoding of new information in memory and the establishment of retrieval cues (Taylor et al., 1990). It has been suggested that slowing of information processing speed may be fundamental to the encoding and recall deficits that are characteristic of memory dysfunction in PD (Cooper & Sagar, 1993a).

3. *Language:* A deficit in naming as assessed by the Boston Naming Test is less consistently observed in PD patients than in Alzheimer's disease patients, with some PD patients showing preserved naming and others exhibiting mild impairment (Goldman *et al.,* 1998; Troster, Stalp, Paolo, Fields, & Koller, 1995b). When the naming total score is either below expectation or impaired, the provision of phonemic cues often facilitates naming in nondemented PD patients, a finding less commonly observed in patients with dementia related to either PD or Alzheimer's disease. However, impaired naming is commonly observed in PD patients with dementia (Troster *et al.,* 1995b).

Even nondemented patients may show impaired letter and category fluency (Auriacombe *et al.,* 1993; Bayles, Trosset, Tomoeda, Montgomery, & Wilson, 1993; Randolph *et al.,* 1993; Taylor *et al.,* 1986a; Troster *et al.,* 1995b). Impairment may be more pronounced in PD patients with dementia, who may perform similarly to patients with Alzheimer's disease (Bayles *et al.,* 1993; Goldman *et al.,* 1998; Troster *et al.,* 1995b).

4. *Visuospatial function:* PD patients often experience impairment in eye movement and spatial contrast sensitivity (Bodis-Wollner *et al.,* 1987), although other aspects of visual sensory abilities may be relatively unaffected. Nondemented patients, especially those in the early phases of the disease, may show preserved performance on tests including the Judgment of Line Orientation (JOLO) and the Benton Facial Recognition Test (Levin *et al.,* 1991; Richards, Cote, & Stern, 1993b). Performance on the JOLO may be particularly resistant to PD, even in patients with advanced disease, although demented patients may perform poorly on this test (Levin *et al.,* 1991). However, with increases in disease duration or cognitive dysfunction, impairment on visuospatial and visuconstructive tests is common (Cummings & Huber, 1992; Levin *et al.,* 1991; Mohr *et al.,* 1990).

Deficits in visuospatial and visuoconstructive performance may to a large extent reflect impairment in frontal lobe function rather than impairment in more posterior brain regions (Bondi *et al.,* 1993; Cummings & Huber, 1992; Ogden, Growdon, & Corkin, 1990). Visuospatial tests are often less familiar than verbal tests, placing greater reliance on frontally dependent abilities such as problem solving and planning. A recent study demonstrated that when statistical analysis was used to control for deficits related to frontal lobe performance, PD patients did not show significant deficits in comparison with control subjects on either visuoconstructive tests (Block Design) or visuoperceptual tests (Benton Visual Form Discrimination) (Bondi et al., 1993).

Variables Affecting Neuropsychological Function in Parkinson's Disease

A number of variables increase the risk of moderate to severe neuropsychological dysfunction in patients with PD. Neuropsychological dysfunction or dementia has been observed to be more common in patients having the following characteristics: later age of disease onset, particularly after age 60 (Caparros-Lefebvre, Pecheux, Petit, Duharnel, & Petit, 1995; Dubois, Pillon, Sternic, Lhermitte, & Agid, 1990b; Hietanen & Teravainen, 1988; Katzen, Levin, & Llabre, 1998); longer disease duration (Biggens et al., 1992; Katzen et al., 1998); a rigid–brady-kinetic presentation rather than predominant tremor (Huber, Christy, & Paulson, 1991; Pillon et al., 1989); and/or a higher, cumulative exposure to dopaminergic therapy or less benefit from dopaminergic therapy (Caparros-Lefebvre et al., 1995; Lieberman et al., 1979; Pillon et al., 1989; Portin & Rinne, 1986; Taylor, Saint-Cyr, & Lang, 1987). It has been proposed that a convergence between disease-related frontal lobe dysfunction and normal age-related decline in frontal lobe function may contribute to the greater frequency and severity of cognitive dysfunction in later-onset patients (Dubois et al., 1990b).

Early in the course of the disease, PD patients often show asymmetric motor symptoms, with either the right or left extremities being more affected, and different patterns of neuropsychological dysfunction have been associated with this asymmetry. Patients with right hemiparkinsonism have been observed to show greater deficits in left hemisphere–mediated verbal abilities than patients with left hemiparkinsonism, whereas left hemiparkinsonism has been associated with more pronounced right hemisphere–mediated visuospatial deficits (Blonder, Gur, Gur, Saykin, & Hurtig, 1989; Starkstein, Leiguarda, Gershanik, & Berthier, 1987; Taylor et al., 1986a), although not consistently (Spicer, Roberts, & LeWitt, 1988). Right hemiparkinsonian patients may also show greater depression than left hemiparkinsonian patients (Starkstein, Preziosi, Bolduc, & Robinson, 1990), which is consistent with evidence that left hemisphere lesions are associated with a higher frequency of depression than right lesions (Robinson & Szetela, 1981; Starkstein & Robinson, 1989).

Dementia in Parkinson's Disease

Between 20 and 40% of PD patients develop cognitive impairment sufficiently severe to meet the criteria for a diagnosis of dementia (Aarsland, Tandberg,

Larsen, & Cummings, 1996; Lieberman, 1998; Mayeux *et al.*, 1990; Rajput, 1992). Older age is a major risk factor (Aarsland *et al.*, 1996), with one study reporting that 65% of a surviving cohort of PD patients over the age of 85 were demented (Mayeux *et al.*, 1990). Patients are also at increased risk for dementia if they are depressed (Aarsland *et al.*, 1996; Marder, Tang, Cote, Stern, & Mayeux, 1995), have masked facies at disease onset, have predominant rigid–akinetic motor dysfunction (rather than tremor), or experience hallucinations (Stern, Marder, Tang, & Mayeux, 1993). Estrogen replacement therapy may protect against the development of dementia in female PD patients (Marder *et al.*, 1998). In nondemented patients, poor performance on tests of word fluency may be predictive of the subsequent development of dementia (Jacobs *et al.*, 1995a). The presence of dementia at disease onset argues against a diagnosis of PD and is more characteristic of other illnesses, including Alzheimer's disease, dementia with Lewy bodies, or Creutzfeldt-Jacob disease.

A number of hypotheses have been proposed to explain why some patients develop dementia. Use of antiparkinsonian medications, particularly levodopa, may produce a long-term neurotoxic effect that compromises brain function, although this hypothesis is controversial (Agid, 1998; Fahn, 1996). While dopamine deficiency in basal ganglia-thalamocortical pathways may contribute to disrupted cognition, there is substantial evidence that more pronounced cognitive dysfunction reflects involvement of nondopaminergic neuronal systems (Pillon *et al.*, 1989). Consistent with this, dopaminergic therapy does not have a reliable effect on neuropsychological measures in patients with advanced disease (Gotham *et al.*, 1988). Neuropathological studies have revealed that the brains of demented PD patients exhibit greater neuronal loss in multiple regions outside of the substantia nigra, including the locus cereleus, ventral tegmentum, nucleus basalis of Meynert, and anterior cingulate gyrus (Zweig, Cardillo, Cohen, Giere, & Hedreen, 1993). Disruption of the cholinergic neurotransmitter system may play an important role in inducing dementia in PD patients (Dubois *et al.*, 1983). Finally, PD patients are at increased risk for other dementing illnesses, notably Alzheimer's disease and dementia with Lewy bodies (Hughes, Daniel, Blankson, & Lees, 1993).

The DSM-IV defines criteria for Dementia Due To Parkinson's Disease. These criteria require the presence of impairment in memory plus impairment in at least one additional neuropsychological domain (e.g., aphasia, apraxia, agnosia, executive dysfunction) that is believed to be related to PD and that causes impairment in social and occupational functioning. Determining whether a PD patient meets these criteria is sometimes challenging because it may be difficult to determine the relative contributions of cognitive deficits versus motor disability to impairment in social and occupational functioning. Many patients with advanced PD experience severe motor disability that limits their ability to work, to care for themselves, and to interact socially, and it may be particularly difficult to determine the extent to which neuropsychological dysfunction accounts for these changes. In addition, the apraxia observed in many PD patients is often a feature of the motor disability. These issues must be carefully considered in determining whether a PD patient meets the criteria for dementia.

Because of the difficulty in assessing the contribution of motor disability to decline in social and occupational functioning, it may be more appropriate to base a diagnosis of dementia in PD mainly on neuropsychological findings, particularly findings that are believed to be relatively uncontaminated by the motor abnormalities of the disease. Cummings and Benson (1992a) have suggested that in general, dementia can be diagnosed on the basis of persistent impairment in at least three neuropsychological domains, such as language, memory, visuospatial skills, emotion or personality, and higher-level cognition (e.g., conceptual abstraction, judgment, calculation, executive function). These criteria can be used to diagnose dementia in patients with PD when there is no other likely cause for the presence of significant neuropsychological function.

Neuropsychiatric Disorder in Parkinson's Disease

Depression is common in PD patients, although its diagnosis may be confounded by an overlap between symptoms inherent to depression and those common in PD that are independent of depression. Parkinson's disease patients often exhibit psychomotor slowing, mild attentional and memory dysfunction, sleep disturbance, reduced participation in usual activities, and other behavioral changes that reflect the cognitive and motor features of the disease rather than depression. Symptoms such as tearfulness, loss of appetite, irritability, or depressive feelings and thoughts (e.g., pessimism, dysphoria) may be more useful in diagnosing depression in PD patients. An instrument that has been helpful in evaluating depression in PD patients is the Beck Depression Inventory (Beck, Ward, Mendelson, Mock, & Erbaugh, 1961; Huber, Freidenberg, Paulson, Shuttleworth, & Christy, 1990; Levin, Llabre, & Weiner, 1988).

Between 30 and 60% of patients do become depressed at some point in the disease (Cummings, 1992a; Gotham, Brown, & Marsden, 1986; Lieberman, 1998; Santamaria & Tolosa, 1992), and in about 25% of patients, symptoms of depression may appear before motor change is apparent (Cummings, 1992a; Mayeux, Stern, Rosen, & Benson, 1983). In about 50% of cases, the depression is mild and does not meet the DSM-IV criteria for diagnosis of major depression (Cummings, 1992a; Sano & Mayeux, 1992). Depression in PD may be distinguished from that associated with other disorders by the presence of a high frequency of anxiety and a low suicide rate, despite the presence of suicidal ideation (Cummings, 1992a). Depression is more common in patients with predominant bradykinesia or rigidity rather than in those with tremor (Cummings, 1992a; Huber, Paulson, & Shuttleworth, 1988).

There is accumulating evidence that the depression associated with PD reflects biochemical alterations fundamental to the disease. The disease often involves deterioration in the raphe nucleus, a brainstem region important to the brain's supply of serotonin, a neurotransmitter critical to the regulation of mood. There are also changes in other mood-regulating systems, including the dopaminergic and noradrenergic systems (Cummings, 1992a; Mayeux *et al.,* 1986; Sano & Mayeux, 1992). There is evidence that even nondepressed PD patients have lowered rates of cerebrospinal fluid 5-hydroxyindoleacetic acid (CSF-5-HIAA), a by-product of serotonin metabolism, suggesting that these patients may be predisposed to developing depression. This reduction has been observed to be even more pronounced in PD patients who are depressed or demented (Mayeux, Stern, Cote, & Williams, 1984; Mayeux, Stern, Sano, Williams, & Cote, 1988). One study found that depressed patients with PD showed reduced metabolism in the caudate nucleus and orbitofrontal cortex as compared with nondepressed patients (Mayberg *et al.,* 1990); this pattern is different from that associated with idiopathic depression, in which dorsolateral frontal hypometabolism has been described (Baxter *et al.,* 1989).

Mild depression may to some extent be reactive to having a serious degenerative disease and associated losses, in which case psychotherapy may be helpful, particularly for nondemented patients. However, in many cases treatment with antidepressant medication may be necessary (Cummings, 1992a; Silver & Yudofsky, 1992). Electroconvulsive therapy has been effective in treating PD patients experiencing severe depression, often with relief of both affective and motor symptoms (Faber & Trimble, 1991; Rasmussen & Abrams, 1992).

Depression often exacerbates neuropsychological dysfunction but usually does not change the overall neuropsychological profile (Kuzis, Sabe, Tiberti, Leiguarda, & Starkstein, 1997; Starkstein *et al.,* 1989a; Taylor, Saint-Cyr, Lang, & Kenny, 1986b; Troster *et al.,* 1995b). Parkinson's disease patients with depression continue to show a relative weakness on tests more sensitive to frontal lobe function, with particular dysfunction on those derived from language and memory tests (Troster *et al.,* 1995a; Troster *et al.,* 1995b). Those PD patients who suffer from major depression may exhibit faster cognitive, functional, and motor decline that those who are mildly or not depressed (Starkstein, Mayberg, Leiguarda, Preziosi, & Robinson, 1992b).

About 40% of PD patients experience anxiety (Stein, Heuser, & Vade, 1990). These patients may also experience panic attacks, particularly during "off" periods when medications are less effective at relieving motor symptoms.

Some PD patients experience visual hallucinations, and prevalence estimates have ranged up to 40% (Cummings, 1992b). The hallucinations are more common at night and often consist of silent, well-formed images of children, people, or animals. Unlike patients with severe psychotic disease, PD patients are often aware that these hallucinations are unreal and do not find them frightening or threatening. Hallucinations may be induced by levodopa therapy, sometimes occurring within the context of a medication-induced delirium (Goodwin, 1971; Tanner, Vogel, Goetz, & Klawans, 1983), and adjustment of medication may relieve these symptoms. There is evidence that patients are at increased risk for experiencing visual hallucinations if they have dementia, longer disease duration, more advanced disease, older age, and sleep disturbance (Sanchez-Ramos, Ortoll, & Paulson, 1996; Tanner, Vogel, Goetz, & Klawans, 1983).

Although this view is controversial, it has been suggested that PD patients may have distinctive, long-standing personality characteristics that are present before clinical symptoms appear. Characteristics observed to be more frequent in individuals who later developed PD include tendencies be self-controlling, to be followers rather than leaders, and to be pedantic, industrious, rigid, and depressed (Poewe, Daramat, Kemmler, & Gerstenbrand, 1990; Ward *et al.*, 1983). A personality style characterized by a low tendency to seek novelty has been observed in PD patients and has been related to abnormally low levels of dopamine (Menza, Golbe, Cody, & Forman, 1993). Although these findings require additional validation and replication, they raise the possibility that personality characteristics may be useful in identifying individuals who may be at increased risk for developing PD.

OTHER PARKINSONIAN SYNDROMES WITH NEUROPSYCHOLOGICAL CORRELATES

In addition to PD, other progressive diseases with parkinsonian features are associated with neuropsychological abnormality. These include progressive supranuclear palsy and multiple system atrophy and are sometimes referred to as the "Parkinson's plus" syndromes. Although their motor symptoms overlap with those of PD, subtle differences can be discerned by neurologists experienced in diagnosing movement disorders. These disorders are distinctive in being minimally responsive or unresponsive to the medications used to treat PD, particularly levodopa therapy.

The neuropsychological profiles of these disorders resemble those of PD, but with distinctive features that may be useful in differential diagnosis. In some, dementia is frequent relatively early in the course of the disease. Accurate diagnosis and assessment of neuropsychological function may also be helpful in determining the patient's need for support and structure in carrying out activities of daily living and other responsibilities.

Each of these disorders and its associated characteristics are briefly described in the following sections. Neurologic symptoms focus on those that may be evident during neuropsychological evaluation. More detailed description of the neurology of each disease can be found in the book by Watts and Koller (1997).

Progressive Supranuclear Palsy

Progressive supranuclear palsy (PSP) was first described by Steele, Richardson, and Olszewski (1964) and is sometimes referred to as Steele-Richardson-Olszewski syndrome (Golbe, 1997). It is the most common Parkinson's plus syndrome, but is still fairly rare, with a prevalence of 1.4 per 100,000 (Golbe, Davis,

Schoenberg, & Duvoisin, 1988). It is usually diagnosed in patients in their late fifties to mid-sixties, and death occurs after 5 to 10 years (Golbe, 1997).

Among the first symptoms of the disease is loss of voluntary vertical eye movements (*vertical voluntary supranuclear gaze palsy* or *supranuclear opthalmoplegia*). When asked to voluntarily track the tip of a pencil moved up and down centrally in front of them without moving the head, PSP patients have difficulty moving their eyes above the horizontal midline. However, they have less difficulty tracking when they are asked to fixate on a visual target, and their head is moved up and down by the examiner. Later in the course of the disease, horizontal gaze also becomes impaired. Other early motor symptoms often include rigidity of the neck and trunk (*axial rigidity*), resulting in postural instability, with falls and impaired gait. Patients may exhibit dysarthria, masked facies, and drooling. Tremor sometimes occurs in PSP but is uncommon. When tremor occurs, it is more likely to involve action tremor (during voluntary movements) than a resting tremor (Golbe, 1997).

Neuropsychological impairment may occur early in this disorder and is often progressive and more severe than that associated with the other Parkinson's plus syndromes. Progressive supranuclear palsy has been described as the prototypical subcortical dementia (Albert *et al.,* 1974). Among the most prominent difficulties are mental slowness and deficits in executive function as assessed by tests such as word fluency and the Wisconsin Card Sorting Test (Grafman, Litvan, Gomez, & Chase, 1990b; Johnson, Litvan, & Grafman, 1991; Litvan, Grafman, Gomez, & Chase, 1989). The ability to switch between different task sets and activities may be particularly impaired. Decline in memory has also been described, particularly increased forgetting with time delay and impaired delayed recall (Litvan *et al.,* 1989). Recognition may be stronger than recall, although still not within normal limits. Naming may be abnormal (Milberg & Albert, 1989). Visuospatial function is often difficult to evaluate because of prominent oculomotor dysfunction. Personality and affective changes, including vagueness, irritability, and apathy, have been described (Albert *et al.,* 1974). Detailed description of the neuropsychological characteristics of PSP is provided elsewhere (Grafman, Litvan, & Stark, 1995).

The occurrence of dementia is more frequent in PSP than in PD but lower than in Alzheimer's disease. One study comparing these patient groups reported dementia in 58% of PSP patients, 93% of Alzheimer's disease patients, but only 18% of PD patients (Pillon, Dubois, & Ploska, 1991). In comparison with Alzheimer's disease patients, PSP patients may show greater impairment in verbal fluency but stronger naming (Milberg & Albert, 1989). Although memory impairment may be present in PSP, it may be less severe than that observed in Alzheimer's disease (Milberg & Albert, 1989).

Multiple System Atrophy

The term multiple system atrophy (MSA) refers to a group of disorders involving the cerebellum, brain stem, and basal ganglia and having the common symptomology of extrapyramidal features (such as motor rigidity and bradykinesia), cerebellar abnormalities (such as gait ataxia and dysarthria), and autonomic dysfunction (often postural hypotension) (Graham & Oppenheimer, 1969; Quinn, 1989; Shulman & Weiner, 1997). Disorders included as MSAs are olivopontocerebellar degeneration (spinocerebellar degenerative disorders) (Dejerine & Thomas, 1900), striatonigral degeneration (atypical parkinsonism) (Van der Eecken, Adams, & van Bogaert, 1960), and progressive autonomic failure (Shy-Drager syndrome) (Shy & Drager, 1960). Symptoms of these disorders usually appear at about age 50, somewhat earlier than PD symptoms.

Because these disorders are rare and difficult to diagnose, their distinctive neuropsychological correlates are not well defined. Mild neuropsychological change, although not dementia, is often present, particularly on tests sensitive to executive function. Patients with mild to moderately advanced MSA may show mental slowness and impaired set shifting (Robbins et al., 1992). However, deficits in executive function may be inconsistent, and one study focusing on striatonigral degeneration revealed deficits on tests of letter/category fluency and the Trail-Making Test, and delayed recall in a relatively unstructured verbal memory test. However, deficits were not observed on a simplified Wisconsin Card Sorting Test, the Stroop Test, or a somewhat more structured verbal learning test (Pillon et al., 1995b). Patients with olivopontocerebellar degeneration may exhibit mild or no change in neuropsychological function, although depression is common (Berent et al., 1990; Kish, El-Awar, Shut, Oscar-Berman, & Freedman, 1988). Where executive function deficits are observed in MSA patients, they may be similar to those associated with PD, but less severe than those associated with PSP (Pillon et al., 1995b). A study focusing on visuospatial abilities found that MSA patients showed significantly impaired performance on Judgment of Line Orientation, although not on the WAIS-R Block Design (Hua & Lu, 1994). Neuropsychiatric changes in MSA may include apathy, depression, and emotional lability.

CORTICOBASAL DEGENERATION

Corticobasal degeneration (CBD) is a rare disorder involving progressive dysfunction in the cerebral cortex and the basal ganglia, with initial symptoms being most common after age 60 (Gibb, Luther, & Marsden, 1989; Riley et al., 1990; Watts, Brewer, Schneider, & Mirra, 1997). The combination of extrapyramidal motor symptoms with focal cortical symptoms distinguishes CBD from PD. Motor symptoms are often asymmetric, with either the right or left side being more affected, and may include rigidity, tremor, and dystonia, abnormal posturing of the limbs (Riley et al., 1990). Symptoms of cortical sensory loss, such as impaired tactile or visual discrimination, are common early in the disorder. Eye movements may be disturbed, with a breakdown of smooth pursuit and saccadic movements.

A feature often distinguishing CBD from PD, other parkinsonian syndromes, and Alzheimer's disease is the presence of severe apraxia, impairment in the voluntary control of movement (Leiguarda, Lees, Merello, Starkstein, & Marsden, 1994; Pillon *et al.*, 1995a). Patients with CBD may have difficulty executing motor commands, either in response to verbal instruction or in imitation of others' movements or postures. A fascinating feature frequently associated with CBD is the "alien limb" syndrome, in which the patient feels as though a limb, often an arm, is moving outside of his control (Doody & Jankovic, 1992).

Recent studies suggest that cognitive dysfunction or dementia may be significant in patients with CBD and is sometimes the presenting symptom (Lerner *et al.*, 1992; Schneider, Watts, Gearing, Brewer, & Mirra, 1997). The pattern of neuropsychological function fits the subcortical pattern, resembling that of PSP except that apraxia may be more severe in CBD. Patients with CBD may show impaired performance on the Dementia Rating Scale, with pronounced impairment in executive functions as exhibited on tests of letter/category fluency or the Wisconsin Card Sorting Test, which is similar to the performance seen in PSP (Pillon *et al.*, 1995a). Memory for new information may be impaired overall, although less severely than in Alzheimer's disease (Massman, Kreiter, Jankovic, & Doody, 1996; Pillon *et al.*, 1995a). Memory often benefits from structure, and a substantial amount of the information initially acquired in immediate memory may be retained after a time delay, which is similar to the findings in PSP but in contrast with Alzheimer's disease (Pillon *et al.*, 1995a). Naming may be impaired in CBD patients, although their naming ability often benefits from phonemic cuing, unlike that of Alzheimer's disease patients (Massman *et al.*, 1996). Patients with CBD are often mildly depressed (Massman *et al.*, 1996).

HUNTINGTON'S DISEASE

Huntington's disease (HD) is an inherited, progressive neurodegenerative disease first described by George Huntington in 1872 (Huntington, 1972). The disease causes impairment in movement and neuropsychological function, often accompanied by psychiatric abnormality. The classic motor symptoms of the disease include involuntary *choreic movement* (an abnormal low-frequency writhing and jerking of the head, limbs, and trunk) and *dystonia* (abnormal posturing). Oculomotor impairments are also prominent early in the course of the disease.

The disease most frequently becomes clinically symptomatic in middle-aged individuals but occasionally is not diagnosed until older adulthood. Therefore, the possibility of HD should be considered in the differential diagnosis of older adults, particularly when the initial symptoms include movement abnormalities or neurobehavioral disorder and there is a strong family history of a similar disorder. The characteristics and neurobehavioral features of HD are briefly reviewed here, and more detailed discussions can be found in other sources (Brandt & Butters, 1996; Bylsma, 1997; Folstein, Brandt, & Folstein, 1991).

It is well established that HD is an inherited disease whose genetic basis has been localized to a defect on chromosome 4 resulting in a DNA mutation producing abnormal repetition of a specific trinucleotide set (Huntington's Disease Collaborative Research Group, 1993; Gusella *et al.,* 1983). The disease is inherited as an autosomal dominant trait, so that each child of a person with HD has a 50% chance of inheriting the abnormal gene and will eventually exhibit symptoms if he or she lives long enough.

Initial clinical symptoms of HD most frequently appear around age 40. However, there is a wide range in the age of disease onset, with some individuals beginning to exhibit symptoms in childhood and others not becoming symptomatic until they reach the seventh or eighth decade. In persons carrying the HD gene, both the age at which the disease becomes symptomatic and the rate of disease progression are genetically determined and therefore similar between family members (Brandt *et al.,* 1996; Duyao *et al.,* 1993). The disease duration averages between 15 and 17 years, with disease progression often being more rapid for those with an early age of disease onset (Myers *et al.,* 1991). The overall prevalence of HD is 5 to 8 per 100,000, increasing to 12 per 100,000 between the ages of 40 and 55 (Conneally, 1984).

Blood tests can now determine with high accuracy whether the gene has been inherited. Because the testing will determine whether an individual will eventually develop a progressive, neurodegenerative, currently incurable disease, it is important that individuals receive counseling in conjunction with undergoing the blood test. Protocols have been developed for helping individuals to appreciate the implications of the possible outcomes of the blood test, to decide whether to undergo the test, and to process psychological and other reactions to the test findings (Codori & Brandt, 1994; Hersch, Jones, Koroshetz, & Quaid, 1994; Jones, 1996; Wiggins *et al.,* 1992).

Dysfunction in basal ganglia-thalamocortical pathways plays a major role in the movement, neuropsychological, and psychiatric abnormalities associated with HD. A major focus of the neuropathophysiology of HD is dysfunction within the striatum, a group of basal ganglia structures receiving neural input from other brain regions (illustrated in Appendix H). Initially, the major affected basal ganglia structures are the caudate nucleus and, to a lesser extent, the putamen (Dom, Malfroid, & Baro, 1976; Vonsattel *et al.,* 1985). Neuropathological studies also provide evidence of neuronal loss in the cerebral cortex, including areas within the dorsolateral prefrontal cortex (Sotrel *et al.,* 1991).

Neuropsychological Features of Huntington's Disease

Neurobehavioral changes are often among the earliest symptoms of HD, although these may be subtle and not apparent on screening tests. Patients may exhibit decline in judgment and planning, and neuropsychiatric symptoms such as increased levels of irritability, anxiety, or apathy may be noted. In patients suspected to have this disease, it may be necessary to administer more challenging tests, such as a full WAIS-III and the Wisconsin Card Sorting Test, to detect subtle deficits that may be present early in the course of the disease.

In formal neuropsychological assessment, among the earliest deficits are difficulties with attention and executive function. Patients with HD often exhibit significant impairment on tests such as the Trail-Making Test, Wisconsin Card Sorting Test, Digit Span Backwards, and WAIS-III Mental Arithmetic (Butters, Sax, Montgomery, & Tarlow, 1978; Josiassen, Curry, & Mancall, 1983). The Brief Test of Attention may be particularly sensitive to subtle deficits in attention (Schretlen, Brandt, & Bobholz, 1996).

Impairment in aspects of memory is also often present. As described in Chapter 5, two major memory systems of the brain are the declarative and nondeclarative (implicit) memory systems (Squire, 1994). In patients with HD, declarative memory may be compromised, and a subcortical neuropsychological profile is often observed, with deficits similar to those observed in Parkinson's disease but distinct from those associated with Alzheimer's disease. In HD patients, deficits in the acquisition of new material in memory and in memory retrieval are more prominent than impairment in memory storage. Memory impairment is particularly apparent in unstructured conditions requiring organization of material to be learned, such as word list learning. Retrieval from verbal declarative memory is often impaired, with deficits apparent on tests of recall memory, while recognition memory is considerably stronger and relatively preserved in mildly affected patients (Butters *et al.*, 1986; Butters, Wolfe, Marone, Granholm, & Cermak, 1985; Delis *et al.*, 1991).

Patients with HD may also show impairment on tests of remote memory (Albert, Butters, & Brandt, 1981). Unlike patients with Alzheimer's disease, HD patients do not show a temporal gradient in their remote memory deficit, and HD patients have equal difficulty retrieving both temporally recent and distant information (Beatty, Salmon, Butters, Heindel, & Granholm, 1988). Awareness of memory deficits may be compromised in HD patients (Brandt, 1985).

Patients with HD also exhibit deficits in aspects of nondeclarative memory, particularly in skill-based procedural learning of visuomotor or nonmotor skills (Bylsma, Brandt, & Strauss, 1990; Heindel *et al.*, 1988; Heindel, Salmon, & Butters, 1991; Heindel *et al.*, 1989; Paulson, Butters, Salmon, Heindel, & Swenson, 1993). Patients with Parkinson's disease also often exhibit deficits in procedural learning, while this aspect of memory may be relatively strong in patients with Alzheimer's disease (Heindel *et al.*, 1991; Heindel *et al.*, 1989).

Early in the course of HD, patients often exhibit impairment on tests of language function. Patients show reduced word fluency, with similar levels of deficit in letter and category fluency. This pattern contrasts with that seen in patients with Alzheimer's disease, who often exhibit greater deficits in category than letter fluency (Butters *et al.*, 1986; Butters *et al.*, 1985). The word fluency deficit in HD may be more closely related to difficulty in initiating and maintaining behavior rather than to the breakdown of semantic knowledge that is more characteristic of Alzheimer's disease. Patients with HD also exhibit fewer perseverative and intrusion errors than patients with Alzheimer's disease. Naming is compromised in HD, with errors often reflecting misperception of stimulus items and inappropriate attention to stimulus detail rather than the semantic paraphasic errors that are more characteristic of Alzheimer's disease (Hodges *et al.*, 1991).

Visuospatial performance is compromised even in mild HD, with deficits evident on tests such as the copying of the clock design, the Rey-Osterrieth Complex Figure (Lezak, 1995; Osterrieth, 1944; Rey, 1941) or the WAIS-III Block Design (Brouwers *et al.*, 1984). If the full WAIS-III has been administered, the Perceptual Organization Index may be dramatically lower than the Verbal Comprehension Index. These visuospatial difficulties may contribute to spatial disorientation in everyday life. They are not attributable to the movement disorder, sometimes appearing even before movement symptoms are pronounced (Josiassen *et al.*, 1983).

Neuropsychiatric Features of Huntington's Disease

Patients with mild HD often suffer from neuropsychiatric and behavioral disorders. Depression is most common, sometimes preceding the appearance of motor symptoms. As with depression in Parkinson's disease, dysfunction in basal ganglia–thalamocortical brain circuits is believed to contribute to the depression associated with HD. The depression tends to run in families, and whether an HD patients develops depression may to some extent be determined by whether other affected individuals in the same family have developed depression. Patients with HD are at increased risk for both attempted and completed suicide (Farrer, 1986). Although less common than depression, other psychiatric and behavioral disorders are often observed in HD patients, including impaired judgment, substance abuse, aggression, and apathy (Shoulson, 1990). Impaired awareness of neuropsychological decline may contribute to disruptive behaviors, including poor judgment.

9

NEUROPSYCHOLOGICAL PROFILES IV

Traumatic Brain Injury, Substance-Related
Disorders, Normal Pressure Hydrocephalus,
Metabolic and Toxic Disorders

TRAUMATIC BRAIN INJURY

Background

It is well established that although traumatic brain injury (TBI) is most common among young adults and children, the elderly comprise the third group at greatest risk, especially after age 65 (Frankowski, 1986; Kraus, 1987; Naugle, 1990). Negative outcomes following TBI are more frequent in older adults, including longer recovery time, need for extended care, and even death (Alberico, Ward, Choi, Marmarou, & Young, 1987; Luerssen, Klauber, & Marshall, 1988; Rothweiler, Temkin, & Dikmen, 1998). However, the variables and underlying mechanisms contributing to these outcomes are not well understood.

Some age-related differences in the correlates of TBI have been observed fairly consistently. In young adults, TBI is most frequently sustained during an automobile accident, whereas in older adults it most commonly follows a fall (Kraus, 1987; Naugle, 1990). Older adults are, in general, at increased risk for falls owing to decline in balance and gait, and those with movement disorders or cerebrovascular disease are at particularly high risk. Among older adults, TBI is equally common among men and women, in contrast to the preponderance of men in younger adult TBI cases. Although the overall rate of alcohol consumption is lower among older as compared with younger adults, alcohol consumption increases the frequency of falls and is more likely to be implicated in fall-related than in automobile accident–related TBI in older adults (Fields, 1997).

Older age also places individuals at increased risk for certain neurologic sequelae following TBI, most notably subdural hematoma, intracranial hemorrhage, and posttraumatic infections (Fogel & Duffy, 1994; Luerssen *et al.,* 1988). Since these sequelae may develop over the course of several days, neurobehavioral correlates of TBI may not be apparent immediately following an accident. Therefore, it is important that older individuals who have suffered a blow to the head be monitored for at least several days to rule out the possibility of a slowly developing abnormality, with particular attention to symptoms such as headache, dizziness, or confusion.

Neuropsychological Correlates of Traumatic Brain Injury in Older Adults

In recent years there has been increasing attention focused on possible differences between younger and older adults in the neuropsychological sequelae of TBI. There has also been greater focus on approaches for differentiating between the neuropsychological sequelae of TBI and abnormalities associated with dementing disorders. While most of the existing studies have included relatively small samples of patients and must be considered preliminary, these have provided intriguing and useful findings, which are providing suggestions for clinical practice as well as a basis for future research.

One of the factors complicating research on TBI in general is variation in the definition of what constitutes a mild, moderate or severe brain injury. Two variables that have been helpful in defining the severity of injury are the Glasgow Coma Scale (GCS) and whether the injury is "uncomplicated" or "complicated." The GCS rates the patient's level of consciousness following a head trauma on a 15-point scale based on the stimulus required to induce opening of the eyes, the highest level of motor response, and the highest level of verbal response (Teasdale & Jennett, 1974). A 15-point score indicates that the patient can spontaneously open the eyes, can follow simple motor commands, and is oriented to time, place, and person. A score of 8 or less is used to define patients in coma. An uncomplicated brain injury is one in which there are no significant findings from structural neuroimaging (e.g., by computed tomography or magnetic resonance imaging) following the accident. A complicated injury is defined as one in which there are positive findings, such as brain contusions or a hematoma. Most of the studies of the neuropsychological correlates of TBI in older adults have examined individuals with mild (GCS of 13 to 15 without complications) to moderate injuries (GCS of 9 to 12 without complications or 13 to 15 with complications).

Several studies have suggested that the pattern of acute neuropsychological deficit in older adult TBI is similar to that seen in young adults (Aharon-Peretz et al., 1997; Fields, 1994; Fields, 1997; Goldstein *et al.,* 1994). In one study evaluating deficits in adults over age 50 sustaining mild to moderate TBI, impairments were observed on tests of memory, naming, word fluency, and conceptualization (Goldstein *et al.,* 1994). In another study comparing older and young adults following mild TBI, neuropsychological performance was not significantly different on most tests of memory and attention (Fields, 1994; Fields, 1997).

There are, however, preliminary findings raising the possibility that neurobehavioral complaints following TBI may be more problematic among older adults. In older adults, these complaints may persist longer and perhaps even increase during the months following an injury. For most young individuals experiencing mild to moderate TBI, neurobehavioral complaints resolve within 3 to 6 months of the accident, including problems with attention and memory, headaches, dizziness, light and noise sensitivity, depression, irritability, and anxiety. In one study comparing post-TBI complaints in individuals over the age of 50 with those in individuals between the ages of 18 and 45 having TBI of comparable severity, the pattern of complaints was similar for the two groups 1 month following the injury. However, at 4 months postinjury, the older patients more frequently endorsed fatigue, difficulty in processing information, mild depression, sensitivity to noise, and dizziness (Taylor, Fields, Starratt, Russo, & Diamond, 1993). In addition, during this time period the older patients perceived increased difficulty with cognition, behavior, and posttraumatic stress, while the younger patients reported improvement. Another study of older patients with mild to moderate TBI reported increased symptoms of depression over 4 to 13 months following the injury (Goldstein *et al.,* 1999). These preliminary findings raise the possibility that neurobehavioral complaints may not resolve as quickly among elderly TBI victims and, in fact, may increase for some symptoms.

Neuropsychological Differences between Traumatic Brain Injury and Alzheimer's Disease

Preliminary studies have also suggested differences in the neuropsychological profiles of older patients with TBI and those with Alzheimer's disease. Several studies have suggested that measures of executive function and memory may be most useful in discriminating between these groups (Goldstein *et al.,* 1996; Young, Fields, & Lovell, 1995). In comparison with elderly TBI patients, mildly affected Alzheimer's disease patients may show more severe and widespread verbal learning deficits, weaker facilitation by category structure when performing word fluency tests, and reduced cognitive flexibility.

SUBSTANCE-RELATED DISORDERS

Background

The DSM-IV provides criteria for substance-related disorders, including those related to the use of a drug (including alcohol), to the side effects of a prescription or over-the-counter medication, or to exposure to toxins (American Psychiatric Association, 1994). The DSM-IV distinguishes between substance use disorders and substance-induced disorders. Within substance use disorders, separate criteria are provided for substance dependence and substance abuse, and within substance-induced disorders, there are separate criteria for substance intoxication and substance withdrawal. These criteria are detailed in the DSM-IV manual (American Psychiatric Association, 1994) and summarized in Table 9.1.

Criteria for specific substance-induced disorders with prominent neuropsychological features are also detailed in the DSM-IV. These include Substance-Induced Persisting Amnestic Disorder and Substance-Induced Persisting Dementia. Patients with milder neuropsychological sequelae may be diagnosed with Substance-Induced Disorder Not Otherwise Specified.

As in younger adults, alcohol-related substance disorders are more common among men than women, but some of the general characteristics of substance-related disorders in older adults are somewhat different from those in younger adults. The prevalence of alcohol abuse and dependence in older adults is generally reported to be about 2% among community-dwelling older adults, lower than that observed among younger adults (Helzer, Burnam, & McEvoy, 1991; Regier et al., 1988). However, the incidence of heavy alcohol consumption in older adults is considerable higher, ranging between 3 and 9% (Liberto, Oslin, & Ruskin, 1992). A significant number of older adults with alcohol-related problems are late-onset drinkers who either begin to abuse alcohol or experience undesirable effects of alcohol use after the age of 65. Late-onset drinking accounts for between 15 and 68% of the alcohol problems seen in older adults (Atkinson, Tolson, & Truner, 1990; Schonfeld & Dupree, 1991). Older widowed women are particularly vulnerable to late-onset alcohol abuse (Gomberg, 1995).

TABLE 9.1   Summary of the DSM-IV Classification of Substance-Related Disorders

1. Substance use disorders

a. *Substance dependence:* A pattern of increased tolerance together with compulsive behaviors to obtain the substance and withdrawal symptoms when it is withheld. These features may interfere with performance of work, social, and other everyday activities.

b. *Substance abuse:* A pattern of maladaptive behaviors in the absence of substance dependence, such as recurrent failure to fulfill work or family responsibilities, use of the substance in dangerous conditions such as when driving, or continued use even when this is detrimental to social or interpersonal relationships.

2. Substance-induced disorders

a. *Substance intoxication:* The development of a reversible syndrome that is physiologically related to recent substance use and adversely affects behaviors such as cognition, mood, and social and occupational functioning.

b. *Substance withdrawal:* The development of a syndrome directly related to cessation of prolonged, heavy use of a substance which includes distressing physiological and behavioral changes interfering with functioning.

Older adults are at increased risk for substance related-disorders associated with the use of prescription and over-the-counter medications. Individuals over the age of 65 consume more than 30% of all prescription medications (Baum, Kennedy, & Forbes, 1984). Medications having potential for causing substance-related disorders include anticholinergic agents, antihistamines, antihypertensive and cardiovascular medications, antiparkinsonian medications, anxiolytic medications, chemotherapeutic agents, corticosteroids, gastrointestinal medications, muscle relaxants, nonsteroidal anti-inflammatory medications, and antidepressant medications. Older adults receive almost 40% of prescriptions for benzodiazepines, a class of drugs used to treat anxiety and insomnia that is frequently involved in substance-related disorders (Thompson, Moran, & Neis, 1983). One study of community-dwelling elderly persons being treated at a mental health clinic found that about 5% of the average case load abused prescription drugs, and the most commonly abused drugs were sedative–hypnotics, anxiolytic agents, and analgesics (Jinks & Raschko, 1990). Because of their slowed metabolism and reduced body weight, older adults may be more sensitive to these medications, making it more difficult to predict both positive treatment effects and undesirable side effects that may affect neuropsychological function and mood.

In addition, while substance abuse in younger adults often reflects intentional behaviors aimed at altering psychological state, there is evidence that abuse in older adults often reflects substance misuse, the maladaptive use of substances due to misunderstanding or errors (Ellor & Kurz, 1982). Older adults may have greater difficulty reading and understanding the instructions written on medication containers, particularly if the instructions are complex or if the patient suffers from cognitive dysfunction. These factors increase the likelihood that older persons may inadvertently develop a substance-related disorder because they have misused a medication.

Assessing Substance-Related Disorders during the Clinical Interview

It is important to query both the patient and the accompanying person about the patient's consumption of alcohol and medications. If the patient is taking medications, either prescription or over-the-counter, it is important to determine who is controlling the medication regimen. If this is under the patient's control, he might be asked to explain the regimen and how he monitors whether he is following it correctly. His ability to explain this clearly may suggest whether the regimen is being correctly followed. The potential for a substance-related disorder is increased if the patient controls his own medications and appears confused about what he is taking and when he should take it. In addition, the potential for undesirable side effects related to drug interactions is increased if the patient is taking multiple medications prescribed by different specialists. If this appears to be an issue, it is recommended that the entire medication regimen be reviewed by a clinician with expertise in the psychopharmacology of older adults.

The patient and family should also be queried about the patient's alcohol consumption. Even if there is no past history of alcohol overuse and the patient's alcohol consumption has not increased, it is important to determine whether there may have been changes in behavior related to this consumption. Because of changes in body mass and metabolism, it is possible for older adults to become more easily intoxicated even if consumption is unchanged or reduced. If they are retired, older adults may not exhibit the obvious changes in occupational and social functioning that are characteristic of substance-related disorders in younger adults, but other changes may suggest a detrimental effect of alcohol consumption, such as decreased ability to care for themselves or social withdrawal. It is not uncommon for older patients to deny that they are experiencing adverse effects of alcohol consumption, while family members express considerable concern. Patients who have been diagnosed with depression, anxiety, or antisocial personality disorder may be at increased risk for alcohol-related disorders (Ross, Glaser, & Germanson, 1988). A number of questionnaires are available to facilitate assessment of alcohol use (Connors, 1995), including the CAGE (Ewing, 1984; Mayfield, McLeod, & Hall, 1974), TWEAK (Chan, Pristach, Welte, & Russell, 1993) and Michigan Alcoholism Screening Test (MAST) (Selzer, 1971).

If the clinical interview strongly suggests that the patient has an alcohol-related disorder, it is important to investigate whether there is a history of other medical or psychiatric conditions with neuropsychological correlates that often co-occur with alcoholism. These include traumatic brain injury, blackouts, hypertension, diabetes, withdrawal seizures, hepatic dysfunction, chronic obstructive pulmonary disease, personality disorders, mood disorders, and anxiety/phobic disorders (Rourke & Loberg, 1996). These conditions may exacerbate any neuropsychological changes associated with alcohol use.

Brain Changes Associated with Alcohol-Related Disorders

Chronic use of alcohol causes changes in brain structure and functioning. Structural imaging of the brains of chronic alcoholics has revealed cortical and subcortical atrophy as well as reductions in white matter (Jernigan *et al.,* 1991b; Pfefferbaum *et al.,* 1992). Structures showing atrophy include the mesial temporal lobe, the frontal lobe (dorsolateral and orbitofrontal), parieto-occipital cortex, the cerebellum, the caudate nuclei, and anterior and posterior diencephalic structures (including the mamillary bodies of the hypothalamus, the dorsomedial nucleus of the thalamus, and the basal forebrain). Cortical changes are reported in alcoholics of all ages, and ventricular enlargement indicative of subcortical atrophy is also common, particularly in older patients with a long history of drinking (Bergman, Borg, Hindmarsh, Idestrom, & Mutzell, 1980; Pfefferbaum, Rosenbloom, Crusan, & Jernigan, 1988). When alcoholics abstain from drinking, the atrophy may reverse to some extent (Artman, Gall, Hacker, & Herrlich, 1981; Carlen, Wortzman, Holgate, Wilkinson, & Rankin, 1978). However, even alcoholics who have been abstinent may continue to exhibit abnormalities in parietal and medial frontal cortex metabolism (Gilman *et al.,* 1990; Volkow *et al.,* 1992), electrophysiologic functioning (Glenn, Parsons, & Sinha, 1994) and synaptic receptors (Freund & Ballinger, 1991). These findings indicate that chronic alcohol abuse may have permanent effects on brain function.

The more severe neurobehavioral syndromes associated with long-term alcoholism are known to cause irreversible changes in brain structure and function. Changes in the mamillary bodies of the hypothalamus, the dorsomedial nucleus of the thalamus, the basal forebrain, and the medial temporal lobe are believed to be critical in the severe amnestic disorder associated with Korsakoff's syndrome (Hata *et al.,* 1987a; Jernigan *et al.,* 1991a).

It is believed that thiamine deficiency plays a major role in these brain changes. Because of poor dietary practices, alcoholics, and particularly older alcoholics are likely to suffer from nutritional deficiencies, and thiamine deficiency can cause hemorrhagic brain lesions (Victor & Adams, 1985). These lesions are believed to contribute to the neuropsychological deficits observed in chronic alcoholics (Bowden, 1990) and play a major role in the more severe and permanent neurobehavioral changes associated with Wernicke's encephalopathy and Korsakoff's syndrome.

The following discussion will focus on neuropsychological changes associated with the use of alcohol, benzodiazepines, and antidepressants, substances associated with disorders that have been most frequently studied in older populations.

Neuropsychological Changes Associated with Alcohol-Related Disorders

A distinction can be made between the mild to moderate neuropsychological deficits observed in detoxified alcoholics and the more severe impairments associated with alcoholic dementia, Wernicke's encephalopathy, and alcoholic Korsakoff's syndrome. Among alcoholics of all ages, only about 10% of those who are detoxified and treated for nutritional deficiencies exhibit severe, irreversible impairments that meet criteria for an amnestic or dementia syndrome (Rourke & Loberg, 1996). Among the remainder, 50 to 85% exhibit mild to moderate neuropsychological deficits (Rourke & Loberg, 1996).

Alcoholics who have been abstinent for 1 to 3 weeks exhibit deficits in a variety of neuropsychological domains. The most prominent deficits may be in visuospatial abilities (e.g., WAIS-III Block Design); attention and executive functions (e.g., Trail-Making Test, Wisconsin Card Sorting Test); challenging memory tasks, particularly visual but also verbal (e.g., Wechsler memory tests, California Verbal Learning Test); and perceptual-motor skills (e.g., WAIS-III Digit-Symbol, Grooved Pegboard, Finger Tapping) (Eckardt & Martin, 1986; Grant, 1987; Parsons, Butters, & Nathan, 1987; Rourke & Grant, 1999; Rourke & Loberg, 1996; Ryan & Butters, 1986). The Wechsler Full-Scale and Verbal IQs may be within normal limits, but the Performance IQ may remain abnormal because of its dependence on visuospatial and visuomotor abilities (Grant, 1987). Certain WAIS tests are particularly sensitive to alcohol-related neuropsychological dysfunction, including Block Design, Digit-Symbol, and Object Assembly (Parsons & Leber, 1981).

One variable contributing to the frequency and severity of neuropsychological deficits is the patient's age. Following a short period of abstinence, younger alcoholics may show mild, circumscribed, or no neuropsychological change, while deficits are more common, widespread, and severe in older alcoholics (Eckardt, Stapleton, Rawlings, Davis, & Grodin, 1995; Grant, Adams, & Reed, 1984; Rourke & Grant, 1999). One study found that after about 4 weeks of detoxification, in comparison with healthy control subjects, younger alcoholics (below age 51) exhibited deficits in executive function (e.g., Trail-Making Test) and visuomotor tasks (e.g., Block Design, Digit-Symbol), while older alcoholics (over age 51) also exhibited deficits in attention, memory (e.g., Wechsler Logical Memory and Visual Reproduction), and perceptual motor tasks (e.g., Grooved Pegboard, Finger Tapping) (Rourke & Grant, 1999). Older patients may also experience more frequent and persistent symptoms of alcohol withdrawal, including confusion, anxiety, restlessness, insomnia, and autonomic symptoms such as sweating and increased heart rate (Brower, Mudd, Blow, Young, & Hill, 1994).

With continued abstinence from alcohol consumption, neuropsychological status may improve, particularly after longer periods of abstinence (4 to 5 years) and in younger patients. After 1 year of abstinence, 10 to 30% of the patients who have deficits immediately following detoxification may continue to have persisting mild deficits (Grant, Reed, & Adams, 1987b; Rourke & Loberg, 1996). With continued abstinence, improvement may continue over the course of 4 to 5 years or longer (Brandt et al., 1983; Fabian & Parsons, 1983). Younger patients are more likely to show complete recovery of neuropsychological function, but older adults may continue to show deficits in visuospatial, visuomotor, and perceptual motor skills even after 1 to 4 years of abstinence (Eckardt et al., 1995; Rourke & Grant, 1999).

The pattern of these mild to moderate deficits is fairly variable, reflecting the multiplicity of factors that may directly or indirectly contribute to neuropsychological status in recently detoxified alcoholics. Alcoholics frequently suffer from other medical or psychiatric conditions that have neuropsychological correlates, such as traumatic brain injury, blackouts, hypertension, diabetes, withdrawal seizures, liver dysfunction, chronic obstructive pulmonary disease, personality disorders, mood disorders, and anxiety–phobic disorders (Rourke & Loberg, 1996). A model detailing the nature of these variables and their impact on neuropsychological function has been developed (Grant, 1987).

A significant proportion of individuals who abuse alcohol will eventually develop cirrhosis of the liver, and there is evidence that this alone may produce neuropsychological dysfunction and may contribute to *hepatic encephalopathy.*

Hepatic encephalopathy refers to generalized brain dysfunction related to liver dysfunction and is characterized by abnormalities in mood, cognition, and level of consciousness. However, even in the absence of hepatic encephalopathy, individuals with liver cirrhosis may exhibit significant neuropsychological change (Moss, Tarter, Yao, & VanThiel, 1992; Tarter, Hegedus, Van Thiel, Gavaler, & Schade, 1986).

Some patients, particularly those with a long history of alcohol abuse, develop a dementia that does not resolve even after long periods of abstinence. This dementia is characterized by impairment in multiple neuropsychological domains, including executive functions (conceptualization, problem solving, judgment), in memory, and in visuospatial abilities (Goldstein, 1985; Lishman, 1986; Salmon *et al.*, 1993). The memory deficit is often severe but not more pronounced than that in other neuropsychological domains. Patients may exhibit mental slowness and often appear apathetic and unconcerned about their deficits (Cutting, 1978; Ryan & Butters, 1986b; Salmon *et al.*, 1993). Language function is often relatively preserved.

Because of poor dietary practices, alcoholics and especially older alcoholics are likely to suffer from nutritional deficiencies, particularly thiamine deficiency (Victor & Adams, 1985), which can cause hemorrhagic brain lesions. This deficiency plays a major role in the development of *Wernicke's encephalopathy* and *Korsakoff's syndrome,* disorders most commonly seen in alcoholics but which may also occur in nonalcoholic illnesses causing thiamine depletion, such as some gastrointestinal disorders (Parkin, Blunden, Rees, & Hunkin, 1991; Shimomura, Mori, Hirono, Imamura, & Yamashita, 1998a).

Wernicke's encephalopathy is a global confusional state characterized by pronounced ataxic motor symptoms, abnormal eye movements, and incoherent speech (Victor *et al.*, 1989). It is often accompanied by Korsakoff's syndrome, a major feature of which is severe memory dysfunction (Victor *et al.*, 1989). With abstinence from alcohol and treatment with large doses of thiamine and other vitamins, the Wernicke's encephalopathy may resolve, but in about 75% of patients, the Korsakoff's syndrome persists (Victor *et al.*, 1989). In some cases, a Korsakoff's-like severe memory deficit may develop even in the absence of an obvious Wernicke's encephalopathy (Blansjaar & van Dijk, 1992).

Traditionally, alcoholic Korsakoff's syndrome (AK) was believed to primarily reflect damage to midline posterior diencephalic brain nuclei, particularly the mamillary bodies of the hypothalamus and the dorsomedial thalamic nucleus. However, more recent evidence suggests that the presence of lesions in other brain regions may also be critical, particularly the anterior diencephalon (the basal forebrain, hypothalamic gray matter), the mesial temporal lobe, and orbitofrontal cortex (Hata *et al.*, 1987b; Jernigan, Schafer, Butters, & Cermak, 1991c). It is notable that the basal forebrain plays a major role in modulation of the cholinergic neurotransmitter system that is critical to the functioning of brain regions important to memory, including medial temporal lobe structures such as the hippocampus.

Major neuropsychological features of AK include both anterograde and retrograde amnesia, deficits in executive functions, and personality changes (Albert *et al.,* 1980; Butters & Cermak, 1980; Salmon *et al.,* 1993; Squire, 1982). Patients with AK show relatively preserved Wechsler IQ scores, but their performance on tests of memory for new information is significantly lower (Butters & Cermak, 1980). The impairment in recent memory may be as severe as that seen in patients with Alzheimer's disease, although less severe than that observed in non-Korsakoff's alcoholics (Delis *et al.,* 1991). Increased interference between different episodes of memory as well as perseverative responding may contribute to the anterograde memory deficit (Butters & Cermak, 1980). Patients with AK also show a temporally graded retrograde amnesia, with poor recall of events in the past 10 to 20 years but better preserved memory for preceding time periods (Albert *et al.,* 1980; Albert, Butters, & Levin, 1979). The presence of retrograde amnesia may be helpful in distinguishing between Korsakoff's and non-Korsakoff's alcoholics, since the latter generally do not have retrograde amnesia. During tests of memory, the recall of AK patients is likely to reflect *confabulation,* the report of material that was not originally presented, often implausible in nature. Patients with AK often have relatively preserved verbal fluency (Weingartner, Grafman, Boutelle, Kaye, & Martin, 1983). Similar to non-Korsakoff alcoholics, AK patients may show mild to moderate deficits in visuospatial abilities, in developing and shifting problem-solving strategies, and in judging temporal order or event frequency (Salmon, Butters, & Schuckit, 1986; Weingartner *et al.,* 1983). However, these deficits may not be as severe as those associated with alcoholic dementia. Although they exhibit a range of deficits, AK patients often appear apathetic, indifferent, and unconcerned and have difficulty in organizing and initiating their own behavior.

In some cases, it may be difficult to distinguish between patients with AK and those with alcoholic dementia. Although both groups of patients have a severe memory deficit, this develops more gradually in patients with alcoholic dementia (Cutting, 1978). In patients with AK, there is often a sudden change in memory function accompanied by Wernicke's encephalopathy. In addition, in patients with AK the memory impairment is pronounced and considerably greater than deficits in other abilities. This contrasts with the more uniform deficits seen in patients with alcoholic dementia.

Neuropsychological Changes Associated with Medication Use

A wide variety of different medications have the potential for causing cognitive impairment. A complete listing of prescription medications, including possible neuropsychological effects, is contained in the Physician's Desk Reference (1999). Medications most likely to affect cognition include those used to treat anxiety, depression, insomnia, movement disorders, psychosis, cardiac arrhythmia, hypertension, pain, bacterial infections, cancer, seizure disorders, gastrointestinal illnesses, and common colds. A listing of specific medications that may affect cognition is found Table 9.2, as presented in the Clinical Practice Guidelines for

TABLE 9.2 Medications That May Cause Cognitive Impairment[a]

Type of medication	Generic name	Common trade name(s)
Anticholinergic agents	Scopolamine	Transderm Scop, Isopto-Hyoscine
	Orphenadrine	Norflex, Norgesic,[b] Norgesic Forte[b]
	Atropine	Various, Lomotil[c]
	Trihexyphenidyl	Artane
	Benztropine	Cogentin
	Meclizine	Antivert, Bonine
	Homatropine	Isopto-Homatropine, Hycodan[c]
Antidepressants	Amitriptyline	Elavil, Endep, Etrafon,[c] Triavil,[c] Limbitrol[c]
	Imipramine	Tofranil
	Desipramine	Norpramin
	Doxepin	Sinequan
	Trazodone	Desyrel
	Fluoxetine	Prozac
Antimanic agents	Lithium	Eskalith, Lithobid, Lithotabs
Antipsychotic (neuroleptic) agents	Thioridazine	Mellaril
	Chlorpromazine	Thorazine
	Fluphenazine	Prolixin
	Prochlorperazine	Compazine
	Trifluperazine	Stelazine
	Perphenazine	Trilafon, Etrafon,[c] Triavil[c]
	Haloperidol	Haldol
Antiarrhythmic agents (oral)	Quinidine	Quinidex, Quinaglute
	Disopyramide	Norpace
	Tocainide	Tonocard
Antifungal agents	Amphotericin B	Fungizone
	Ketoconazole	Nizoral
Sedative/hypnotic agents		
Benzodiazepine derivatives	Diazepam	Valium, Valrelease
	Chlordiazepoxide	Librium, Libritabs, Librax[c]
	Lorazepam	Ativan
	Oxazepam	Serax
	Flurazepam	Dalmane
	Triazolam	Halcion
Barbituric acid derivatives	Alprazolam	Xanax
	Phenobarbital	Various, Donnatal[c]
	Butabarbital	Butisol
	Butalbital	Fiorinal,[b,c] Fioricet,[c] Esgic[c]
	Pentobarbital	Nembutal
Chloral and carbamate derivatives	Chloral hydrate	Notec, Aquachloral
	Meprobamate	Miltown, Equanil, Equagesic[b]
Antihyperintensive agents		
Beta-adrenergic antagonists	Propranolol	Inderal, Inderide[c]
	Metoprolol	Lopressor
	Atenolol	Tenormin
	Timolol	Timoptic

(continues)

TABLE 9.2 *(continued)*

Type of medication	Generic name	Common trade name(s)
Alpha-2 agonists	Methyldopa	Aldomet, Aldoril[c]
	Clonidine	Catapres, Catapres-TTS, Combipres[c]
Alpha-1 antagonists	Prazosin	Minipress
Calcium channel blockers	Verapamil	Calan, Isoptin
	Nifedipine	Procardia, Adalat
	Diltiazem	Cardizem, Cardizem CD
Inotropic (cardiotonic) agents	Digoxin	Lanoxin, Lanoxicaps
Corticosteroids	Hydrocortisone	Cortef, Cortisporin,[c] Neo-Cortef[c] Cortaid
	Prednisone	Deltasone, Prednisone Intensol
	Methylprednisone	Medrol, Solu-Medrol
	Dexamethaszone	Decadron, Neo-Decadron[c]
Nonsteroidal anti-inflammatory agents	Ibuprofen	Motrin, Rufen, Advil, Nuprin, Medipren
	Naproxen	Naprosyn, Anaprox, Aleve
	Indomethacin	Indocin
	Sulindac	Clinoril
	Diflunisal	Dolobid
	Choline magnesium trisalicylate	Trilisate, Tricosal
	Aspirin	Various
Narcotic analgesics	Codeine	Tylenol with Codeine,[c] Robitussin AC,[c] Brontex,[c] other codeine cough preparations
	Hydrocodone	Lortab,[c] Lorcet,[c] Vicodin,[c] Hycodan,[c] Hycomine,[c] Tussionex[c]
	Oxycodone	Percodan[b], Percotcet[c], Tylox[c], Roxicet[c]
	Meperidine	Demerol, Mepergan[c]
	Propoxyphene	Darvon, Darvon-N, Darvocet-N,[c] Wygesic,[c] Darvon Compound[b]
Antibiotics	Metronidazole	Flagyl, Metrogel
	Ciprofloxacin	Cipro
	Norfloxacin	Noroxin
	Ofloxacin	Floxin
	Cefuroxime	Zinacef, Ceftin
	Cephalexin	Keflex
	Cephalothin	Keflin
Radiocontrast media	Metrizamide	Amipaque
	Iothalamate	Conray
	Diatrizoate	Hypaque, Renovist
	Iohexol	Omnipaque
H_2 receptor antagonists	Cimetidine	Tagamet, Tagamet HD
	Ranitidine	Zantac
	Famotidine	Pepcid
	Nizatidine	Axid

(continues)

TABLE 9.2 *(continued)*

Type of medication	Generic name	Common trade name(s)
Immunosuppressive agents	Cyclosporine	Sandimmune
	Interferon	Intron A, Roferon A, Actimmune
Antineoplastic agents	Chlorambucil	Leukeran
	Cytarabine	Cytosar-U
	Interleukin-2	
	Spirohydantoin mustard	Spiromustine
Anticonvulsants	Phenytoin	Dilantin
	Valproic acid	Depakene, Depakote
	Carbamazepine	Tegretol
Antiparkinsonian agents (see also anticholinergic agents)	Levodopa	Larodopa
	Levodopa/carbidopa	Sinemet
	Bromocryptine	Parlodel
	Pergolide	Permax
Antiemetics	Prochlorperazine	Compazine
	Metoclopramide	Reglan
	Hydroxyzine	Atarax, Vistaril
	Promethazine	Phenergan
	Trimethobenzamide	Tigan
	Diphenhydramine	Benadryl, Dramamine
	Meclazine	Antivert
Skeletal muscle relaxants	Cyclobenzaprine	Flexaril
	Methocarbimol	Robaxin
	Carisoprodal	Soma, Soma Compound[b]
	Baclofen	Lioresal
	Chlorzoxazone	Parafon Forte, Paraflex
Antihistamines/decongestants	Diphenhydramine	Benadryl, Tylenol PM,[c] Sominex, other OTC cough/cold preparations
	Chlorpheniramine	Chlor-Trimeton, Deconamine,[c] Contac,[c] Tylenol Cold,[c] Hycomine, [c] other OTC cough/cold preparations[c]
	Brompheniramine	Dimetane, Dimetapp,[c] Drixoral,[c] other OTC cough/cold preparations[c]
	Pseudoephedrine	Sudafed,[c] Actifed,[c] Robitussin PE,[c] Dimetapp,[c] Entex,[c] Drixoral,[c] Tylenol Cold,[c] Claritin-D,[c] other OTC cough/cold preparations[c]
	Phenylpropanolamine	Ornade,[c] Triaminic,[c] Poly-Histine,[c] Hycomine,[c] other OTC cough–cold and appetite suppressant preparations[c]

OTC = over-the-counter.

[a] These are examples only; new medications appear regularly. [b]These compounds contain aspirin. [c]These compounds may contain other active ingredients.

Adapted from *Clinical Practice Guidelines for Recognition and Initial Assessment of Alzheimer's Disease and Related Dementias (1996). U.S. Department of Health and Human Services.*

Recognition and Initial Assessment of Alzheimer's Disease and Related Dementias, published by the U.S. Department of Health and Human Services (Costa et al., 1996). Among these medications, those whose neuropsychological correlates have received the most study are the benzodiazepines, a class of sedative-hypnotics, and antidepressants, particularly tricyclic antidepressants having anticholinergic properties. The focus of most studies has been on memory function.

Benzodiazepines are prescribed for treatment of anxiety, agitation, or insomnia. They may to lead to dependence after only several days of use, and increased tolerance may develop after long-term use, resulting in the desire for increased dosages to maintain treatment effects. Use of these medications in older adults requires particular caution because treatment effects are less predictable, undesirable side effects are more common, and withdrawal symptoms may be heightened. Symptoms of withdrawal may include irritability, anxiety, insomnia, fatigue, headache, dizziness, poor concentration, muscle twitching, tremor, weakness, nausea, depression, seizures, delirium, confusion, and tinnitus. These symptoms may be more pronounced when short-acting medications are discontinued abruptly, and gradual tapering over 4 to 6 weeks is recommended (Hommer, 1991; Woods & Winger, 1995). It has been recommended that long-acting benzodiazepines such as chlordiazepoxide (Librium), diazepam (Valium), and flurazepam (Dalmane) not be prescribed for adults over age 65 (American Psychiatric Association, 1990).

The impact of benzodiazepines on memory function has been most widely studied in healthy volunteers. These studies suggest that benzodiazepines may have an acute, deleterious effect on memory within several hours of initial administration, but that these deficits may resolve somewhat with continued use. Relatively low dosages of long-acting benzodiazepines such as diazepam (2 mg) and even short-acting benzodiazepines such as oxazepam (Serax, 30 mg), lorazepam (Ativan, 2 mg) or midazolam (Versed, 3 mg) have been shown to impair both explicit and implicit memory performance within 5 hours after administration (Buffett-Jerrott, Stewart, & Teehan, 1998; Curran, Pooviboonsuk, Dalton, & Lader, 1998; Legrand et al., 1995; Loke, Hinrichs, & Ghoneim, 1985; Stewart, Rioux, Connolly, Dunphy, & Teehan, 1996). Lorazepam (Ativan, 2 mg) may also produce significant abnormalities in electrophysiological measures related to attention and memory (Curran et al., 1998). The acute effects of benzodiazepines on memory appear to be independent of their sedative effects (Ghoneim & Hinrichs, 1997; Veselis, Reinsel, Feshchenko, & Wronski, 1997), and lorazepam may have more detrimental effects on memory than oxazepam in dosages that produce similar sedative effects (Curran, 1991). In healthy adults, the acute deleterious effects of diazepam may decrease somewhat with continued drug administration and may disappear following withdrawal (Ghoneim, Mewaldt, Berie, & Hinrichs, 1981). It has been suggested that diazepam disrupts the acquisition of new information in memory rather than reducing the ability to retain newly acquired information over time delays (Ghoneim et al., 1981; Hinrichs, Mewaldt, Ghoneim, & Berie, 1982; Lister, Weingartner, Eckardt, & Linnoila, 1988).

While transient deficits have been observed in studies involving healthy volunteers, chronic treatment of patients with benzodiazepines may be associated with more persistent memory deficits, which remain even after the medication has been discontinued and the patient detoxified (Lister *et al.,* 1988; Rummans, Davis, Morse, & Ivnik, 1993; Tata, Rollings, Collins, Pickering, & Jacobson, 1994). In a study of detoxified benzodiazepine-dependent patients over 54 years of age, deficits in verbal learning and immediate and delayed memory were observed in testing conducted within 6 to 10 days after detoxification (Rummans *et al.,* 1993). Patients who have undergone long-term benzodiazepine treatment may experience neuropsychological deficits persisting for some time after the medication has been discontinued. In one study, patients undergoing long-term treatment with benzodiazepines and then 6 months of abstinence showed neuropsychological deficits before withdrawal. These patients continued to show some improvement following withdrawal, although at 6 months they continued to exhibit significant impairment in multiple neuropsychological domains, including verbal learning and memory, psychomotor skills, and visuomotor and visuoconceptual abilities (Tata *et al.,* 1994).

Studies focusing on older adults confirm that benzodiazepines may have acute effects on memory. Low doses of either alprazolam or lorazepam administered to older volunteers have been observed to impair immediate memory recall and increase intrusion errors, and higher doses may also impair delayed recall and aspects of visual perception (Pomara *et al.,* 1998). With continued use for up to 3 weeks, partial tolerance may develop and deficits decrease, although not to pretreatment levels (Pomara *et al.,* 1998). Even low doses of diazepam may produce memory and psychomotor deficits in normal older adults (Pomara *et al.,* 1984), and higher dosages (10 mg) may produce memory deficits similar to those seen in patients with Alzheimer's disease (Block, DeVoe, Stanley, Staley, & Pomara, 1985). Although it is not clear that the magnitude of the acute changes in memory are larger in healthy older adults than in younger adults (Block *et al.,* 1985; Hinrichs & Ghoneim, 1987; Pomara *et al.,* 1985), the pretreatment memory performance of older adults is often lower than that of younger adults. This raises the possibility that older adults being treated with benzodiazepines may be at increased risk for deficits in everyday memory functioning if they suffer even mild compromise related to medication use.

Another class of medications with potential for affecting the neuropsychological function of older adults are antidepressants. Some antidepressants have anticholinergic or sedating effects that may degrade neuropsychological function. Of particular concern are the older generation tricyclic antidepressants (TCAs), whose relatively strong anticholinergic properties may affect memory. The TCAs include imipramine (Tofranil), clomipramine (Anafranil), amitriptyline (Elavil), desipramine (Norpramin), trimipramine (Surmontil), and doxepin (Sinequan). The newer generation antidepressants have reduced or no anticholinergic effects, including the selective serotonin-reuptake inhibitors (SSRIs, e.g., fluoxetine (Prozac), fluvoxamine (Luvox), paroxetine (Paxil), setraline (Zoloft) and the atypical antidepressants such as buproprion (Wellbutrin), nefazodone (Serzone), vanlafaxine (Effexor), and trazedone (Desyrl). Among the newer generation medications, fluoxetine and trazodone have minimal anticholinergic effects, while paroxetine is more anticholinergic. However, trazodone has sedating effects that may affect episodic memory (Curran, Sakulsripring, & Lader, 1988).

Studies of healthy adults, including healthy older adults, have demonstrated mild decrements in memory, attention, and psychomotor speed in the period immediately following administration of TCAs (Curran *et al.,* 1988; Danion *et al.,* 1990). The impact of TCAs on the neuropsychological function of patient groups has, however, been more inconsistent. In general, where detrimental effects are seen, these are in the acute period immediately following initiation of the medication and may resolve over time. In patients whose depression is relieved, mild deficits related to the anticholinergic properties of the medication may be counterbalanced by an improvement in cognition related to beneficial treatment effects. Thus, patients treated with TCAs, especially those who show relief of depression, may show no change or mild improvement in memory (Glass, Uhlenhuth, Hartel, Matuzas, & Fischman, 1981; Siegfried & O'Connolly, 1986).

However, some studies have reported decrements in memory associated with TCA use (Lamping, Spring, & Gelenberg, 1984). One study focusing on older adults observed that a depressed group being treated with antidepressant medications that were largely TCAs showed a small, but statistically significant deficit in memory in comparison with an unmedicated depressed group (Marcopulus & Graves, 1990).

If a patient exhibits increased confusion following initiation of a TCA or a change in dosage, several possibilities might be considered. First, the medication may be ineffective, and the patient's depression may have worsened. Second, the patient may be experiencing medication toxicity or a medication interaction, which can cause global confusion and disorientation (Preskorn & Jerkovich, 1990). Finally, the patient may have already experienced a subtle decline related to a dementing illness, which makes him more sensitive to the anticholinergic effects of standard doses of the antidepressant (Petracca, Teson, Chemerinski, Leiguarda, & Starkstein, 1996). In patients with Alzheimer's disease, the cholinergic neurotransmitter system is already compromised. While use of TCAs in these patients may improve functioning somewhat, this may be accompanied by a mild decline in cognition (Petracca *et al.,* 1996), although this is not always the case (Reifler *et al.,* 1986).

Thus, while antidepressant medications may not necessarily compromise neuropsychological function in older adults, it is important to be alert to this possibility, particularly in the oldest old and in patients who may already be experiencing mild deficits related to neurodegenerative disease.

NORMAL PRESSURE HYDROCEPHALUS

Normal pressure hydrocephalus (NPH) is a disorder in which the production of cerebrospinal fluid (CSF) within the brain ventricles exceeds absorption, resulting in distention of the ventricles and reduced blood flow to periventricular white matter (Jeffreys, 1987; Stambrook, Gill, Cardoso, & Moore, 1993). Common causes of NPH are subarachnoid hemorrhage, severe head trauma, and central nervous system infection such as meningitis or encephalitis. Normal pressure (or communicating) hydrocephalus is distinguished from obstructive (or non-communicating) hydrocephalus in which CSF reabsorption is abnormal because of a physical blockage of fluid movement between the ventricles. Obstructive hydrocephalus can be caused by conditions such as congenital malformations or tumors. Structural imaging reveals ventricular enlargement in the absence of overall atrophy in both communicating and noncommunicating hydrocephalus, with the cause of the obstruction sometime evident in the latter case. In NPH, neurobehavioral changes may be more critical to the diagnosis because other structural abnormalities are not present. It has been suggested that hydrocephalus may contribute to between 2 and 12% of cases of dementia (Clarfield, 1989; Strub & Black, 1988).

The classic symptoms of NPH are the triad of abnormal gait, urinary incontinence, and cognitive decline (Adams, Fisher, Hakim, Ojemann, & Sweet, 1965; Fisher, 1977; Fisher, 1982; Strub & Black, 1988). Patients often exhibit disturbed balance, unsteadiness while walking, and a short, wide-based gait. Incontinence may be characterized by either abnormal frequency of urination or sudden urgency in the need to urinate. During examination of reflexes, patients often exhibit "frontal release" signs, such as grasping and rooting.

Although cognitive change is among the classic NPH symptoms, this is typically mild early in the course of the disorder, but it may become more severe if the disorder is untreated. In contrast to other dementing illnesses, the neuropsychological correlates of NPH have not been well defined, although certain findings are generally reported (Caltagirone, Gainotti, Masullo, & Villa, 1982; Fisher, 1977; Lezak, 1995; Stambrook et al., 1988; Stambrook *et al.,* 1993). Patients often exhibit a behavioral and cognitive syndrome suggestive of frontal lobe dysfunction, including apathy, lack of spontaneity, mental slowing, perseverative responding, and akinesia. They may fail to show concern about urinary accidents. Deficits in abilities to maintain attention and resist distraction are often among early neuropsychological abnormalities, and these may contribute to impairment in memory. Word fluency may be deficient. Language functions may remain relatively preserved, including naming, comprehension, reading, and writing, although apathy and affective flatness may contribute to sparse and aprosodic verbal output. Psychomotor speed may be slowed.

Neuropsychiatric changes associated with NPH have also been described (Price & Tucker, 1977; Pujol, Leal, Fluvia, & Conde, 1989). Behaviors suggestive of depression may be apparent, although in some cases these behaviors may reflect other symptoms such as apathy and reduced movement. Agitation or psychotic behaviors have occasionally been described, particularly in patients with NPH induced by head injury.

The symptoms of NPH, unlike those of other dementing disorders, may be reversible if the disorder is detected early and appropriately treated (Black, 1980;

Stambrook *et al.,* 1988). The most common treatments are lumbar puncture or surgical installation of a ventricular shunt, both of which normalize CSF flow and pressure within the ventricles. Lumbar puncture can be performed in an outpatient clinic and is often used to help establish the diagnosis of NPH and the potential benefit of the more invasive shunting procedure. In lumbar puncture, a small amount of CSF is removed to see if there is a transient improvement in symptoms, suggesting that shunting may be appropriate. A brief neuropsychological evaluation focusing on assessment of attention, memory, and mental speed is often performed before and after the lumbar puncture to help monitor whether there is an improvement in mental status. Shunting involves the placement of a device in the brain ventricle to divert CSF so that it will be absorbed more efficiently. Following shunting, there may be substantial improvement in gait and continence and also in neuropsychological function, particularly in patients with only mild cognitive decline. Recent reports of the proportion of cases showing clinical improvement following shunting have ranged between 40 and 80% (Black, Ojemann, & Tzouras, 1985; Peterson, Mokri, & Laws, 1985; Shenkin, Greenberg, Bouzarth, Gutterman, & Morales, 1973). Improvement is more likely when the disease is treated early in its course, when the classic triad of symptoms appear relatively suddenly related to a specific etiology, and when cognitive decline is minimal (Caltagirone *et al.,* 1982; Thomsen, Borgesen, Bruhn, & Gjerras, 1986).

METABOLIC AND TOXIC DISORDERS

Metabolic disorders involve disturbances in the body's chemistry that affect the functioning of organ systems, including the brain and central nervous system, and thus may affect neuropsychological function. These disorders often occur in conjunction with medical illnesses, which have an elevated frequency among older age groups. Among community-dwelling individuals over the age of 65, 86% have at least one chronic medical illness, and 50% have at least two (Jarvik & Perl, 1981; Levenson & Hall, 1981). Metabolic disorders may be a direct expression of a specific disease or may reflect an undesirable side effect of the treatment selected for the disease. Some medications used to treat common illnesses or interactions between these medications have the potential to disrupt metabolism, and older individuals are particularly vulnerable to these disruptions. In addition, because of reduced body weight, older individuals are particularly sensitive to the toxic effects of medication regimens and to metals and solvents found in some occupational settings. Table 9-2 lists common medications that potentially may disrupt cognitive function.

Metabolic disorders can result in significant abnormality in neuropsychological function, affecting attention, mental speed, mood, memory, and arousal. Since treatment for these disorders may halt and sometimes even reverse cognitive decline, the role of metabolic disturbance should be carefully considered as a possible etiology. This can be accomplished by ensuring that the patient has recently received a comprehensive medical evaluation, including appropriate laboratory tests (Cummings & Benson, 1992b). The following laboratory tests are often included: complete blood count (CBC) and chemistry profiles (e.g., sodium, calcium, niacin, thiamine, BUN and creatinine), syphilis serology (rapid plasma reagin [RTA], fluorescent treponemal antibody [FTA]) thyroid-stimulating hormone (TSH) for hypothyroidism, T_3 and T_4 for hyperthyroidism, and vitamin B_{12}. The review of medical records will indicate whether the patient has experienced illnesses that may compromise metabolic function. The background history obtained during the clinical interview can be used to determine if the patient may have been exposed to toxic agents in the workplace.

Conditions associated with metabolic and toxic disorders that may compromise neuropsychological function are listed in the remainder of this chapter. More detailed description of these conditions can be found in other sources (Cummings & Benson, 1992a; Lee & Loring, 1993).

Chronic anoxia (oxygen deprivation): This may be associated with chronic pulmonary insufficiency, sleep apnea, chronic cardiac disease, or anemia.

Acute anoxia: This may result from cardiopulmonary arrest (heart attack), carbon monoxide intoxication, strangulation, or hanging.

Chronic renal (kidney) failure: This condition alone may result in a *uremic encephalopathy*, resulting in compromise of intellectual function (Bremer, Wert, Durica, & Weaver, 1997; Souheaver, Ryan, & DeWolfe, 1982). In addition, some treatments for renal failure, including dialysis and immunosuppressant drugs used in conjunction with renal transplantation, are associated with significant neuropsychological decline.

Hepatic (liver) disease: Alcohol-induced cirrhosis of the liver as well as other chronic liver disease can produce a *hepatic encephalopathy* associated with pronounced neuropsychiatric disorder. Even in the absence of hepatic encephalopathy, individuals with liver cirrhosis may exhibit significant neuropsychological change (Moss *et al.,* 1992; Tarter *et al.,* 1986). Hepatic disorder can result in disruption of the production of porphyrins, resulting in porphyria, which is also associated with neuropsychiatric disorder.

Pancreatic disorders: These include hypoglycemia (low blood sugar), hyperglycemia (elevated blood sugar), and acute pancreatitis (Draelos *et al.,* 1995; Mooradian, Perryman, Fitten, Kavonian, & Morley, 1988; Reaven, Thompson, Nahum, & Haskins, 1990; Ryan & Williams, 1993; Wredling, Levander, Adamson, & Lins, 1990).

Electrolyte abnormalities: These include hyponatremia and hypernatremia (abnormally low and high blood sodium, respectively) and abnormality in serum calcium or magnesium. Elevated serum calcium levels *(hypercalcemia)* are often associated with the presence of cancer or thyroid disorder.

Extracerebral cancers: Cancers outside of the brain may produce metabolic disturbance, generate infections or deposits within the nervous system, or produce a "limbic encephalitis," each of which may compromise neuropsychological function. In addition, treatments for cancer may have toxic effects on brain function.

Deficiencies in vitamins or organ function: Deficiencies in certain vitamins, particularly B_1 (thiamine), B_{12}, niacin, and folate are associated with impairment in cognitive function. In older individuals, it is particularly important to exclude the possibility of a B_{12} deficiency because this can be easily treated with B_{12} injections, often reversing cognitive deficits to some extent. Chronic alcoholics often experience a thiamine deficiency and may develop Wernicke-Korsakoff's syndrome, described earlier in the section on Substance-Related Disorders. Individuals with other disorders causing nutritional deficiencies, such as gastrointestinal disturbances, are also at increased risk for developing this syndrome (Parkin *et al.,* 1991; Shimomura *et al.,* 1998a).

Hyper or hypothyroidism. Either abnormally high or abnormally low thyroid activity can compromise neuropsychological function, which may improve with treatment (Baldini *et al.,* 1997; Dugbartey, 1998; Mennemeier, Garner, & Heilman, 1993; Osterweil *et al.,* 1992; Prinz *et al.,* 1999).

Hypo or hyperparathyroidism: These disorders are associated with dysfunction of the parathyroid gland, which is adjacent to the thyroid, and may also result in hypo- or hypercalcemia (abnormally low or high levels of blood serum calcium, respectively), which may be an additional source of change in mental status. These disorders are often accompanied by decline in neuropsychological status, which may be reversed with treatment (Lorusso, Poli, & Casmiro, 1994; Numann, Torppa, & Blumetti, 1984; Stuerenburg, Hansen, Thie, & Kunze, 1996).

Cushing's disease, Addison's disease: These disorders are caused by abnormal production of glucocorticoids and are associated with change in neuropsychological and neuropsychiatric function (Johnstone, Rundell, & Esposito, 1990; Starkman, Gebarski, Berent, & Schteingart, 1992). Cushing's disease involves an excess of cortisol, most often due to abnormal function of the adrenal medulla or occurring as an undesirable side effect of treatment with steroids. Addison's disease results from abnormally low production of cortisol. The cognitive change associated with each of these disorders may be reversed with appropriate treatment.

Panhypopituitarism: This disorder of the pituitary gland is commonly caused by hypothyroidism in conjunction with adrenal insufficiency and can be reversed with appropriate treatment.

Medication-induced confusion: As was discussed earlier in the section on Substance-Related Disorders, older individuals are at increased risk for developing cognitive confusion related to side effects of medication as well as to its overuse or misuse. Patients taking benzodiazepines (a class of sedative–hypnotics) or antidepressants are at increased risk for medication-induced confusion. Particularly when patients use multiple medications, it is important that the regimen be reviewed by a clinician expert at geriatric psychopharmacology to evaluate the role of medication toxicity or interactions in cognitive confusion. Such confusion may be ameliorated once the medications are appropriately adjusted.

Toxic exposure to metals and solvents: Prolonged exposure to certain metallic agents and solvents sometimes used in occupational settings have been associated with dysfunction in cognition and affect (White, Feldman, & Travers, 1990; White & Proctor, 1993). Metallic agents of concern include lead, mercury, manganese, arsenic, thallium, aluminum, gold, tin, bismuth, and nickel. Solvents associated with behavioral dysfunction include trichloroethylene, trichlorethane, perchloroethylene, toluene, carbon disulfide, methyl alcohol, carbon tetrachloride, ethylene glycol, ethyl chloride, and acrylamide.

10

ASSESSMENT OF DEPRESSION DURING THE NEUROPSYCHOLOGICAL EVALUATION

Neuropsychological evaluation often contributes to the assessment of affective disorders in older adults. An issue frequently motivating this evaluation is the question of dementia versus depression. In many cases, the patient or the family has become concerned when the patient has exhibited behavioral changes such as loss of interest in usual activities, reduced spontaneity, apathy, irritability, or cognitive confusion. Since such changes may be initially interpreted as symptoms of depression, the patient is often first referred for psychiatric evaluation. This may be followed by a request for neuropsychological evaluation.

In such cases, an important diagnostic issue is whether the patient has neuropsychological dysfunction and if so, whether this is likely to be related to depression alone, to depression in combination with a neurodegenerative disorder, or to a neurodegenerative disorder alone. Distinguishing between these alternatives is critical, since they are associated with different treatment strategies and prognostic outcomes. Individuals with pure depression may be less able to care for themselves and to engage in social interaction, and effective treatment may largely restore independent functioning. For individuals with depression and significant cognitive dysfunction possibly related to a neurodegenerative brain disease, treatment for depression may help improve mood and functional abilities but may have less impact on neuropsychological performance. Such patients may continue to require considerable support and structure and should be closely tracked to evaluate the possibility of a neurodegenerative disease. For patients found to have neurodegenerative disease without depression, treatment alternatives may be aimed at slowing or preventing further cognitive decline, providing support, and relieving disruptive behaviors.

CRITERIA FOR DIAGNOSING DEPRESSION

The DSM-IV defines separate criteria for major depressive episode, major depressive disorder, and dysthymic disorder (American Psychiatric Association, 1994). A major depressive episode is defined as an interval lasting at least 2 weeks during which the patient exhibits depressed mood or loss of interest or pleasure in usual activities. The interval must represent a change for the patient and must include multiple symptoms such as sadness, tearfulness, disturbance of appetite and/or sleep, motor slowness or agitation, fatigue, low self-esteem, guilt, difficulty in concentrating or making decisions, or thoughts of death. A major depressive disorder is diagnosed when there is a history of one or more depressive episodes in the absence of other psychiatric disorders such as schizophrenia or mania. A dysthymic disorder is diagnosed when the patient chronically experiences symptoms of depression for at least 2 years, but these do not meet the criteria for major depressive episode or major depressive disorder.

PREVALENCE, RISK FACTORS AND CHARACTERISTICS OF DEPRESSION IN OLDER ADULTS

Among community-residing adults over age 65, the prevalence of major depression is lower than among younger adults, with most estimates falling between 1 and 5% (Blazer, 1993). However, the prevalence of milder depressive symptoms in older adults is much higher, ranging between 10 and 25% (Blazer, 1993). The prevalence of both major depression and dysthymic disorder is even greater for older individuals who are hospitalized or living in long-term care facilities.

Variables increasing the risk of depression both for individuals over age 65 and for younger adults include female sex, unmarried (particularly widowed) status, the occurrence of stressful life events, and the absence of a supportive social network (National Institutes of Health Consensus Development Conference, 1993). Older adults are likely to experience a number of stressful life cycle changes, such as the retirement from work, moving from a long-time family home, or the severe illness or death of a spouse. Coexisting medical illnesses increase the risk of depression, particularly thyroid disorders, cancer, cerebrovascular disease, Parkinson's disease, myocardial infarction, and chronic obstructive pulmonary disease. Medications used to treat medical conditions may have side effects predisposing the patient to depression. For example, one class of hypertensive medications, the beta blockers, includes depression as a possible side effect. Limited education has been associated with increased risk of depression in older adults (Gallo, Royall, & Anthony, 1993). In individuals over age 65 suffering their first major depressive episode, a family history of depression is less common than is the case for younger adults experiencing the onset of depression (Caine, Lyness, & King, 1993; Maier *et al.,* 1991; Mendlewicz & Baron, 1991).

Considerable research has focused on whether late-life depression, the onset of an initial major depressive episode after age 65, has characteristics distinguishing it from depression occurring earlier in life. If such differences exist, they may have important implications for predicting which individuals may develop depression and for treatment recommendations. Although many studies have examined these issues, the findings have been variable and conflicting, in part because of methodological differences in important features such as the severity of the patients' depression, the research setting (e.g., outpatient clinic versus psychiatric hospital), the variables measured, and the degree and nature of any concurrent medical illness (King & Caine, 1995; Nussbaum, 1997).

In an effort to facilitate research, the National Institutes of Health sponsored a conference on the diagnosis and treatment of depression in late life (National Institutes of Health Consensus Development Conference, 1993). The conference panel noted that depression is underdiagnosed and undertreated in older adults owing to a combination of factors. Depressive symptoms in older adults may be somewhat different from those observed in younger adults, with depressed mood being less prominent. Vegetative symptoms (poor appetite, insomnia, lack of energy, absence of pleasure) may be more indicative of depression and more helpful in making diagnostic decisions. Although changes in sleep patterns and reduction in energy often occur with normal aging, insomnia accompanied by anxiety, obsessive sad thoughts, and reduced interest in usual activities are often symptomatic of depression. Depressed older adults may not exhibit the loss of self-esteem and guilt that are characteristic of depression in younger adults but are more likely to appear apathetic, agitated, anxious and preoccupied with physical complaints (Avery & Silverman, 1984; Bieliauskas, 1993; Blazer, 1993). The possible role of medical conditions in causing depression-like symptoms must be carefully considered because these may be very treatable. For example, patients with untreated thyroid dysfunction may exhibit decreased energy or apathy, which is relieved when the thyroid disorder is effectively treated.

ASSESSING DEPRESSION DURING THE CLINICAL INTERVIEW

Assessment of depression in older adults during neuropsychological evaluation depends on three major activities: (1) information and impressions gathered during the clinical interview, (2) the use of questionnaires for assessing the presence and severity of depressive symptoms, and (3) findings from neuropsychological testing. Each of these activities is discussed in the following sections.

The clinical interview is most critical when evaluating depression during a neuropsychological evaluation (National Institutes of Health Consensus Development Conference, 1993). Some psychologists prefer to use a structured interview (e.g., the Structured Clinical Interview for Diagnosis for the DSM-III-R) or a rating scale, for example, the Hamilton Depression Rating Scale (Hamilton, 1967) to quantify their impressions. Although these procedures may be useful in some cases, they are time-consuming and may be unneccessary when a well organized and detailed interview can be conducted.

First, the presence of depressive symptoms is carefully examined. When asked directly, older adults often do not describe themselves as depressed but will report depressive symptoms when specifically queried. The patient can be asked about his experience of daily life, particularly changes in interest in daily activities, the frequency of pleasurable activities, the nature and quality of social interactions, and thoughts about the future. The possibility of changes in mood can be examined, particularly whether there have been increased episodes of irritability, impatience, or anger. Depressed patients often spontaneously report concerns about memory and attention, even when formal testing reveals that changes in these abilities are not significant (Kahn, Zarit, Hilbert, & Niederehe, 1975; Larrabee & Levin, 1986). Although older adults may be aware of cognitive changes, they may not realize that such symptoms can be associated with depression. It is critical to query the patient about the presence of vegetative symptoms, particularly insomnia and loss of appetite.

In addition to interviewing the patient, it is important to interview a close family member or friend about changes in the patient's behavior. Specific questions can be used to discern the presence of depressive symptoms. However, informant perspectives must be interpreted cautiously, because these individuals are not trained in psychological assessment. On the one hand, overreporting of patient symptoms of depression is particularly likely in caregivers who are depressed themselves or in caregivers of patients with Alzheimer's disease, who may interpret unusual patient symptoms as reflecting depression. On the other hand, underreporting of depressive symptoms may occur because older informants may be unaware of the unique characteristics of depression in older adults.

If depressive symptoms are present, their relationship to other variables must be carefully examined, particularly to life cycle changes and medical conditions. The relatively sudden onset of depressive symptoms and cognitive decline after major life cycle changes (e.g., the death of a significant other, the loss of one's home, retirement from work, a recent illness in the patient or a spouse or close family member) may reflect reactive depression. However, if behavioral changes such as apathy and cognitive confusion were present before such life cycle changes or persist for a prolonged interval after other depressive symptoms have receded, this raises the possibility of an underlying medical or neurodegenerative disorder. The relationship of behavioral changes to medical conditions that are associated with depression-like symptoms, such as thyroid dysfunction, cancer, anemia, and hypertension, must be carefully explored.

The psychologist's impression of the patient's mood during the clinical interview and the formal testing is also critical. Patients who appear withdrawn, lacking in energy, easily tearful, sad, or anxious are more likely to be depressed. Irritability or difficulty in sustaining effort during the testing is also suggestive of depression.

When evaluating depressed patients, it is particularly important to use the clinical interview to initially engage and motivate the patient's involvement in the entire evaluation process. Depressed patients may be withdrawn, fatigued, and disinterested, and these characteristics may limit their ability to exert their best effort in a consistent fashion throughout the evaluation. The evaluation will be facilitated if the examiner makes a special effort to establish and maintain rapport with the patient, to exhibit empathy with the patient's concerns, to provide encouragement as appropriate, and to allow opportunities for rest breaks.

In patients who are already being treated for depression, the nature of that treatment must be carefully determined because this may affect cognitive function. Some antidepressant medications have anticholinergic properties that may contribute to memory impairment or confusion. Medications that may contribute to confusion have been discussed in Chapter 9. The possible impact of electroconvulsive therapy on neuropsychological function is reviewed later in this chapter.

INSTRUMENTS FOR SCREENING FOR DEPRESSION

A second source of data useful in evaluating depression is the patient's response to a self-report questionnaire assessing symptoms of depression. For older adults, commonly used instruments include the Beck Depression Inventory (BDI) (Beck *et al.*, 1961) and the Geriatric Depression Scale (GDS) (Yesavage *et al.*, 1983).

The BDI includes 21 items assessing depressive symptoms such as sadness, guilt, tearfulness, appetite, and fatigue. The patient responds to each item by choosing among four response alternatives designed to reflect increasing severity of that symptom and scored on 4-point scale (0 to 3 points). Patients are instructed that if several of the alternatives seem to apply to them, they are allowed to mark all that apply. The total score is computed by summing the individual item scores and is interpreted on the basis of cutoff scores. Probable depression is suggested by scores of 9 or below, mild to moderate depression by scores between 10 and 18, moderate to severe depression by scores from 19 to 29, and severe depression by scores of 30 or above. The accuracy of the BDI for correctly classifying depressed patients and nondepressed individuals is relatively high, usually exceeding 80% for outpatients although somewhat lower for inpatients (Norris *et al.*, 1987; Rapp *et al.*, 1988). There is also a 13-item short form of the BDI. This instrument has been less well studied but appears to have only slightly lower accuracy than the total BDI (Foelker, Schewchuk, & Niederehe, 1987; Scogin, Hamblin, Beutler, & Corbishley, 1988).

Although the BDI has strong psychometric properties and is widely used, it was not specifically developed for use with older adults and has several disadvantages for this population. Its multiple-choice format may be confusing to older adults, particularly patients whose cognition is mildly compromised. The response alternatives for each item are not mutually exclusive, and some are relatively lengthy. Patients may have difficulty remembering each alternative when trying to choose between them, which will slow their reponses, increase the possibility that they may become frustrated, and extend the length of time necessary to complete the instrument. In addition, the BDI includes a number of items assessing somatic complaints (e.g., problems with general health, appetite, libido). These problems are common in nondepressed older adults and may be related to variables such as concurrent medical conditions or even normal age-related changes.

The Geriatric Depression Scale (GDS) was specifically designed for evaluating depression in older adults. It includes 30 items, each of which is responded to in a yes–no format. Although patients sometimes complain that having only two choices restricts their response, the yes–no format is generally easier to complete than that of the BDI. The GDS places greater emphasis on cognitive complaints (e.g., concerns about memory, concentration) than on somatic symptoms as compared with the BDI. Responses consistent with depression are summed to yield a total score, and the test developers suggest that total scores above 10 are indicative of depression. The accuracy of the GDS for correctly classifying both outpatients and inpatients as well as nondepressed individuals is at least comparable with that of the BDI (Olin, Schneider, Eaton, Zemansky, & Pollock, 1992; Rapp *et al.,* 1988). A 15-item short form of the GDS has also been developed, although its psychometric properties are less well understood than those of the standard GDS (Sheikh & Yesavage, 1986).

In evaluating depression in patients with dementia, although self-report questionnaires can be used, the findings must be interpreted more cautiously and greater reliance must be placed on other sources of data. In patients with Alzheimer's disease, the accuracy of the GDS may be reduced, particularly in patients lacking awareness of cognitive change or with moderate to severe dementia (Burke *et al.,* 1998; Feher, Larrabee, & Crook, 1992; Gilley & Wilson, 1997). An alternative questionnaire is the Neuropsychiatric Inventory, an interview form that queries informants familiar with the patients on the presence of depressive symptoms (Cummings *et al.,* 1994). The Neuropsychiatric Inventory was specifically designed to evaluate patients with Alzheimer's disease and to distinguish symptoms of depression from nondepressive neuropsychiatric symptoms common in these patients, such as apathy. The Neuropsychiatric Inventory and depression in Alzheimer's disease have already been discussed in Chapter 6.

In older patients, symptoms of anxiety often accompany depression. Instruments available for evaluating anxiety include the Beck Anxiety Inventory (Beck & Steer, 1990) and the Spielberger State/Trait Anxiety Inventory (Spielberger,

Gorsuch, & Lushene, 1970). However, the validity of these instruments for evaluating older adults has not been well established.

It is important to note that, as with all test data, the findings from self-report instruments are best interpreted within the context of the clinical interview findings and behavioral observations of the patient. The test score on the GDS or BDI represents only one part of the data necessary to evaluate mood during the neuropsychological evaluation. So, for example, even if a patient's GDS score is below 10, he may be diagnosed as depressed on the basis of other data, and the converse is also true.

NEUROPSYCHOLOGICAL PROFILES OF DEPRESSION

A third source of data for evaluating depression is neuropsychological test performance. Several major patterns of neuropsychological findings are commonly seen in older patients who are depressed. The first is a pattern of relatively severe neuropsychological dysfunction, most often seen in patients who are more severely depressed, hospitalized, with limited education, from low socioeconomic status, with bipolar disorders, and males (Raskin, 1986). In a study of severely depressed older inpatients (50 to 85 years) who were carefully screened to exclude those with a possible history of neurodegenerative brain disease or confounding medical illness including cerebrovascular disease, widespread deficits were observed on measures of attention, word generation, verbal immediate and delayed recall, and visuospatial ability (King, Cox, Lyness, & Caine, 1995). These findings suggest that severe depression may compromise multiple neuropsychological domains to produce a dementia syndrome.

A second pattern more often observed in older patients with mild to moderate depression, typically receiving outpatient treatment, is one of milder and more circumscribed neuropsychological deficits, which may not achieve clinical significance. Mild to moderately depressed outpatients are more likely to express concern about cognitive dysfunction than are patients with other disorders or nondepressed, healthy older adults. In some cases, these complaints are more closely related to a tendency to focus on negative experiences than to true neuropsychological deficits. However, in some cases the deficits may be real, although so subtle that they may not be clinically significant. In one study comparing mild to moderately depressed outpatients averaging 61 years of age with healthy control subjects, the presence of depression was associated with deficits on measures of visual memory and nonverbal intelligence (WMS-R Visual Reproduction, WAIS-R Performance IQ) but not on a wide variety of other tests of attention, executive function, verbal abilities, and verbal memory, including the WAIS-R Digit Span or Digit-Symbol, WMS-R Logical Memory, Boston Naming Test, Controlled Oral Word Association, Wisconsin Card Sorting Test, Stroop Test, or Rey-Osterrieth Complex Figure (Boone *et al.*, 1995). In contrast, the severity of the patients' depression (mild versus moderate) affected measures of executive function and psychomotor speed. Another study comparing mild to moderately depressed older outpatients (ages 60 to 75) with control subjects found deficits only on timed visuomotor tests (e.g., the Trail-Making Test) but not on a wide array of other tests of memory, fluency, or visuospatial ability (Lyness, Eaton, & Schneider, 1994).

It is important to emphasize that while some research studies have found statistically significant deficits in groups of depressed patients as compared with nondepressed control groups, individual patients may not show clinically observable deficits. The neuropsychological dysfunction in individual depressed outpatients is often so small that the clinical test scores fall largely within the expected range (Bieliauskas, 1993; Boone et al., 1995; Lesser et al., 1996). Where deficits are clinically significant, they are most common on tests sensitive to visual memory, executive function, and timed visuomotor performance, resulting in an overall neuropsychological profile resembling that of a subcortical dementia (Massman, Delis, Butters, Dupont, & Gillin, 1992) or of focal right hemisphere dysfunction (Boone et al., 1995; Lesser et al., 1996). When this profile is seen, the possible contribution of subcortical cerebrovascular disease or focal right hemisphere disease must be carefully considered.

The performance of mildly depressed patients is often characterized by inconsistency within and across neuropsychological domains, reflecting difficulty in sustaining concentration or mental effort. Performance may be somewhat stronger in more structured or mildly challenging conditions. On memory tests, depressed patients often perform substantially better in structured conditions, for example, in recognition as compared with recall. Such conditions may stimulate the patient to mobilize and maintain mental effort. On tests of verbal memory, errors are more likely to reflect omission of material than intrusion or confabulation of unpresented material.

DEPRESSION AND BRAIN DISEASE

There is accumulating evidence that depression in older adults, particularly the initial onset of severe depression in late life (after age 50), may be related to the presence of neurodegenerative brain disease. Among individuals initially referred for evaluation of depression, between 25 and 30% are ultimately diagnosed with a progressive neurodegenerative brain disease (Siegel & Gershon, 1986).

Older inpatients with severe late-onset depression have an elevated frequency of pronounced structural abnormalities in comparison with nondepressed older individuals or older patients with initial depressive episodes beginning earlier in life. Although healthy older people often have some structural abnormalities, these are more severe in patients with late-life depression, often consisting of lesions in the deep white matter, periventricular regions, the basal ganglia and other subcortical structures (Coffey et al., 1990; Figiel et al., 1991; Lesser et al., 1996; Salloway et al., 1996). The presence and severity of neuropsychological change may reflect the degree of structural abnormality (Lesser et al., 1996; Salloway et al., 1996).

Depressed patients with large amounts of white matter disease are particularly vulnerable to deficits in executive function (Lesser *et al.*, 1996).

Thus, the onset of late-life depression may be closely related to subcortical abnormalities that are often consistent with cerebrovascular disease. In such patients, it is particularly important that the findings from brain structural imaging be reviewed. While a computed tomography scan is a less expensive and less uncomfortable approach to brain imaging, magnetic resonance imaging is often more sensitive to subcortical lesions and periventricular abnormalities.

Among older patients, those with depressed mood are at increased risk for developing Alzheimer's disease. In a study of older adults initially diagnosed with major depression or dysthymia without cognitive impairment, 22% developed a progressive dementia consistent with Alzheimer's disease within 2 years (Nussbaum, Kaszniak, Allender, & Rapcsak, 1995). The presence of deep white matter or subcortical structural abnormalities at the initial evaluation was predictive of which individuals would later develop dementia. In a longitudinal study of community-dwelling older adults initially without dementia, the risk of later developing a dementing illness, primarily Alzheimer's disease, was twice as high for those with depressed mood at baseline (Devanand *et al.*, 1996).

THE CONCEPT OF PSEUDODEMENTIA

A number of different terms have been used to label the neuropsychological change sometimes observed in older depressed patients. These terms include pseudodementia (Kiloh, 1961), dementia syndrome of depression (Folstein & McHugh, 1978), and depression related cognitive dysfunction (Stoudemire, Hill, Gulley, & Morris, 1989). One purpose of these terms is to distinguish the neuropsychological change associated with depression from that associated with neurodegenerative brain diseases, highlighting the possibility that some of the cognitive dysfunction associated with depression may be reversible if treatment is effective.

Terms such as pseudodementia continue to be useful in reminding clinicians of the importance of considering depression as a factor contributing to cognitive change and of the possibility that effective treatment may ameliorate this change. The term is best applied to patients with major depression who do not have significant neurodegenerative disease. However, it must not be assumed that effective treatment of depression will necessarily reverse cognitive deficits. One large-scale study found reversible cognitive dysfunction in only 11% of demented inpatients with depression aged 45 to 64 years and in fewer than 4% of those over age 64 (Smith & Kiloh, 1981). As previously discussed, the cognitive impairment observed in some older individuals experiencing late-life depression may primarily reflect underlying structural abnormalities rather than reversible deficits (Coffey *et al.*, 1990; Figiel *et al.*, 1991; Lesser *et al.*, 1996; Salloway *et al.*, 1996). Even depressed patients with dementia whose cognitive dysfunction improves somewhat with treatment are at increased risk for a dementing illness (Alexopoulos, Meyers, Young, Mattis, & Kakuma, 1993a; Alexopoulos, Young, & Meyers, 1993b). Thus, although treatment for depression may help some demented patients feel and function better, it may not produce a large and permanent improvement in neuropsychological performance.

DIFFERENTIATING DEPRESSION FROM ALZHEIMER'S DISEASE

Research examining the neuropsychological differences between patients with depression and those with Alzheimer's disease has suggested that these two groups often have distinctive profiles. The neuropsychological deficits seen in patients with depression are often less widespread and milder than those seen in patients with Alzheimer's disease or other dementing illnesses. Memory function may be particularly helpful in differentiating depression from Alzheimer's disease. Depressed patients without dementia often do not exhibit a uniform, dense memory impairment (Burt, Zembar, & Niederehe, 1995; Hill, Stoudemire, Morris, Martino-Saltzman, & Markwalter, 1993; Kaszniak, 1987; Niederehe, 1986), and the presence of consistent impairment across memory tests is more suggestive of Alzheimer's disease than of depression (Dannenbaum, Parkinson, & Inman, 1988; DesRosiers, Hodges, & Berrios, 1995; Hart, Kwentus, Hamer, & Taylor, 1987). On tests of memory for new information, Alzheimer's disease patients often have a more pronounced deficit in storing new information in memory over time, while depressed patients have a greater weakness in the initial acquisition of new material in memory. Thus, Alzheimer's disease patients often show deficient immediate recall and a large decline between immediate and delayed recall, while depressed patients show less decline over a time delay even when immediate recall has been deficient (Hart *et al.*, 1987). In patients with Alzheimer's disease, both recall and recognition may be impaired, whereas recognition memory may be relatively preserved in patients with depression even when recall is impaired (Nussbaum, Kaszniak, Swanda, & Allender, 1988). The presence of intrusion errors during verbal memory tests is more characteristic of depressed patients with Alzheimer's disease than of depressed patients not diagnosed with Alzheimer's disease (Hill *et al.*, 1993). Mildly to moderately depressed patients may not exhibit impairments in other neuropsychological domains including naming, word fluency, and visuoconstructive ability (Hart *et al.*, 1987; King, Caine, Conwell, & Cox, 1991a).

The patient's insight with regard to neuropsychological dysfunction may be helpful in distinguishing depression from Alzheimer's disease, the latter group often denying that they have experienced neuropsychological change, including memory deficits (Green *et al.*, 1993; McGlynn & Kaszniak, 1991). In contrast, patients with depression often report a variety of cognitive complaints, particularly in memory and attention, and may do so even when formal testing does not reveal significant neuropsychological dysfunction (Kahn et al., 1975; Larrabee & Levin, 1986).

The response style of depressed patients with neuropsychological dysfunction and those with Alzheimer's disease is often qualitatively different. In depressed patients, deficits may reflect difficulty in exerting effort and failure to respond, including errors of omission and "don't know" responses. Performance within a neuropsychological domain may be highly variable in depressed patients, and structure and cuing may substantially facilitate performance. In contrast, patients with Alzheimer's disease often exert excellent effort during testing, are more likely to make intrusion and false positive errors, show less variability within neuropsychological domains, and benefit less from structure and cuing.

ELECTROCONVULSIVE THERAPY AND NEUROPSYCHOLOGICAL CHANGE

One approach to the treatment of severely depressed patients, particularly those who are suicidal or who refuse to eat, is the use of electroconvulsive therapy (ECT) (Abrams, 1992). Because this treatment is often effective quickly and avoids the side-effects of antidepressant medications, it has been increasingly applied to older patients.

An important issue in evaluating an older patient who has been treated with ECT is the possible impact of this treatment on neuropsychological function. Neuropsychological evaluation is sometimes requested for depressed patients who have been treated with ECT to help determine whether the patient may be suffering from cognitive dysfunction apart from depression. Therefore, it is important to understand how ECT in itself may affect neuropsychological status.

Most of the research concerning the impact of ECT on neuropsychological function has examined middle-aged, hospitalized patients rather than adults over the age of 60. One set of factors modulating the impact of ECT on cognitive status are the parameters of the ECT treatment. Although bilateral (rather than unilateral) ECT may offer the fastest and greatest relief of depression, this approach may be associated with more pronounced and persistent neuropsychological deficit (Sackheim *et al.,* 1993; Sobin *et al.,* 1995; Weiner, Rogers, Davidson, & Squire, 1986). Neuropsychological deficits are likely to be milder in patients who receive unilateral rather than bilateral and brief pulse rather than sine-wave ECT, delivered to the nondominant brain hemisphere, usually the right hemisphere (Sackheim *et al.,* 1993; Sobin *et al.,* 1995; Weiner *et al.,* 1986). Cognitive effects may also be smaller when there are larger time intervals between the treatments (Lerer *et al.,* 1995).

Patients typically receive a course of 10 to 12 ECT treatments administered on a weekly or biweekly basis. Immediately following an ECT treatment, patients are often disoriented, inattentive, and confused and may show deficits in multiple neuropsychological domains (Daniel & Crovitz, 1986). However, within several days following the end of a treatment course, neuropsychological performance in most domains may return to the pre-ECT level or may show improvement if the depression has been relieved (Coleman *et al.,* 1996; Stoudemire, Hill, Morris, & Dalton, 1995).

A possible exception to this recovery is the persistence of deficits in memory. Patients may continue to have impairment in retrograde memory (memory for information known prior to the ECT treatment), particularly for autobiographical information, and to a lesser extent in anterograde memory (memory for new information) (Sackheim, 1992; Squire, 1986; Steif, Sackheim, Portnoy, Decina, & Malitz, 1986). However, even these deficits are often resolved by 1 to 2 months following the end of the treatment course, even in patients receiving bilateral ECT (Calev *et al.,* 1991; Devanand, Verma, Tirumalasetti, & Sackheim, 1991; Sackheim *et al.,* 1993).

Pretreatment cognitive status and the duration of disorientation immediately following treatment may be predictive of the duration of memory deficits following ECT. One study of middle-aged inpatients found that deficits in retrograde memory for autobiographical information 2 months following the end of a treatment course were more likely to be present in patients having preexisting cognitive impairment or in those who had experienced prolonged post-treatment disorientation, even when these patients showed improvement on a measure of overall mental status (Sobin *et al.,* 1995). However, complaints of memory change in some patients may be more reflective of residual depression than of neuropsychological change related to the treatment (Coleman *et al.,* 1996; Freeman, Weeks, & Kendell, 1980; Pettinati & Rosenberg, 1984).

Few studies have focused on whether the neuropsychological changes associated with ECT in older adults are different from those described for younger and middle-aged adults. There are relatively few data focusing on the neuropsychological impact of ECT on patients with late-life depression, although there is some evidence that memory deficits following ECT may increase with age (Zervas *et al.,* 1993). Older age groups are more likely to include a greater number of individuals with preexisting cognitive dysfunction, who may be more vulnerable to neuropsychological decline following ECT. However, ECT has been used to effectively treat depression in patients with dementing disorders, including Alzheimer's disease (Abrams, 1992).

Because ECT-related cognitive compromise is most likely during an ECT course, it is recommended that neuropsychological evaluation occur at least 1 month following the end of a treatment course, when even memory deficits are likely to have resolved. If the evaluation must be performed within a treatment course, it is recommended that this occur at least 3 to 4 days following a treatment, when it is likely that posttreatment confusion and disorientation have subsided. It is important to note that the relapse rate following an ECT course is relatively high even when patients are maintained on antidepressant medication. In one large-scale well-designed study, 59% of patients treated with either unilateral or bilateral ECT relapsed within 1 year (Sackheim *et al.,* 1993). Thus, in evaluating patients previously treated with ECT, the possibility of a depression relapse and its impact on neuropsychological function must be considered.

11

ORGANIZING AND INTERPRETING TEST FINDINGS

This chapter will begin to address one of the most challenging and critical phases of the evaluation—interpreting the test findings to reach a conclusion about the patient and to address the issues motivating the neuropsychological evaluation. Taken alone, the test scores are merely numbers without meaning. They become informative only when they are first, interpreted with respect to expectations about how the patient should perform and second, integrated with each another and with the wealth of other information gathered during the evaluation. All of this information influences how the test scores are organized and interpreted and, thus, the conclusions of the evaluation.

Successful evaluation is a challenging task involving multiple levels of analysis, which ultimately merge to yield the major outcomes of the evaluation. A detail-oriented level of analysis initially focuses on the objective test findings. These are subsequently integrated to form an impression of the patient's overall neuropsychological profile. The neuropsychological profile is a pattern identifying the patient's strengths and weaknesses. Identification of this pattern (or its absence), rather than individual test scores, is critical in developing final conclusions about the patient.

A more abstract level of analysis begins with the initial impression of the patient that is inferred on the basis of background information and the clinical interview. This analysis generates overall hypotheses about the patient, which can be applied to tailor the formal testing and to organize and interpret the test findings. As the psychologist becomes more experienced with different clinical disorders and types of patients, abstract levels of analysis are more quickly achieved, and they more strongly direct the evaluation. Hypotheses concerning possible outcomes of the evaluation develop more quickly and accurately, and meaningful associations between different sources of data are recognized more easily.

This chapter is organized to reflect a sequence of activities that can be applied to organizing and interpreting the test findings, as outlined in Table 11.1. These activities include computing the raw test scores, comparing the test scores with normative data to obtain standardized scores, compiling the data summary sheet, determining estimates of premorbid abilities, interpreting test scores, identifying the neuropsychological profile and disorders associated with this profile, and identifying change on reevaluation.

However, this material cannot serve as a substitute for supervised training in neuropsychological evaluation. As with the remainder of the book, this chapter is meant as a guide to be initially used in conjunction with supervised training or to convey to nonpsychologists the procedures and logic of neuropsychological evaluation. Before attempting to independently evaluate older individuals, it is necessary to obtain supervision from a neuropsychologist who is experienced with this patient group.

COMPUTING RAW TEST SCORES

Total raw scores for each test are computed by use of the standardized instructions provided in the test manuals. The scoring guidelines must be followed carefully so that valid scores will be computed. On some tests, even a 1-point error in scoring raw data may change the interpretation of the test score. If the tests are administered and scored by a technician, then it is the psychologist's responsibility to ensure that the technician is familiar with administration procedures and scoring guidelines. Even with experienced technicians, it is recommended that

TABLE 11.1 Steps in Organizing and Interpreting Test Findings

1. Compute raw test scores
2. Compute standardized scores corresponding to each test score
3. Compile the data summary sheet
4. Determine estimates of premorbid abilities
5. Interpret test findings
6. Identify the neuropsychological profile
7. Identify change on reevaluation

the psychologist rescore random samples of patient data on a periodic basis to validate the scoring accuracy.

Attentive and precise scoring of protocols is particularly important when relatively unstructured verbal responses are required, for example, on several of the Wechsler verbal intelligence tests, such as the WAIS-III Similarities. Test manuals provide guidelines and illustrations for scoring typical patient responses. It is recommended that the examiner be highly familiar with these guidelines because they determine not only how the test protocol is scored but also how it is administered. For example, on some tests such as the WAIS-III Similarities, if the patient gives a vague or suboptimal response, the examiner is required to query the patient further. If the examiner is unfamiliar with the scoring guidelines, the patient may not be queried, resulting in an artifically low test score. Several of the WAIS-III verbal tests are terminated only when the patient has made a specified number of zero-point responses. Lack of familiarity with scoring guidelines may result in premature test termination, thereby invalidating the total test score. Thus, knowledge of scoring guidelines contributes to the validity of both test administration and test scoring.

COMPUTING Z-SCORES

After the raw test scores are computed, they are compared with the normative data to determine if the scores are within normal limits for the sample from which the normative data were derived. The choice of normative data is critical because it heavily influences how the test data are interpreted. In choosing normative data for a particular test, it should first be determined whether and how test scores are affected by patient characteristics, such as age and education, and the manner in which alternative sets of normative data adjust for the effects of these variables. Over the course of clinical practice, the psychologist's choice of normative data may change as sets of data more appropriate to the patient population being served become available.

The patient's performance relative to the normative data set is inferred by converting the raw test score into a standard score, typically a z-score, percentile, scaled score, or T score. Characteristics of these scores and conversions between scores are indicated in Table 11.2. Although there is some variation in the nature of the standard scores provided in different test manuals, use of a common standard score across tests facilitates appreciation of the overall profile of the patient's neuropsychological strengths and weaknesses.

The z-score is often preferred as a common standard test score. This score represents the number of standard deviation (SD) units between the patient's test score and the mean of the normative sample. It is computed by calculating the difference between the test score and the mean of the normative sample and then dividing that difference by the SD of the normative sample. The z-score computation is illustrated in Table 11.3.

TABLE 11.2 Conversions between Standard Scores

Percentile	T	SS	z	Percentile	T	SS	z
	20	1	−3.00	24			−0.71
	21		−2.90		43	8	−0.70
	22		−2.80	25			−0.67
	23	2	−2.70	26			−0.64
	24		−2.60	27			−0.61
	25		−2.50		44		−0.60
	26		−2.40	28			−0.58
1			−2.33	29			−0.55
	27	3	−2.30	30			−0.52
	28		−2.20		45		−0.50
	29		−2.10	31			−0.50
2			−2.05	32			−0.47
	30	4	−2.00	33			−0.44
	31		−1.90	34			−0.41
3			−1.88		46		−0.40
	32		−1.80	35			−0.39
4			−1.75	36			−0.36
	33	5	−1.70	37			−0.33
5			−1.65	38			−0.31
	34		−1.60		47	9	−0.30
6			−1.56	39			−0.28
	35		−1.50	40			−0.25
7			−1.48	41			−0.23
8			−1.41	42			−0.20
	36		−1.40		48		−0.20
9			−1.34	43			−0.18
	37	6	−1.30	44			−0.15
10			−1.28	45			−0.13
11			−1.23	46	49		−0.10
	38		−1.20	47			−0.08
12			−1.18	48			−0.05
13			−1.13	49			−0.03
	39		−1.10	50	50	10	0.00
14			−1.08	51			0.03
15			−1.04	52			0.05
	40	7	−1.00	53			0.08
16			−0.99	54	51		0.10
17			−0.95	55			0.13
18			−0.92	56			0.12
	41		−0.90	57			0.18
19			−0.88		52		0.20
20			−0.84	58			0.20
21			−0.81	59			0.23
	42		−0.80	60			0.25
22			−0.77	61			0.28
23			−0.74		53	11	0.30

(continues)

TABLE 11.2 *(continued)*

Percentile	T	SS	z	Percentile	T	SS	z
62			0.31	87			1.13
63			0.33	88			1.18
64			0.36		62		1.20
65			0.39	89			1.23
	54		0.40	90			1.28
66			0.41		63	14	1.30
67			0.44	91			1.34
68			0.47		64		1.40
69			0.50	92			1.41
	55		0.50	93			1.48
70			0.52		65		1.50
71			0.55	94			1.56
72			0.58		66		1.60
	56		0.60	95			1.65
73			0.61		67	15	1.70
74			0.64	96			1.75
75			0.67		68		1.80
	57	12	0.70	97			1.88
76			0.71		69		1.90
77			0.74		70	16	2.00
78			0.77	98			2.05
	58		0.80		71		2.10
79			0.81		72		2.20
80			0.84		73	17	2.30
81			0.88	99			2.33
	59		0.90		74		2.40
82			0.92		75		2.50
83			0.95		76		2.60
84			0.99		77	18	2.70
	60	13	1.00		78		2.80
85			1.04		79		2.90
86			1.08		80	19	3.00
	61		1.10			20	3.30

TABLE 11.3   Computation of the z-Score

$z = (x - X)/SD$
where x is the patient's raw score,
  X is the mean of the normative sample
  SD is the standard deviation of the normative sample
Example: raw score = 90
      normative mean = 100
      normative SD = 15
$z = (90 - 100)/15 = -0.67$

The z-score describes the patient's performance relative to the normative sample. Thus, a z-score of +1 indicates that the patient's score is one SD above the normative mean, while a z-score of −1 indicates that the patient's score is one SD below the normative mean. The larger the z-score, the more divergent is the patient's score from the mean of the normative sample. For example, if Patient A obtains a z-score of + 0.5 and Patient B obtains a z-score of + 1.6, this means that Patient B's performance is more divergent from the normative mean. In most cases, larger, more positive z-scores indicate that the patient is performing better than the average of the normative sample. This is true for all tests in which the total number of points increases with better performance such that higher total test scores represent better performance than lower test scores. For example, higher raw scores on the WMS-III Logical Memory or on each of the WAIS-III tests represent better performance than lower scores.

However, for some tests, larger raw data scores represent weaker performance. This is true when raw data represent the number of errors (e.g., number of errors on the Wisconsin Card Sorting Test) or the performance time (e.g., time to complete Trails A). In such cases, the larger the test score, the worse the performance. Tables of standardized scores often make adjustments such that large, more positive standardized scores, such as z-scores, consistently represent performance that is better than the mean of the normative sample. However, this issue must be carefully considered when using a new set of normative data so that the meaning of standardized scores is clear.

COMPILING THE NEUROPSYCHOLOGY DATA SUMMARY SHEET

The next step is to summarize the raw test and standard scores by entering them in a data sheet. A sample Neuropsychology Data Summary Sheet is included as Appendix E. The data sheet includes columns for entering the raw scores, the standard scores provided in the test manual (e.g., percentile, T, z, age-scaled scores), the z-score conversions of the standard scores, premorbid estimates of abilities, interpretations of test scores and qualitative comments concerning test performance. Approaches to estimating premorbid abilities and interpreting test scores are described in the following sections.

APPROACHES TO ESTIMATING PREMORBID ABILITIES

Premorbid ability refers to the patient's characteristic level of ability prior to possible neurologic, psychiatric, or other disorders affecting behavior. Actual information about the patient's premorbid ability, such as an intelligence quotient obtained in elementary or high school, is rarely available, so this ability must be estimated based on information gathered during the evaluation. Determining an estimate of premorbid ability is a critical step, since this estimate is used as a standard to determine whether the patient has experienced significant decline in neuropsychological function. If the patient's current performance is significantly lower than his estimated premorbid ability, this supports the hypothesis that he has experienced neuropsychological change.

As discussed in Chapter 3, when evaluating older individuals, the assessment of specific abilities (memory, attention, etc.) may be more important than formal assessment of overall intelligence. Although a number of different approaches for assessing premorbid intelligence have been suggested, approaches for estimating premorbid levels of specific abilities are less well developed. As will be detailed later in this chapter, it is recommended that estimates of premorbid intelligence be applied as one basis for estimating abilities within specific neuropsychological domains.

Approaches for estimating premorbid intelligence are indicated below. More detailed discussion of each of these approaches can be found in other sources (Lezak, 1995; Vanderploeg, 1994).

Best Performance Method

Lezak (1995) has suggested that data concerning the highest level of the patient's performance, either in the past or currently, can be used to estimate premorbid ability. So, for example, the highest test score from the WAIS-III or another intelligence test could be used to estimate premorbid ability.

The best test approach has, however, been criticized because even among normal individuals there is variability between intelligence test scores, and an individual's best score may not be representative of overall intelligence or of specific abilities. Use of this approach has been observed to overestimate intelligence even in normal individuals (Mortensen, Gade, & Reinisch, 1991). In individuals with diffuse brain disease, such as Alzheimer's disease, most, if not all, of the patient's scores may be below the premorbid level, and even consideration of the best test score is likely to result in underestimation of premorbid ability.

"Hold" Scores

The method of "hold" scores bases estimates of premorbid intelligence on test scores that tend to be relatively resistant to neurobehavioral disease. Scores on the Vocabulary and Information tests from the Wechsler scales remain relatively stable with normal aging and have been described as hold tests for estimating the premorbid Verbal IQ (VIQ). Similarly, the Picture Completion test has been described as a hold test for estimating the premorbid Performance IQ (PIQ).

Use of these Wechsler tests as hold tests has been criticized because they are sometimes sensitive to subtle brain damage, although typically less so than other tests, such as the Digit-Symbol test. Wechsler intelligence test scores may therefore underestimate the premorbid ability in individuals with mild brain disease.

This is particularly likely in language-impaired patients, in whom verbal test scores are likely to be compromised.

Another type of hold test is word reading performance, and several word reading tests have been proposed for estimation of premorbid ability, particularly Verbal IQ. The National Adult Reading Test (NART) was developed in England as an approach for estimating intelligence quotients in patients with dementia (Nelson, 1982; Nelson & O'Connell, 1978). Prediction equations have been developed for using NART scores to predict Verbal, Performance, and Full-Scale Wechsler IQ scores (Crawford, Parker, Stewart, Besson, & DeLacey, 1989). As might be predicted given its verbal test demands, the NART score is more accurate in predicting Verbal and Full-Scale IQ than in predicting Performance IQ.

Because the NART includes some British words whose pronounciation is unfamiliar to Americans, the American National Adult Reading Test (AMNART) was developed. The unfamiliar words were replaced with words of similar frequency that occur in American English (Schwartz & Saffran, 1987). The NART-R is a modified version of the NART developed for use with Canadians and North Americans (Blair & Spreen, 1989).

Grober and Sliwinski (1991) have developed a regression-based method for applying a version of the AMNART and years of education to predict premorbid Verbal IQ in older healthy and mildly demented adults. Five of the AMNART items were excluded because they produced unreliable findings, so the version of the AMNART included in the regression equation includes only 45 items instead of the 50 in the original AMNART. The 45-word AMNART used by Grober and Sliwinski and the regression equation are included in Table 11.4. Normative data for this modified 45-word AMNART are provided by the Mayo's Older Americans Normative Studies (MOANS) (Ivnik et al., 1996).

Use of reading scores to estimate premorbid ability has been criticized because even these scores may be degraded by the presence of dementia (Patterson, Graham, & Hodges, 1994; Storandt, Stone, & LaBarge, 1995; Taylor *et al.,* 1996). However, decline in reading scores is minimal or absent in mildly demented patients (Maddrey, Cullum, Weiner, & Filley, 1996). In patients with pronounced language deficits or more severe dementia, reading performance may decline more dramatically and is more likely to underestimate intelligence (Paque & Warrington, 1995; Stebbins, Gilley, Wilson, Bernard, & Fox, 1990). In more severely demented patients, it may be appropriate to apply a modification of the Grober and Sliwinski equation that corrects for mental status using scores on the Mini-Mental Status Examination (MMSE) (Taylor *et al.,* 1996). This formula is indicated in Table 11.5.

Demographic Equations

These equations use demographic variables that correlate with intelligence to predict premorbid IQ scores. Barona, Reynolds, and Chastain (1984) applied statistical regression to develop one widely used set of equations for predicting

TABLE 11.4   Modified AMNART Word List and Equation for Predicting Verbal IQ Based on AMNART Score and Education

VIQ = 118.56 − 0.88 (AMNART errors) + 0.64 (years of education)

Modified AMNART word list

ache	chassis
aisle	cellist
capon	algae
debt	superfluous
chord	chamois
heir	thyme
deny	apropos
bouquet	virulent
caprice	zealot
gauge	façade
worsted	cabal
depot	abstemious
nausea	détente
naïve	scion
subtle	papyrus
pugilist	quadruped
fetal	prelate
blatant	epitome
placebo	beatify
hiatus	hyperbole
simile	imbroglio
meringue	syncope
sieve	

Adapted from Grober & Sliwinski, 1991.

WAIS-R VIQ, PIQ, and Full-Scale IQ (FSIQ). Their equations include the demographic variables of age, sex, race, education, occupational status, urban-rural residence, and geographic region of residence.

Approaches using demographic variables to estimate premorbid ability are attractive because they do not depend on patient performance and therefore will

TABLE 11.5   Equation for Predicting Verbal IQ in Patients with Dementia, Correcting for Mental Status

Corrected premorbid VIQ = 118.56 − 0.88 (AMNART errors) + 0.64 (years of education) + 0.63 (30 − MMSE[a] score)

[a] MMSE = Mini-Mental Status Examination.
Adapted from Taylor *et al.*, 1996.

be unaffected by the presence of cognitive deficits. In the evaluation of older individuals, an attractive feature of demographic equations is that although they were originally developed for groups up to age 74, Helmes (1996) has developed modified equations to allow age coding for groups up to age 99, based on a large Canadian sample. These equations are included in Table 11.6.

There are, however, a number of limitations to estimating premorbid intelligence on the basis of demographic equations. As is common with predictive equations based on statistical regression, they tend to underestimate the abilities of above-average individuals and overestimate abilities of below-average individuals because of a statistical phenomenon known as regression toward the mean (Anastasi & Urbina, 1997). Thus, the accuracy of prediction is compromised.

TABLE 11.6 Formulas for Estimating Verbal IQ (VIQ), Performance IQ (PIQ), and Full-Scale IQ (FSIQ) Based on Demographic Variables

VIQ = 54.2 + 0.49 (age) + 1.92 (sex) + 4.24 (race) + 5.25 (education) + 1.89 (occupation) + 1.24 (region)

PIQ = 61.58 + 0.31 (age) + 1.09 (sex) + 4.95 (race) + 3.75 (education) + 1.54 (occupation) + 0.82 (region)

FSIQ = 54.96 + 0.47 (age) + 1.76 (sex) + 4.71 (race) + 5.02 (education) + 1.89 (occupation) + 0.59 (region)

Age: 1 = 16–17   9 = 70–74
2 = 18–19   10 = 75–79
3 = 20–24   11 = 80–84
4 = 25–34   12 = 85–89
5 = 35–44   13 = 90–94
6 = 45–54   14 = 95–99
7 = 55–64   15 = ≥100
8 = 65–69

Sex: 1 = female; 2 = male

Race: 3 = white; 2 = black; 1 = other

Education (years):   1 = 0–7
2 = 8
3 = 9–11
4 = 12
5 = 13–15
6 = 16+

Occupation: 6 = professional/technical
5 = managerial/office/clerical/sales
4 = skilled labor
3 = not in labor force
2 = semiskilled labor
1 = unskilled labor

Region: 2 = urban (>2500 population); 1 = rural (<2500 population)

Adapted from Helmes, 1996.

One approach that has been proposed to increase the accuracy of demographic equations is to incorporate a measure of the individual's general ability by including scores from hold tests in the equation (Krull, Scott, & Sherer, 1995; Vanderploeg, Schinka, & Axelrod, 1996). This approach has been validated in studies using WAIS-R hold tests involving predominantly younger individuals. It has the disadvantage that it requires administration of time-consuming tests, which might not otherwise be included. However, it may be useful in estimating the premorbid abilities of more severely demented patients.

Historical Data

Another approach to estimating premorbid ability involves the use of historical data about the patient. The ideal historical data are scores from intelligence or achievement tests taken when the patient was a young adult, but these are rarely available. However, data concerning the patient's history, such as the highest level of academic achievement, work history, and avocational interests can often be obtained and used in developing a clinical judgment concerning premorbid ability. Information concerning the education and occupations of the patient's children may be informative, particularly for older individuals whose educational achievement may have been limited by financial hardship or social conditions. For example, it is likely that an individual who was a successful attorney or physician has at least high average intelligence. An older African-American woman who completed the seventh grade and did domestic work but whose two children are both college professors might be predicted as having at least average intelligence. However, a weakness in using historical data to estimate premorbid intelligence is that this approach is relatively subjective, with the accuracy of the estimate depending on the quality of the clinical judgment.

GUIDELINES FOR ESTIMATING PREMORBID ABILITIES

Each of the common methods for estimating premorbid intelligence has strengths and weaknesses. One concern about all of these approaches is that they were developed and validated in comparison with previous versions of the Wechsler intelligence scales rather than with reference to the recently published WAIS-III. However, this is unlikely to significantly change their accuracy, since the IQ scores derived from the WAIS-R and the WAIS-III correlate highly and differ by an average of less than 3 points (*WAIS-III WMS-III Technical Manual,* 1997).

Rather than depending on a single approach, it is recommended that information be integrated from several of them. The following sections describe and illustrate an approach for estimating premorbid intelligence and neuropsychological abilities.

1. *Compute initial estimates of premorbid IQ.* It is recommended that two estimates of premorbid IQ be computed initially. The first can be derived from

the Helmes demographic equations with extended age coding to estimate VIQ, PIQ, and FSIQ (Table 11.6). A second estimate of VIQ can be derived from the 45-word AMNART using the Grober and Sliwinski equation (Table 11.4).

2. *Choose between the AMNART and demographic estimates of VIQ:* This choice depends on comparison between the two estimates and the patient's characteristics. For example, if the estimate of VIQ based on the demographic equation is higher than that based on the AMNART for a patient with significant dementia or language dysfunction, the demographic estimate may be more accurate. However, if the AMNART-based estimate is higher, particularly for a patient with only mild cognitive dysfunction, this estimate may be more accurate because it is less affected by regression toward the mean.

3. *Classify each estimated IQ score:* The classifications suggested by Wechsler (1981) are used to label each IQ score, as indicated in Table 11.7.

4. *Consider adjusting the IQ classifications in view of the patient's background characteristics:* In some cases, the patient's estimated IQ scores will seem discrepant with the impression of the patient gained during the clinical interview, and adjustment of the estimates may be appropriate. The most common condition for considering such adjustment is when the estimates of the patient's intellectual level are lower than is implied by the patient's behavior and the educational and occupational achievement of other family members. If the achievement of the patient's children is considerably advanced, particularly for a patient who may have had limited opportunities, this raises the possibility that demographic equations may underestimate the patient's true intellectual level. The presence of an AMNART-estimated Verbal IQ that is higher than the demographic estimate is also consistent with this possibility. For example, the opportunities available to older women and to African-Americans may have been more limited than those available to Caucasian men.

In such cases, the classifications of the IQ estimates may be modified. The most common case is when the demographic estimates fall within the average range, but the patient's behavior and family background suggest that it is appropriate to elevate these classifications to at least the high average range (see Example 2 below).

TABLE 11.7 Classifications for Estimated IQ Scores, Based on Wechsler

Score	Classification
130 and above	Very superior
120–129	Superior
110–119	High average
90–109	Average
80–89	Low average
70–79	Borderline
69 and below	Mentally retarded

Adapted from Wechsler, 1981.

5. *Determine initial predictions of average performance within each neuropsychological domain:* Within each individual, there may be characteristic variability in premorbid abilities associated with different neuropsychological domains. For example, some individuals have relatively stronger verbal than visuospatial abilities, whereas others show the opposite pattern. The identification of neuropsychological change is facilitated to the extent that the estimates of premorbid abilities reflect these individual differences in strengths and weaknesses.

It is recommended that initial prediction of verbal abilities and verbal memory be based on the estimated VIQ and that prediction of visuospatial abilities and visual memory be based on the estimated PIQ. This recommendation is based on the fact that the VIQ is more strongly correlated than the PIQ with verbal abilities and verbal memory, and the opposite is true for visuospatial abilities and visual memory (*WAIS-III WMS-III Technical Manual,* 1997). It is recommended that the estimated Full-Scale IQ be used to estimate premorbid attention and executive function.

Thus, if the classifications of the estimated Verbal, Performance and Full-Scale IQs were high average, average, and average, respectively, it would be estimated that test scores within the domains of verbal abilities and verbal memory would fall within the high average range, and test scores within the domains of visuospatial abilities, visual memory, attention, and executive functions would all fall within the average range.

6. *Consider adjusting estimates for each neuropsychological domain based on the patient's individual characteristics:* As with the estimates of premorbid IQ, it is sometimes necessary to adjust estimates of abilities for specific neuropsychological domains on the basis of other information gathered during the evaluation. The patient's history of professional and avocational activities may suggest possible neuropsychological strengths and weaknesses, which require adjustment of the premorbid estimates. For example, if the patient was successful in a profession heavily dependent on memory (e.g., law or medicine), verbal memory might be predicted as a relative strength. If a patient successfully managed both a household and a responsible professional position outside the home, executive function might represent a relative strength. If a patient was a successful painter or architect, visuospatial abilities might represent a relative strength. However, if the patient reported that he always had difficulty reading maps and frequently became lost, visuospatial abilities may represent a relative weakness.

It is best to be conservative in making decisions about neuropsychological strengths and weaknesses. Many patients will not have obvious strengths, and for these patients adjustments of the initial estimates of premorbid abilities will be unnecessary. However, when the clinical history strongly supports the presence of particular neuropsychological strengths that are not reflected in the initial premorbid estimates, it is recommended that the estimates be adjusted as follows. For neuropsychological strengths, the classification of that domain can be elevated one level. So, for example, if it is initially estimated that the patient's premorbid visuospatial abilities and visual memory fell within the average range, but the patient was successful at an occupation heavily dependent on these abilities, the premorbid estimate might be raised from average to high-average (see Example 3 below).

The following examples illustrate the recommended approach for estimating premorbid general intellectual function and abilities within specific neuropsychological domains.

EXAMPLE 1

The patient is an 80-year-old Caucasion woman with 18 years of education who formerly worked as a nurse. She lives in an urban area. Based on the Helmes' demographic equations (Table 11.6), her FSIQ, VIQ, and PIQ were estimated as 119 (high average), 120 (high average), and 114 (high average). The AMNART estimate of her Verbal IQ was 116 (high average). Based on these estimated IQ scores, it was further estimated that scores within each neuropsychological domain (attention and executive function, verbal abilities, visuospatial and visuoconstructive abilities, visual memory, verbal memory) should fall within the high average range. Adjustment of these estimates was not considered necessary based on the patient's other characteristics.

EXAMPLE 2

The patient is a 75-year-old African-American man with a 12 years of education who formerly worked as a farmer. He lives in a rural area in the southeastern United States. Based on the demographic equations, his FSIQ, VIQ, and PIQ were estimated as 97 (average), 97 (average), and 96 (average). The AMNART estimate of his VIQ was 90 (average).

However, the patient's behavior as well as background information suggested that the intellectual level of the patient and his family was somewhat higher than these estimates. During the clinical interview, the patient's speech included use of sophisticated vocabulary and logic. The patient and his wife had five children, four with college degrees, and three with advanced graduate degrees in law or social work. The patient's wife had obtained a nursing degree in middle age after raising her children.

Therefore, the classifications of the estimated FSIQ and VIQ scores were elevated to the high average range. Since neither the patient nor family members exhibited obvious strengths in visuospatial abilities, the classification of the PIQ was not changed. Abilities within the neuropsychological domains of attention, executive function, verbal abilities, and verbal memory were estimated to fall within the high average range. Visuospatial abilities and visual memory were estimated to fall within the average range.

EXAMPLE 3

The patient is a 78-year-old, Caucasian man with 16 years of education, who formerly worked as a successful architect and lives in an urban area. Based on the demographic equations, his FSIQ, VIQ, and PIQ were estimated as 120 (superior), 121 (superior) and 115 (high average). The AMNART estimate of his VIQ was also 120 (superior). Given the visuospatial demands of being a successful architect, the classification of the estimated PIQ was elevated to the superior range. Therefore, premorbid abilities within each neuropsychological domain were estimated to fall within the superior range.

INTERPRETING TEST FINDINGS

After premorbid estimates of abilities have been inferred, the next step involves assigning meaning to the test findings. Each test score is interpreted at several different levels, as indicated in Table 11.8. First, each test score is interpreted by itself, both with respect to the normative data and with respect to the patient's premorbid ability. Then the test scores are considered as a whole, to infer the profile of test scores identifying patient strengths and weaknesses. Neuropsychological profiles associated with common disorders affecting older adults have been described in Chapters 6 through 10. If the patient is being reevaluated, comparison is made between the current and previous test scores to determine if there has been significant change. An approach to each of these levels of test score interpretation is described in the following sections.

Interpreting Each Test Score

Each test score is first interpreted within the context of the normative data. For some tests, conventional labels for test scores falling within specified ranges are recommended in the test manual. However, these labels are not consistent across all tests. For example, it is recommended that a WAIS-III VIQ of 85 ($z = -1.0$) be labeled low average (*WAIS-III WMS-III Technical Manual,* 1997). In contrast, it is recommended that a WCST scaled score of 85 ($z = -1.0$) be labeled as below average (Heaton *et al.,* 1993).

This variation in labeling conventions can complicate appreciation of the overall profile of test findings and communication of test results. Therefore, it is recommended that, where possible, a uniform system be applied to labeling all scores from neuropsychological tests. A suggestion for such a classification system is indicated in Table 11.9. This system is similar to that suggested for labeling Wechsler IQ scores, with the exception that the cutoffs and labels for

---

TABLE 11.8   Levels for Interpreting Test Scores

---

1. Specific test score
   a. Relative to normative data
   b. Relative to premorbid ability
2. Profile of test scores (relative strengths and weaknesses)
3. If reevaluation, presence of change

TABLE 11.9 Labels for Classifying Specific Test Scores

Classification	z-score
Very superior	+1.66 and above
Superior	+1.3 to 1.65
High average	+0.6 to 1.3
Average	−0.6 to +0.6
Low average	−0.6 to −1.3
Borderline	−1.3 to −1.65
Impaired	−1.66 and below

extreme scores have been slightly modified. Most importantly, z-scores below −1.65 or above +1.65 (corresponding to the 5th and 95th percentiles, respectively) are used to define scores that are labeled impaired or very superior. Use of the 5th percentile cutoff for defining impairment corresponds to conventionally acceptable levels of alpha error commonly used in scientific statistical analysis. The alpha error refers to the probability of falsely rejecting the null hypothesis, the hypothesis of no difference between the obtained and hypothesized score. In clinical evaluations, using a cutoff z-score of −1.65 to define impairment means that there is less than a 5% chance that the patient's obtained test score is not significantly below the mean of the normative sample. In other words, there is less that a 5% chance that the patient will be classified as impaired when in fact he is unimpaired. This cutoff score has been recommended by others (Lezak, 1995; McKhann et al., 1984). However, some clinicians prefer to use a more conservative cutoff to define abnormality or impairment and require that performance be at least two standard deviations below the normative mean ($z = > -2.05$, 98th percentile).

Interpreting Test Scores Relative to Premorbid Ability

A second way in which each test score can be interpreted is within the context of the patient's premorbid abilities. For example, if a patient obtains a test score that is average relative to the normative population, is this score within expectation for this patient?

Obviously, if a previously well functioning patient obtains a score that is impaired relative to the normative population, this score can also be interpreted as below expectation for that patient. More difficult decisions arise when the obtained test score falls within one of the intermediate ranges relative to the normative population (e.g., borderline impaired, low average, average), particularly for patients suspected to have been relatively high functioning. In such cases, the clinician must decide to what extent an obtained score must be divergent from the premorbid estimate to be labeled below expectation.

A conservative approach would be to require a relatively large divergence between the obtained score and the premorbid estimate for the obtained score to be labeled below expectation. A less conservative approach might require that obtained scores be only slightly below the premorbid estimate. In clinical practice, the choice between these two approaches depends in large part on the consequences. The more conservative strategy will increase the probability of a *miss*, a failure to identify a patient who may have subtle abnormality. In contrast, the less conservative approach will increase the probability of a *false positive error*, incorrectly identifying a normal patient as having abnormality.

In interpreting individual test scores relative to premorbid ability, it is recommended that a less conservative approach be used, particularly when other data, such as the patient's history, strongly raise the possibility of significant change. Although the presence of a single test score that is below expectation may not be alarming, the presence of multiple scores that are below expectation strongly increases the possibility of neuropsychological dysfunction. The pattern of scores that are below expectation may contribute to diagnosis of an underlying disorder that might be missed if a more conservative approach were applied.

Therefore, it is recommended that the following classification system be used for labeling an obtained test score relative to its premorbid estimate (Table 11.10).

1. A score is interpreted as *within expectation* if its classification matches that of the premorbid estimate for that neuropsychological domain. Thus, for example, if an obtained verbal memory score falls within the high average range and the premorbid estimate for that domain is high average, then the obtained score is labeled within expectation.
2. A score is interpreted as *mildly below expectation* if its classification falls one level below that of the premorbid estimate. For example, if the obtained verbal memory score falls within the average range but the premorbid estimate is high average, the obtained score would be labeled as mildly below expectation.
3. A score is interpreted as *well below expectation* if its classification is two or more levels below that of the premorbid estimate. So, for example, if the obtained verbal memory score falls within the low average range but

TABLE 11.10   System for Interpreting Test Scores Relative to Premorbid Ability

Within expectation: Classification of the obtained score matches that of premorbid estimate.

Mildly below expectation: Classification of the obtained score is one level below the premorbid estimate.

Well below expectation: Classification of the obtained score is two or more levels below the premorbid estimate.

the premorbid estimate is high average, the obtained score would be labeled well below expectation.

This approach may be particularly helpful in detecting subtle change in individuals estimated to have premorbid abilities that were high average or greater. When such individuals experience mild but significant neuropsychological decline, their test scores may remain within the average to low average range. The interpretation of such scores as mildly or well below expectation will highlight the need for the patient to be tracked so that any further change can be detected. For example, if the retired architect described in Example 3 obtained a high average score on the WMS-III LM II, this score would be interpreted as mildly below expectation, given the premorbid estimate that verbal memory should fall within the superior range. This classification of his obtained score would increase the likelihood that he would return for reevaluation. As more effective treatments for dementing disorders, particularly Alzheimer's disease, become available, detection of subtle disease will allow these treatments to be offered earlier in the course of the disease.

When a less conservative approach is used to interpret test scores as below expectation, it is critical that the evaluation report reflect the tentativeness of such findings and the need for reevaluation to aid in their interpretation. In many cases, abnormal test findings are not surprising to the family and patient, but particularly if such abnormalities are subtle, they must be described in a manner that is not unnecessarily alarming.

Identifying the Neuropsychological Profile

Identifying the neuropsychological profile involves comparing the classifications of the obtained test scores to identify neuropsychological strengths and weaknesses. This comparison is most valid when the z-scores for each test are derived from normative data based on performance of the same sample of healthy individuals.

However, this condition is rarely achieved. Although a common normative sample is available for tests from the WAIS-III and WMS-III, normative data for other tests have been derived from different samples. As the normative samples for different tests become less comparable, the validity of directly comparing test score classifications based on z-scores becomes more problematic. However, most normative samples are relatively large, have attempted to exclude individuals with cognitive dysfunction, and have adjusted for critical variables affecting test scores, notably age. When these conditions are met, scores can be compared across tests to provide clinically useful information.

The profile of strengths and weaknesses can be identified as follows. Test scores falling within the highest classification category for that patient based on the normative data are identified as relative strengths. Those scores falling in lower classification categories are identified as relative weaknesses. This approach is illustrated in the case studies in Appendix G.

After the profile of neuropsychological strengths and weaknesses has been identified, it is compared with the neuropsychological profiles associated with common disorders affecting older adults. Disorders most consistent with the obtained profile are identified. In many cases, the neuropsychological profile will raise the possibility of a number of different disorders and, taken alone, is not strongly suggestive of a single disorder. For example, the neuropsychological profile might be consistent with a number of different disorders having what has been described as a subcortical profile, such as subtle cerebrovascular disease, Parkinson's disease, and normal pressure hydrocephalus.

However, when the details of the neuropsychological profile are considered within the context of the wealth of other data gathered during the evaluation, this often directs attention to a specific disorder as most likely. For example, if a patient with a neuropsychological profile suggestive of a subcortical disorder (Table 6.1) has experienced recent urinary incontinence and gait abnormality as well as emotional flatness, this would be more consistent with normal pressure hydrocephalus (Chapter 9). If these characteristics are absent but the patient shows impaired cognitive flexibility and self-structuring and has a history of uncontrolled hypertension or diabetes, then this would be more consistent with cerebrovascular disease than normal pressure hydrocephalus, particularly if neuroimaging has revealed lesions consistent with this disease (Chapter 7). If the patient has an abnormal gait and other movement abnormalities that have been responsive to dopaminergic medication as well as significant concern about cognitive change, this would be more consistent with Parkinson's disease (Chapter 8).

Identifying Change on Reevaluation

For patients who are being reevaluated, a critical decision is whether test scores have changed significantly since the previous evaluation. As was discussed in Chapter 3, scores observed on different testing occasions are unlikely to be identical because the observed test score reflects a combination of the true test score and error variance, the impact of randomly occurring variables. Thus, the challenge is to decide whether a discrepancy between an initial score and a reevaluation score reflects a meaningful change or just random variation.

One approach to making this decision is to determine whether the reevaluation score falls within the *confidence interval* of the initial score. This confidence interval can be calculated by using the test's standard error of measurement, a measure of random error that was described in Chapter 3. The confidence interval reflects a range of scores around the observed score that contains the true score with some known probability.

However, for many tests, the best normative data set for older adults does not provide the information necessary to compute the confidence interval. Where this is the case, it is recommended that the z-scores corresponding to the initial and reevaluation test scores be directly compared. Following logic suggested by Lezak (1995), the following rules can be applied to interpret whether there is change: if the z-score change is less than 1, this is labeled as unchanged performance; z-score changes exceeding 1 suggest possible change; and z-score changes exceeding 2 represent significant change.

12

WRITING THE
EVALUATION REPORT

The evaluation report summarizes the information gathered during the evaluation and the conclusions about the patient derived from this information. It is critical that this report be clear, well organized, readable, and relevant to the referral question. The value of even the best evaluation is lessened if the written report fails to fully address the referral question and to clearly elucidate the evaluation findings and the impression of the patient. Since the patient or his family members may read the report, it is important that the content of the report be written in a nonjudgmental and constructive fashion, particularly the descriptions of the patient's behavior and the psychologist's overall impression of him.

This chapter outlines the major features of the evaluation report. Much of the report can be generated from information included on the Neuropsychological Interview form, the Behavioral Observations form, and the Neuropsychology Data Summary Sheet (included as Appendices C through E, respectively). An outline of the evaluation report is included as Appendix F.

REPORT HEADER

The report begins with a header identifying the clinical practice within which the evaluation took place and its address. Following this, in a prominent location, is a statement indicating the confidentiality of the report. This statement reminds appropriate readers of the need to maintain the patient's confidentiality and signals others that it is inappropriate for them to continue reading the report. The next line can include a title identifying the nature of the evaluation, either an Initial Neuropsychological Evaluation or a Neuropsychological Reevaluation. This is followed by information identifying the patient, typically his name, his date of birth, his medical record number, and the date of the evaluation.

REFERRAL AND BACKGROUND INFORMATION

Referral justification: This section begins by summarizing the referral source, referral question and the reason for the evaluation. The first sentence indicates the patient's name, age, sex, and handedness and the referral source, for example: "Mr. Jones is a 65-year-old, right-handed gentleman who was referred by Jane Gray, M.D."

Next, the justification for the referral is summarized. If the patient has previously being diagnosed with a major medical or neurologic condition associated with neurobehavioral change, this can be indicated in the justification, as well as alternative conditions that are being considered. In some cases, reimbursement may depend on adequate justification for the evaluation, and the psychologist may gradually become familiar with critical words or phrases required by different reimbursement agencies. In many cases, justification of the evaluation in terms of its contribution to diagnosis and treatment planning is sufficient, for example:

> Mr. Jones has a 5-year history of Parkinson's disease (or Alzheimer's disease, cerebrovascular disease, etc.) and was referred for neuropsychological evaluation to help determine the etiology of recent behavioral change (or memory change, hallucinations, etc.) and to contribute to diagnosis and treatment planning.

Description of symptoms: The next several paragraphs summarize the information gathered during the clinical interview and the review of medical records to describe the symptoms of concern and their course. This summary includes the nature of cognitive, behavioral, affective, psychotic, motor, and other symptoms; when they were initially observed; their course, progression, and responsiveness to treatments that have been offered; and their possible relationship to other significant variables, such as personal losses or medical illnesses.

Medical history: Next, the patient's medical history is summarized, highlighting conditions that may be related to current or past neurobehavioral change. The patient's current medication regimen is detailed. Relevant family medical history is described, particularly of disorders associated with neurobehavioral disease.

Social and educational history: The patient's education and occupational history are described. If the patient is retired, the date of and reasons for retirement are important to mention. The patient's current living and support system are outlined, including where he lives and the availability of other support, such as adult children living nearby or a religious organization or other social networks. The patient's characteristic interests and hobbies can be indicated.

BEHAVIORAL OBSERVATIONS

The patient's behavior during the clinical interview and formal testing are described.

TESTS ADMINISTERED

This section includes a listing of the tests administered during the evaluation. For some health care providers, additional information may be required to facilitate reimbursement, such as the time required per test, including the total time necessary for test administration, scoring, and interpretation. On a separate line, the names of the examiners, often the psychologist and a technician, may be indicated.

TEST RESULTS

The description of the test results is organized by neuropsychological domain: general intellectual function, attention, executive function, motor behavior, verbal abilities, visuospatial and visuoconstructive abilities, memory, and affect/personality. The interpretation of each test score is reported, relative both to appropriate normative data and to expectations for that patient. Statements such as the following may be made:

> Naming of pictured items was within the low-average range but only mildly below expectation.
> On a test of verbal memory for structured material in the form of stories, immediate recall was in the high-average range and within expectation.

IMPRESSIONS AND RECOMMENDATIONS

This section can begin with a restatement of the reasons for the evaluation. Next, a description of findings relevant to the referral question is provided. Often, this includes a summary of the neuropsychological profile, indicating relative strengths and weaknesses in neuropsychological domains as well in specific abilities within a domain, for example:

Mr. Jones exhibited a relative strength in attention and executive function and a relative weakness in memory and verbal abilities. He exhibited impaired ability to initially acquire new information in memory although ability to store that information over a time delay was stronger. Within the verbal domain, naming was within expectation but letter fluency was impaired.

Conclusions with regard to the referral question are next indicated. If a diagnostic issue was important, the impression regarding disorders associated with the observed changes is indicated. It is not uncommon to mention a number of different possibilities suggested by the test findings and the patient's history. An opinion concerning the most likely underlying disorder may be offered, highlighting data supporting this choice. Follow-up procedures that might provide confirmatory information and exclude other possibilities may be suggested.

It is often useful to offer an opinion regarding the adequacy of the patient's current level of support and the need for additional support. The impression of the patient's competence for performing important functions such as cooking, driving, and financial management might be suggested. The method for providing feedback to the patient and appropriate family members and the nature of any follow-up services to be provided by the psychologist might be indicated. Recommendations for other types of evaluations or services may be offered. The need for neuropsychological reevaluation may be indicated, with a suggestion as to when this might be useful.

The report ends with the psychologist's signature and the names and addresses of the persons who will receive copies of the report.

13

PROVIDING FEEDBACK AND PLANNING FOLLOW-UP SERVICES

This chapter discusses the final stage of the neuropsychological evaluation, the provision of feedback to the patient and others concerning the findings of the evaluation and the planning of treatment interventions and follow-up services. In some ways, this phase is one of the most challenging aspects of the evaluation. A number of important goals must be accomplished, usually in a limited amount of time. A successful session requires not only that the psychologist apply expertise in neuropsychology but also more general clinical skills, often including methods derived from individual and family psychotherapy. The feedback session may be emotionally charged, and the psychologist may find it necessary to manage not only the emotional responses of the patient and others but also her own reactions to the issues facing them.

The following common objectives of the feedback session are discussed in this chapter:

1. To describe the patient's neuropsychological strengths and weaknesses and the relation of these to the neuropsychological, personality, and other behavioral changes that have been observed
2. To provide information concerning the reason for the changes
3. To discuss treatment and support interventions that may relieve the symptoms of concern and contribute to the patient's independence, safety, and comfort

4. To identify psychological issues affecting both the patient and others that may be exacerbated by or emerge from the patient's illness and to plan interventions for relieving these.

ORGANIZING THE FEEDBACK SESSION

During the clinical interview, the psychologist describes approaches to providing feedback on the findings of the evaluation. In most cases, the feedback is provided by the neuropsychologist during a follow-up session occurring several weeks after the evaluation has been conducted. Ideally, this occurs after the evaluation report has been written, since this report includes the formal record of the outcomes of the evaluation. Holding the feedback session before the report is completed has the potential of creating confusion if the feedback that is provided is somewhat different from what the psychologist ultimately decides to include in the report.

It is recommended that the patient attend the feedback session accompanied by significant persons in his support system. This typically includes family members but may also involve close friends or companions. It is important that the feedback session include those who attended the initial evaluation and that patients with significant neuropsychological dysfunction, particularly memory dysfunction, be accompanied by another person whose memory is intact. It is least desirable if the patient is accompanied by a set of individuals entirely different from those who attended the clinical interview. When this occurs, the perception and account of the patient's history or difficulties may differ from those previously described, sometimes resulting in confusion. If major members of the patient's support system are present, this allows the opportunity for the psychologist to help resolve any differences of opinion, to address individual questions, and to facilitate the interaction between the patient and the family. From a practical point of view, meeting with the patient and all critical family members or close companions at once may avoid the need for additional meetings and phone conversations with those who did not attend the feedback session.

Occasionally, the feedback session will be disrupted by distressed, agitated, or argumentative behavior by one individual, most often the patient, but occasionally an accompanying family member. Such behavior may signal that this individual is already feeling overwhelmed by the feedback that has been provided. In such cases, it may be appropriate to separate the disruptive individual from the rest of the family. The disruptive person can be taken to a separate room, where the psychologist tries to identify and address the reason for the disruption and completes the feedback to him. This often can be accomplished relatively quickly, and then feedback can be completed with the others. Possible reasons for the disruptive behavior can be discussed, including approaches to addressing that individual's concerns and relieving this behavior in the future.

In some cases, however, it may be appropriate for feedback on the neuropsychological findings to be presented by another professional, most often a person who initially referred the patient for evaluation and who is experienced with neurobehavioral disorders. This often occurs when the referral source is a physician (typically an internist, neurologist, or psychiatrist), the neuropsychological evaluation is one of a set of diagnostic tests that have been ordered (perhaps including laboratory tests or a brain scan), and the patient lives at a considerable distance from the evaluation site. In such cases, the physician may present the results of the neuropsychological evaluation within the context of the overall test findings and the diagnosis and treatment plan that have emerged.

If the patient chooses to receive feedback from another qualified professional, it is particularly important that the psychologist clearly communicate the neuropsychological findings to that professional. Ideally, the physician should have a copy of the final report, and the psychologist may also want to speak with the physician about other issues not mentioned in the report that may have an impact on the feedback session, such as variables affecting the patient's support system. If feedback is provided by another professional, the patient can be encouraged to contact the psychologist later if he would like additional information concerning the findings of the neuropsychological evaluation.

CLINICAL CONSIDERATIONS IMPORTANT TO PROVIDING FEEDBACK

The psychologist's clinical skills play a critical role in the success of the feedback session. Although the psychologist leads the session, it should be interactive such that the patient and family feel comfortable responding to the psychologist's comments, asking questions, and voicing their concerns. Although rapport may have been established during the evaluation session, it is important to reinforce the connection with the patient and those accompanying him. As during the evaluation session, it is important to maintain an alliance with the patient. However, for patients who have been determined to have significant dementia and require the support of others, the psychologist's rapport with the family becomes critical, including establishing rapport with individuals who did not attend the initial evaluation. For the patient's best interests to be served, the patient and members of his support system must be trusting of and confident in the psychologist.

Careful listening and checking are important to ensure that the information is being presented in a manner that those attending the feedback session are able to understand and accept. In many cases, the language of neuropsychological reports will not be well understood by nonprofessionals. The test findings may be better understood if the psychologist explains them in terms of the questions that initially motivated the evaluation and their implications for resolving problems associated with changes in the patient's behavior. So, for example, if the patient was initially referred for evaluation of forgetfulness but the test findings indicate that attentional dysfunction plays a major role in this behavior, this can be explained together with possible strategies for improving attention. The psychologist should be alert to verbal and nonverbal signs indicating that the feedback is being understood and may even want to check this understanding by asking questions such as, "To make sure that I've explained what I meant to say, would you like to summarize your understanding of what I've described?"

The psychologist must also be sensitive to the kind and amount of information the patient and family are ready and able to hear and their reaction to this. In many cases, they may be prepared to hear a circumscribed set of information, for example, a description of the neuropsychological weaknesses that may help explain unusual behaviors and likely reasons for the change. The patient and family often feel relieved when they are able to better understand the nature and reasons for these changes because this information returns to them some control over a previously confusing situation, allowing better care of the patient and planning for the immediate future. Ideally, the feedback session should allow the patient and family to feel better informed and able to deal with future challenges.

However, some patients and families are not prepared to hear details of how a dementing illness is likely to progress over time such that the patient ultimately becomes both mentally and physically incompetent. When the diagnosis is Alzheimer's disease, some families prefer to obtain precise information about the effectiveness (or limited effectiveness) of current medication treatments, whereas others prefer to receive less detailed information about this. It is critical that the feedback not be presented in a manner that leaves the family and patient feeling hopeless, overwhelmed, and powerless.

One way of gauging what those attending the feedback session are able and ready to hear is to begin the session by summarizing the purpose for the evaluation and its goals. The patient and/or family can be queried concerning what they hoped to learn from the evaluation and how that would help them. If there are several persons attending the session in addition to the patient, each can be queried separately so that all agendas are considered. However, if the patient's needs are significantly different from those of the family, the psychologist must remember that the patient's stated needs are primary, except perhaps for cases in which it has been determined that these needs may not serve his best interests, as may occur when the patient has a significant degree of dementia. In addition to helping the psychologist determine what feedback is provided, this initial questioning draws the patient and family into the session and encourages a more interactive process throughout the session.

As Knight (1994, 1996) has discussed, the success of the feedback session may be affected by the psychologist's personal characteristics and concerns. Some psychologists find it difficult to provide feedback on the outcomes of neuropsychological evaluation because this often involves discussion of decline in the patient's functioning for reasons that are not totally clear. The psychologist may feel that she is perceived as the bearer of bad news, a difficult role to assume.

Furthermore, although the evaluation may determine that a significant decline has occurred, the psychologist may anticipate that the family expected to hear a more definitive diagnosis for these changes than can in fact be provided. The inability to provide a definitive diagnosis may make some psychologists vulnerable to feeling less competent. These feelings on the psychologist's part may make it more difficult to plan and lead an effective feedback session.

However, it is important to remember that while the patient's deficits are discussed during the feedback session, description of the patient's strengths may empower the patient and family to be more effective in managing what may have been a previously distressing and confusing situation, which they were unsure how to improve. In many cases, when detailing the patient's deficits, the psychologist confirms what the patient and family have already suspected, that there has been behavioral change. However, it is often the case that the psychologist can also clarify specific neuropsychological strengths and explain that deficits are not pervasive. This information may be comforting to the family and to the patient. The patient and family also often suspect that a disease process is involved, and they may welcome any information concerning the possible nature of that disease. The planning of treatment and support interventions during the feedback session empowers the patient and family to move forward and to begin making plans for the future.

The psychologist's success in leading a feedback session may also be affected by her own personal reactions to the patient's condition. Evaluating and providing feedback to an older patient often heightens the psychologist's awareness of negative aspects of the aging process, including the possibility of developing dementia. For older neuropsychologists, these evaluations may exacerbate their own personal concerns about the changes in physical and psychological abilities associated with aging and their own possible need for support in the future. The psychologist's ability to provide feedback in a constructive and caring manner may also be compromised if the psychologist strongly identifies the patient with someone she personally cares about, such as an aging parent or other relative. The delivery of feedback concerning the patient's cognitive decline may heighten her concerns about what the future holds for this relative as well as the help he or she may require and how that will be provided. If the psychologist has such reactions, she may develop an unconstructive emotional involvement in the patient's case, and this involvement may become particularly apparent during the feedback session, which is often less structured than the clinical interview or the formal testing. The psychologist may find it necessary to expend considerable internal resources trying to manage her own personal feelings. It often becomes more difficult to maintain the professional perspective necessary to attend to the patient and family's reactions and needs and to facilitate their interaction and planning. Therefore, it is important for the psychologist to be aware of her personal feelings and reactions throughout the evaluation process and to seek appropriate supervision or counseling if this is needed.

DESCRIBING NEUROPSYCHOLOGICAL STRENGTHS AND WEAKNESSES AND REASONS FOR CHANGE

A major purpose of most neuropsychological evaluations is to quantify the nature of strengths and weaknesses in attention, executive function, verbal abilities, visuospatial abilities, and memory. During the feedback session, the psychologist clarifies the relative integrity of different neuropsychological domains, mentioning not only relative weaknesses but also relative strengths. She describes the relationship of these strengths and weaknesses to the patient's behavioral changes. For example, if the patient repeats questions that have already been answered or manages his medication regimen unreliably, these behaviors may be explained if the patient has significant memory dysfunction. The irresponsible use of money and other unwise behaviors may be explained in terms of a deficit in executive function. It is common for families to become concerned when the patient exhibits decreased activity, such as a lack of interest in previously enjoyable hobbies, and it is often important to clarify to what extent this change may reflect a deficit in executive function (e.g., inability to initiate behavior) as compared to the onset of depression.

When describing dysfunction within a neuropsychological domain, it may be important to clarify the nature and severity of the dysfunction, particularly if this has practical implications for improving the patient's functioning and comfort. It is usually not sufficient to simply say that memory or visuospatial function is impaired. Description of the nature and severity of the dysfunction within a neuropsychological domain often has implications for understanding the patient's behavior and for possible compensatory aids. Elucidation of the difference between long- and short-term memory is often helpful in explaining why the patient can remember distant personal history but cannot remember the responses to his own questions or keep track of the date. It is often important to explain whether memory dysfunction primarily reflects a deficit in the initial acquisition of new information in memory or the retrieval of that information, as compared to a major deficit in memory storage. In the former case, characteristic of subcortical disorders such as Parkinson's disease, the use of structure, cuing, and repetition at the time of memory acquisition may facilitate remembering. In the latter case, more typical of cortical disorders such as Alzheimer's disease, these aids may have little benefit.

However, even when a storage deficit is prominent in memory dysfunction, description of the severity of this deficit may be helpful. The functioning of patients with a milder storage deficit may be improved if they can remember to record important information in a single small notebook that they carry with them at all times in the same location, for example, in a pocket or a handbag. For patients with a more severe storage deficit, it may be necessary to share important information with other family members since the patient may be unable to recall whether or where this information has been recorded.

Most patients and their families also want to gain some idea about the likely cause of the behavioral change. The psychologist can provide feedback concerning the possible diagnoses, the relative certainty of the different alternatives, and additional information that would be useful in finalizing the diagnosis. For example, when family members are told that the patient's memory dysfunction may reflect Alzheimer's disease, they may want to know how this disease is definitively diagnosed and that additional memory decline in the absence of other illness increases the likelihood that the patient has the disease. The patient and/or family may request information concerning reading materials or support services that provide additional descriptions of the disease, and the psychologist should be prepared to provide these resources. However, as was noted earlier, the psychologist must be sensitive to the family's needs and capacity for information so as not to overwhelm them.

DISCUSSING TREATMENT ALTERNATIVES, PATIENT CARE, AND FOLLOW-UP SERVICES

After the nature and possible reasons for neuropsychological change have been discussed, treatment alternatives and follow-up services can be planned. For patients diagnosed with possible or probable Alzheimer's disease, medication and other treatments (e.g., Vitamin E therapy) can be discussed in general terms. Patients who are interested in medications can be referred to a physician experienced in administering these treatments. The possibility that rehabilitation programs may improve functioning can be discussed, particularly for patients with focal deficits without widespread neuropsychological dysfunction. Some patients, particularly those with mild cognitive dysfunction accompanied by depression or anxiety, may benefit from some form of psychotherapy or medication. A behavior management program may be helpful in encouraging agitated or aggressive patients to reduce the frequency of these behaviors. If the neuropsychologist is not able to provide these services, the patient can be referred to another professional.

One issue that often arises is the implication of the neuropsychological findings for the quality of the patient's everyday functioning and for his competence to continue assuming positions of responsibility. Neuropsychological test findings have limited value for predicting the quality of everyday functioning (Dunn, Searight, Grisso, Margolis, & Gibbons, 1990; Heaton & Pendleton, 1981). Other instruments are available for assessing both activities of daily living and instrumental activities of daily living (Fillenbaum & Smyer, 1981; Katz, Ford, Moskowitz, Jackson, & Jaffee, 1963; Lawton, 1971; Lawton, Moss, Fulcomer, & Kleban, 1982; Loewenstein *et al.,* 1981).

However, the neuropsychological findings as well as a review of the patient's recent behaviors may be helpful in inferring the patient's competence for assuming specific responsibilities, such as driving a car, managing financial assets, controlling a firearm, following a medication regimen, maintaining adequate nutrition and personal hygiene, caring for grandchildren, or using a stove. Errors in handling these responsibilities may have grave implications not only for the comfort and health of the patient but also for the safety of others. Because they care about the patient and want to plan for his future well-being, it is not uncommon for family members to suggest that it is necessary to relieve the patient of all responsibilities. This is often an overreaction, except in the case of a patient who has been determined to have a severe and global dementia. The psychologist may play an important role in helping the patient and his family determine how a balance can be maintained between allowing the patient to remain independent as long as possible and preventing him from endangering himself or others.

In most cases, the patient's competence to handle each responsibility should be considered separately, with the exception of patients who have been determined to be severely and globally demented. Most patients are able to continue to handle some responsibilities but are better relieved of others. The neuropsychological test findings may be somewhat helpful in inferring the nature of responsibilities in which errors are likely and those which the patient can continue to perform adequately. For example, a patient with an amnestic syndrome is likely to have difficulty performing responsibilities dependent on consideration of new information, such as the management of investments. However, this patient may still be competent to handle responsibilities dependent on overlearned skills, such as driving on limited and familiar routes. Consideration of the patient's recent functioning may be helpful. A history of previous mistakes within a specific area of responsibility is often predictive that future errors are likely to occur, particularly for patients diagnosed with dementia. So, for example, if an amnestic patient has already caused minor automobile accidents or has become lost while driving, it is probably unwise for him to continue driving.

In some cases, a formal competency evaluation may be necessary, particularly if the patient disagrees with the family concerning his ability to continue assuming a particular responsibility. Grisso (1994) discusses issues related to the evaluation of competence, including the need to determine the type of competence to be assessed, the nature of state regulations, and the use of evaluation instruments specific to different aspects of competence. Competency evaluations are often needed when the patient disagrees with his family about his continued ability to manage his own financial and legal affairs or to drive.

Decisions concerning the continued competence to drive are often particularly complex and emotional. In our car-oriented society, the implications of taking away the car and car keys cannot be underestimated. Patients who can no longer drive may also become unable to independently perform important activities such as grocery shopping, attending doctor's appointments, and participating in social activities. These changes may represent a major blow to the patient's self-esteem and sense of efficacy. On the other hand, unsafe use of a car can easily cause serious injury or even death.

Although older individuals with cognitive dysfunction or dementia are at increased risk for driving poorly and having accidents (Friedland *et al.,* 1988; Hunt *et al.,* 1997; Lucas-Blaustein, Filipp, Dungan, & Tune, 1988), a diagnosis of dementia does not necessarily imply that the patient should stop all driving. Some patients with very mild or mild dementia may continue to drive safely (Hunt, Morris, Edwards, & Wilson, 1993; Hunt *et al.,* 1997; Kapust & Weintraub, 1992; Trobe, Waller, Cook-Flannagan, Teshima, & Bieliauskas, 1996), particularly if they reduce the extent of their driving and confine themselves to familiar, low-traffic routes. However, as the severity of cognitive dysfunction or dementia increases, the patient is at increased risk for poor driving performance and accidents (Hunt *et al.,* 1993; Hunt *et al.,* 1997; Stutts, Stewart, & Martell, 1998; Tuokko, Tallman, Beattie, Cooper, & Weir, 1995b). An international consensus conference has recommended that patients with moderate to severe dementia not be allowed to drive (Johansson & Lundberg, 1997).

Variables that may be useful in evaluating the patient's driving safety include recent driving history, certain neuropsychological findings, and the presence of movement disorder (Logsdon, Teri, & Larson, 1992). A recent history of driving accidents or near accidents, episodes of getting lost while driving, or poor judgment may be predictive of unsafe driving in the future. Patients with deficits in attention (particularly visual attention), in visuospatial and visuoconstructive abilities, or in mental speed are at increased risk for automobile accidents (Fox, Bowden, Bashford, & Smith, 1997; Hunt *et al.,* 1993; Logsdon *et al.,* 1992; Lundberg, Hakamies-Blomqvist, Almkvist, & Johansson, 1998; Owsley, Ball, Sloane, Roenker, & Bruni, 1991; Parasuraman & Nestor, 1991, 1993). Patients with movement disorders, such as Huntington's or Parkinson's disease, are also more likely to drive poorly (Heikkila, Turkka, Korpelainen, Kallanranta, & Summala, 1998; Rebok, Bylsma, Keyl, Brandt, & Folstein, 1995). In some cases, the administration of a formal driving test, available in some medical centers, may be useful in clarifying the patient's continued ability to drive. Even when it is determined that it is likely to be safe for the patient to continue to drive, it is important that his driving be monitored carefully and that reassessment occur on a regular basis, particularly if there is evidence of increased cognitive dysfunction.

Another major decision that may be addressed during the feedback session involves the patient's continued ability to remain in his current living environment. It is important not to make assumptions about the patient's willingness to consider a change. On the one hand, some patients who have been living in their own homes may already be feeling overwhelmed by this responsibility. They may be relieved by the prospect of moving into an environment that provides more support, such as a retirement or assisted living community or personal care home. However, other patients find it emotionally traumatic to consider moving into an unfamiliar setting. For some, this possibility heightens awareness that they are approaching the last phase of their life and is perceived as involving difficult choices between many treasured possessions and abandoning rooms filled with happy memories in order to live in a smaller, unfamiliar space. Adjustment to a new environment may be particularly confusing for a patient with mild dementia. The manner in which the patient has reacted to change in the past may be predictive of how well he will like a new living environment. Individuals who have always been flexible and made friends easily are more likely to adapt well to future change.

If it is determined that the patient needs additional support and structure but would prefer not to move, approaches to strengthening his support system can be considered. If the support system consists of several individuals, they may benefit from counseling to help determine how different responsibilities in supporting the patient will be distributed. For example, if the patient is no longer able to drive, a schedule for taking him to the grocery store or providing groceries can be devised. Other social services, such as senior day care or services providing food, can also be discussed, and a referral to a social worker familiar with the community's social service resources may be helpful. Ways of restructuring the patient's environment to help maintain his independence can be considered. For example, a patient may be able to continue controlling even a complex medication regimen if a family member organizes the medications and places them in labeled pill boxes clearly indicating what should be taken and when. A patient may be able to keep better track of his own appointments and social engagements if a family member helps him record them on a large calendar displayed in a prominent location. A patient who has caused fires while cooking may be able to continue cooking if he can remember to always use a loud timer or to rely on his microwave oven. Alternately, community resources for providing meals can be considered. For patients requiring considerable care at home, health insurance coverage for such care can be considered. For example, some insurance plans provide in-home nursing care to assist with performance of activities of daily living such as dressing and bathing.

ADDRESSING INTERPERSONAL AND FAMILY SYSTEM ISSUES

Although neuropsychological evaluation focuses on the evaluation and treatment of an individual patient, family system and interpersonal issues often emerge during the feedback session. The patient usually functions as a member of a system including family members, often a spouse and adult children, as well as other individuals, such as close friends or a companion. The qualities of the interactions between the persons attending the feedback session, as well as the roles that each has historically assumed, may be important factors in determining the dynamics and outcome of the session. Knight (1994, 1996) provides discussions of how family system issues may impact the feedback session.

Decline in the neuropsychological functioning of an elder member of the family may have implications for the roles and responsibilities of each member of the family system. If an elderly parent who develops dementia has played a major role in nurturing and counseling the rest of the family, perceptions of his decreased ability to perform these roles may cause a shift in the roles of other family members. Family members who have been emotionally dependent on the patient may experience a major psychological crisis and may require treatment themselves. In some cases, the family overreacts to the patient's illness and begins to make sudden, drastic changes in family roles, when this may not yet be necessary or appropriate. During the feedback session, it is important that the psychologist reinforce the family's perception of the patient as a family member with an illness, who can still assume important roles and responsibilities within the family.

If the patient needs support and structure, the process of deciding how this will be provided may highlight the nature of interactions between other family members. Discussion of how these responsibilities will be handled may revive long-standing or unspoken conflicts. Alliances and tensions between sibling pairs may be exacerbated. Where necessary, the need for family counseling may be suggested.

In many cases, the major responsibility for supporting the patient appears to fall on a single individual, often a spouse or an adult daughter. The patient's primary caregiver may become depressed or overwhelmed when confronted with knowledge of the patient's illness, and the psychologist may offer to meet with the caregiver separately to discuss his or her needs. Brief self-report instruments such as the Zarit Burden Inventory (Zarit, Reever, & Back-Peterson, 1980; Zarit, Tood, & Zarit, 1986) or the Brief Symptom Inventory (Derogatis & Spencer, 1982) may be helpful in assessing the nature and severity of caregiver distress. In their concern for caring for a family member, some caregivers neglect their own well-being, failing to maintain adequate levels of sleep, nutrition, and social activity. They may fail to appreciate that they will be better able to offer support for a longer period of time if they also continue caring for themselves.

Primary caregivers may benefit from an opportunity to talk frankly about their feelings concerning the patient's illness, to discuss better approaches for coping with these feelings, and to consider additional sources of support for the patient. If the primary caregiver is a spouse, the extent to which adult children can provide some support can be discussed. It is often the case that the patient's spouse has not revealed the need for additional support to adult children because of the fear of burdening them, when in fact the children are very willing to provide some help. Some caregivers benefit from support groups that allow them to share their emotional responses with other caregivers and to work together to develop strategies for dealing with common issues and problems. It should be noted, however, that support groups are not necessarily helpful to all caregivers. For caregivers of patients with mild to moderate cognitive dysfunction, support group discussions of the problems associated with more severe disease may be depressing rather than supportive.

APPENDIX **A**

PREEVALUATION LETTER

(office address)
(date of letter)

(patient's name and address)

Dear (patient's name),

Dr./Ms./Mr. (name of referring professional) has referred you for neuropsychological evaluation. We have scheduled you to see Dr. (clinician's name) on (date) at (time). The evaluation will take place at (location), and we have enclosed a map indicating the exact location of our office. The neuropsychological evaluation will include a background interview as well as a series of pencil and paper tests and activities. Many individuals find the evaluation process pleasant and interesting. The evaluation may take several hours, and you will be given short rest breaks as needed.

We have developed a list of things that you can do to make the evaluation more efficient and useful in supporting your health:

1. Please try to arrive well rested and well fed. You may want to bring a snack if your appointment runs through the lunch hour.

2. Please bring a list of prescription medications that you are currently taking.
3. Please bring any eyeglasses or hearing aids that you may use.
4. We recommend that you attend the evaluation with a close family member or friend who can provide another perspective on your concerns and background history.
5. Please review your health insurance coverage for neuropsychological evaluation so that you understand your possible financial responsibilities in paying for the evaluation. If you have Medicare, this currently covers a large portion of the evaluation costs.
6. Please look over the enclosed Informed Consent form, which we will ask you to sign. Your signature gives us your permission to perform the evaluation, to discuss your case with other professionals involved in your care, and to release the evaluation report to your health insurance company, if they request this in order to pay for services. The form indicates the approximate cost of the evaluation and your financial responsibility for it.

If you are unable to attend your appointment, we would greatly appreciate being notified at least 48 hours in advance.

We look forward to meeting you. If we can be of further assistance, please feel free to contact us.

Sincerely,
(neuropsychologist's name and title)

INFORMED CONSENT FOR NEUROPSYCHOLOGICAL EVALUATION

You have been scheduled for a neuropsychological evaluation with_____. This evaluation typically includes a clinical interview during which your history is reviewed and formal tests of memory, concentration, and other abilities. Your previous medical records will also be reviewed. The nature and length of the formal testing will depend on the nature of your concerns and difficulties.

You or your guardian will be responsible for the costs of the services provided. The cost of neuropsychological testing, scoring of data, and report preparation is_____ per hour, and the total cost of the evaluation is likely to range between_____ and_____. These costs will apply except in cases where other fees have been previously negotiated with health care providers, such as health maintenance organizations (HMOs) or other managed care providers. We do (or do not) accept reimbursement directly from Medicare. Payment is required at the time of service unless other arrangements have been made.

The results of the evaluation are considered confidential and cannot be released without your permission. Your signature below gives us permission to release the evaluation findings to other professionals that you designate as involved in your care, to specified family members, and to your health insurance provider, if it requires this for reimbursement. Records may be released without your permission if so ordered by the courts. If you were referred by an attorney or by a workers' compensation carrier, the evaluation findings will be released to that person or company.

I have read the information above and consent to receive neuropsychological evaluation. I give permission for the individuals listed below to receive the results of the evaluation.

_____   _____

Patient signature   Date

_____   _____

Signature of family member or guardian   Date

Individuals to
receive results: Name   Address   Phone

_____

_____

_____

NEUROPSYCHOLOGICAL INTERVIEW

Patient name: Referral source:
Medical Record #:   DOB: Age:
DOE: Handedness:
Vision: (glasses?)   Hearing: (aid?)
Accompanying person:
I. Concerns motivating evaluation
General inquiry (symptoms, duration, antecedents)

Specific inquiry (description, duration, antecedents)

1. Attention
2. Judgment/decision making
3. Verbal abilities

   4. Driving, sense of direction
   5. Memory: recent, remote
   6. Personality change
   7. Psychiatric symptoms (hallucinations, depression, anxiety)
   8. Other neurologic and/or medical symptoms:

II. Medical history (for each endorsed, description and duration)

   1. Head injury
   2. Strokes
   3. Hyper- or hypotension
   4. Diabetes
   5. Cancer
   6. Seizure disorder
   7. Huntington's disease
   8. Parkinson's disease
   9. Amyotrophic lateral sclerosis (Lou Gehrig's disease)
  10. Multiple sclerosis
  11. Alzheimer's disease (or senility)
  12. Substance use: tobacco, alcohol
  13. Psychiatric history
  14. Current medications:
  15. CT/MRI findings
  16. Other laboratory test findings
  17. Family history of disease

III. Educational, occupational, and family history

   1. Education and work history
   2. Marriages, current spouse, children
   3. Hobbies, social activities
   4. Current living/support system

Behavioral observations:

Neuropsychological Evaluation of the Older Adult: A Clinician's Guidebook
Copyright © 2000 by Academic Press. All rights of reproduction in any form reserved.

BEHAVIORAL OBSERVATIONS

Patient name: **Observer:**   **Date:**

Answer each question yes/no. Elaborate and provide specific examples when possible.

Appearance:
    Weight: over/under/normal
    Age-appropriate
    Neat, clean

General Behavior:
    Alert
    Cooperative
    Able to concentrate
    Able to exert appropriate effort
    Able to establish set
    Able to maintain set
    Slow response rate
    Impulsive
    Inconsistent
    Perseverative

Language:
Adequate auditory acuity
Adequate speech comprehension
Halting speech
Adequate speech prosody
Dysnomic speech
Circumlocutory or tangential responses

Affect:
Appropriately variable
Exhibited sense of humor
Able to establish rapport
Anxious
Tense body posture
Sad
Euphoric
Crying spells
Irritable
Restless, agitated
Aware of deficits
Concerned about deficits

Motor Behavior:
Tremorous
Slow
Stiff
Masked facial expression
Speech abnormality (dysarthyric, hypophonic)

Other Impressions:

NEUROPSYCHOLOGY DATA SUMMARY SHEET

Patient: _____ DOB: _____ Age: _____ Sex: _____

Race: _____ Yrs Educ: _____ Occup: _____ Region: _____

Hand: _____ Audition: good/marginal/poor   Hearing aid: Y/N/didn't bring

DOE: _____ Vision: good/marginal/poor   Acuity = / Glasses: Y/N/didn't bring

Examiners:

GENERAL INTELLECTUAL FUNCTION

WAIS version =   WMS version =

	Obtained	Obtained z	Premorbid	Premorbid z	Interpret. (Norms/Pt)	Comments
FSIQ	_____	_____	Demo=_____	_____	/	
VIQ	_____	_____	Demo=_____	_____	/	
	_____	_____	AMNART=_____	_____	/	
PIQ	_____	_____	Demo=_____	_____	/	
					/	
VC Index	_____	_____	_____	_____	/	
PO Index	_____	_____	_____	_____	/	
DRS Total	_____	_____	_____	_____	/	
DRS Attention	_____					
DRS I and P	_____					
DRS Construction	_____					
DRS Concept	_____					
DRS Memory	_____					

ATTENTION:

	Raw score	Norm (%, T Age SS, SS, z)	z score	Interpret. (Norms/Pt)	Comments
WMS Mental Control	_____	_____	_____	/ _____	
Digit span total	_____	_____	_____	/ _____	
Forward span	_____	_____	_____	/ _____	
Backward span	_____	_____	_____	/ _____	
Arithmetic	_____	_____	_____	/ _____	
Other tests:	_____	_____	_____	/ _____	
	_____	_____	_____	/ _____	
	_____	_____	_____	/ _____	

EXECUTIVE FUNCTION:

Trails

	Raw score	Norm	z score	Interpret.
Part A #errs=	_____	_____	_____	/ _____
Part B #errs=	_____	_____	_____	/ _____
WCST #decks=	_____	_____	_____	/ _____
# cats	_____	_____	_____	/ _____
# loss of set	_____	_____	_____	/ _____
# errors	_____	_____	_____	/ _____
# PSV errors	_____	_____	_____	/ _____
WAIS Similarities	_____	_____	_____	/ _____
Other tests:	_____	_____	_____	/ _____
	_____	_____	_____	/ _____
	_____	_____	_____	/ _____

MOTOR ABILITIES:

		Raw score	Norm	z score	Interpret.
Tapping	right	_____	_____	_____	/ _____
	left	_____	_____	_____	/ _____
Pegboard	right	_____	_____	_____	/ _____
	left	_____	_____	_____	/ _____
Other Tests:		_____	_____	_____	/ _____
		_____	_____	_____	/ _____
		_____	_____	_____	/ _____

VERBAL ABILITIES:

	Raw score	Norm (%, T Age SS, SS, z)	z score	Interpret. (Norms/Pt)	Comments
Boston Naming Test	_____	_____	_____	___/___	
Letter Fluency	_____	_____	_____	___/___	
Category Fluency	_____	_____	_____	___/___	
WAIS Vocabulary	_____	_____	_____	___/___	
WAIS Comprehension	_____	_____	_____	___/___	
Other Tests:	_____	_____	_____	___/___	
	_____	_____	_____	___/___	
	_____	_____	_____	___/___	

VISUOSPATIAL/VISUOCONSTRUCTIVE ABILITIES:

DRS: letter scanning= ___/11 design matching= ___/4

DRS: ramparts: _0 or 1_ embedded design: _0 or 1_

Clock Drawing	Spont.	Comments	Copy	Comments
Circle	_____		_____	
Numbers	_____		_____	
Time setting	_____		_____	
Time memory	_____		_____	
Total	_____		_____	

	Raw score	Norm (%, T Age SS, SS, z)	z score	Interpret. (Norms/Pt)	Comments
JOLO	_____	_____	_____	___/___	
WAIS Pict. Comp.	_____	_____	_____	___/___	
WAIS Pict. Arrange.	_____	_____	_____	___/___	
WAIS Block Design	_____	_____	_____	___/___	
WAIS Digit Symbol	_____	_____	_____	___/___	
WAIS Matrix Reas.	_____	_____	_____	___/___	
Other Tests:	_____	_____	_____	___/___	
	_____	_____	_____	___/___	
	_____	_____	_____	___/___	

MEMORY AND LEARNING:

Information and Orientation (1 or 0, from WMS or DRS)

Age _____ Year _____ City

DOB _____ Month _____ Day

Current Pres _____ Date _____ Time

Prev Pres _____ Place/Hospital _____

	Raw score	Norm (%, T Age SS, SS, z)	z score	Interpret. (Norms/Pt)	Comments
WAIS Information	_____	_____	_____	/ _____	
WMS I and O	_____	_____	_____	/ _____	
	_____	_____	_____	/ _____	
LM I 1st recall total	_____	_____	_____	/ _____	
LM I recall total	_____	_____	_____	/ _____	
LM learning slope	_____	_____	_____	/ _____	
LMII recall total	_____	_____	_____	/ _____	
LM II % retention	_____	_____	_____	/ _____	
LM II recog. total	_____	_____	_____	/ _____	
LM I thematic total	_____	_____	_____	/ _____	
LM II thematic total	_____	_____	_____	/ _____	
WL 1st recall total	_____	_____	_____	/ _____	
WL recall total	_____	_____	_____	/ _____	
Contrast 1 (PI)	_____	_____	_____	/ _____	
Learning slope	_____	_____	_____	/ _____	
Contrast 2 (RI)	_____	_____	_____	/ _____	
WL II recall total	_____	_____	_____	/ _____	
WL II recognition total	_____	_____	_____	/ _____	
WL II percent retention	_____	_____	_____	/ _____	
VR I recall total	_____	_____	_____	/ _____	
VR II recall total	_____	_____	_____	/ _____	
VR II recog total	_____	_____	_____	/ _____	
Copy total	_____	_____	_____	/ _____	
Discrimination total	_____	_____	_____	/ _____	
% retention	_____	_____	_____	/ _____	
Other Tests:	_____	_____	_____	/ _____	
	_____	_____	_____	/ _____	
	_____	_____	_____	/ _____	

AFFECT/PERSONALITY

GDS = _____ BDI = _____

OVERALL IMPRESSION:

OUTLINE OF THE REPORT OF THE NEUROPSYCHOLOGICAL EVALUATION

Report Header
Confidential: For Professional Use Only

Initial Neuropsychological Evaluation
Name:
Date of birth:
Medical record #:
Date of evaluation:

Referral and Background Information
Referral justification
Description of symptoms
Medical history
Social and educational history

Behavioral Observations

Tests Administered
Names of tests and examiners

Test Results
General intellectual function
Attention
Executive function
Motor function
Verbal abilities
Visuospatial and visuoconstructive abilities
Memory
Affect/personality

Impressions and Recommendations
Restatement of reason for referral
Summary of test findings
Conclusions regarding referral question
Recommendations concerning need for support, competence
Recommendations concerning follow-up services, including need for reevaluation

Psychologist's signature

cc:

APPENDIX G

PATIENT CASES

The following case reports describe the history and neuropsychological findings associated with a variety of neurodegenerative disorders affecting older adults. In most cases, the diagnosis was verified by autopsy or biopsy of brain tissue. Some of the neuropsychological instruments used to assess these patients are older tests that have now been updated and revised. The abbreviations used to identify the tests and diseases are identified in Appendix I.

The following case reports are included:

1. Amnestic syndrome evolving to probable Alzheimer's disease
2. Alzheimer's disease (visuospatial subtype)
3. Early-onset Alzheimer's disease with cortical Lewy bodies
4. Vascular dementia
5. Parkinson's disease with mild cognitive dysfunction
6. Parkinson's disease with Alzheimer's pathology
7. Parkinson's disease with cortical Lewy bodies and hippocampal gliosis
8. Multiple system atrophy (olivopontocerebellar degeneration)
9. Dementia with Lewy bodies
10. Frontotemporal dementia (Pick's disease)
11. Depression without dementia

The author would like to acknowledge the contributions of many colleagues to the clinical history and pathological findings described here. These include Felicia Goldstein, Ph.D., Vicki Roberts, Ph.D., John Woodard, Ph.D., Suzanne Mirra, M.D., Marla Gearing, Ph.D., Julie Schneider, M.D., Bruce Wainer, M.D., Mahlon R. Delong, M.D., Ray L. Watts, M.D., Jerrold L Vitek, M.D., Ph.D, Jorge Juncos, M.D., Marian Evatt, M.D., Allan I. Levey, M.D., Ph.D., Alexander P. Auchus, M.D., Robert C. Green, M.D., Kenneth Walker, M.D., Thomas Thompson, M.D., William McDonald, M.D., Herbert Karp, M.D., Brett E. Sirockman, B.S., Karen E. D'Lauro, M.A., Rebecca Bone, M.A., Kenneth Graap, M.Ed., Stella Harper, B.A, Kathleen Grimes, Ph.D., Laura Flashman, Ph.D., Michael Horner, Ph.D., Denise Mumley, Ph.D., Frank Wolkenberg, M.S., Susan Bowen, Ph.D., Julie Hill, Ph.D., and Pamela Frey, Ph.D. While effort has been devoted to ensuring the accuracy of the descriptions, the author bears any responsibility for possible misrepresentation of the cases.

CASE 1: AMNESTIC SYNDROME EVOLVING TO PROBABLE ALZHEIMER'S DISEASE

At initial evaluation, the patient was a 79-year-old, right-handed man, who had exhibited gradually increasing forgetfulness over the previous 2 years. He had difficulty remembering comments he had made, information that he had read, and the date. He described some mild depression, generally when the weather was cold and gray. However, he denied any tearfulness and stated that he slept and ate well. The patient's past medical history was largely unremarkable. He had completed high school and retired from a career as a salesman.

During the clinical interview, the patient was pleasant and alert. His spontaneous speech was mildly dysnomic, and his affect was brightly anxious. He exhibited some awareness of change but was not overly concerned about this. He was fully cooperative with the formal testing and had no difficulty following test instructions.

Major neuropsychological findings included the following:

1. General intellectual function: Premorbid general intellectual function was estimated to be average. He obtained a score of 131/144 on the DRS, which was interpreted as being within expectation.
2. Attention: Performance of mental control items was unimpaired (WMS-R Mental Control). The auditory digit spans of 7 forward and 7 backward were in the very superior range and within expectation (WMS-R Digit Span).
3. Executive function: On the Trail-Making Test, performance was mildly inconsistent, with Part A being borderline impaired and Part B within the average range. Ability to infer similarity between named items was within the average range and within expectation (WAIS-R Similarities).
4. Verbal abilities: Naming of pictured items was in the low average range, mildly below expectation (BNT). Letter and category fluency were each in the average range and within expectation.

5. Visuospatial abilities: Judgment of line orientation and completion of block designs were each within the average range and within expectation (JOLO, WAIS-R Block Designs).
6. Memory: The patient was oriented in year, day, place, city, and day. He was mildly disoriented in time. He was able to recall the name of the current president, but could not recall the names of the current vice-president or previous president even when phonemically cued. Immediate verbal memory, in either structured or unstructured conditions, was impaired (WMS-R LM, CVLT). Ability to retain that limited memory over a time delay was also impaired. Both immediate and delayed visual memory were impaired (WMS-R VR).
7. Responses to a questionnaire screening for depression did not suggest that he was clinically depressed (GDS).

The patient was initially diagnosed with an amnestic syndrome. One year later he returned for reevaluation. He remained in generally good health, except that he was exhibiting signs of increased forgetfulness, confusion, and social withdrawal. At reevaluation, the following test findings were obtained:

1. General intellectual function: The DRS score had declined to 116/144.
2. Attention: Both performance of mental control tasks and the auditory digit spans continued to be within the average range and within expectation.
3. Executive function: Performance on Trails B had become impaired. In a variety of different tests, the patient exhibited difficulty in establishing and maintaining task sets.
4. Verbal abilities: Conversational speech had become mildly halting and dysnomic. However, in formal testing naming of pictured items continued to be within the average range and within expectation. Category fluency had declined to the borderline impaired range.
5. Visuospatial and visuoconstructive abilities: These continued to be within the average range.
6. Memory: Both verbal and visual memory had declined. The patient showed greater difficulty in retaining even limited information over a time delay.

The patient was diagnosed with probable Alzheimer's disease. Characteristic of this disorder was the early presence of an amnestic syndrome followed by increasing memory dysfunction and the development of deficits in other neuropsychological domains, particularly executive function and verbal abilities. The patient's medical history was not suggestive of other etiologies for the increasing neuropsychological dysfunction.

CASE 2: ALZHEIMER'S DISEASE (VISUOSPATIAL SUBTYPE)

At the initial evaluation, the patient was a 63 year-old, right-handed man with a college education, who had worked as a high school English teacher. He had been concerned about cognitive change occurring over the past 2 years. He reported a variety of visuospatial difficulties, including spatial disorientation when trying to find his car in a parking garage or when walking in his neighborhood, difficulty writing within the appropriate lines when filling out a check, confusion in locating the gas cap on his car, and errors in recognizing common objects in his home. He also expressed concern about decline in word finding. Medical history was notable only for occasional alcohol intoxication. The patient was unaccompanied to the evaluation, and his behavioral presentation was notable mainly for mild anxiety.

Major neuropsychological findings included the following:

1. General intellectual function: Premorbid general intellectual function was estimated to be at least high average. The DRS score of 131/144 points was interpreted as being mildly below expectation.

2. Attention: Performance of WMS-R Mental Control items was largely within expectation, with the exception of an error of omission in reciting the months backward. The forward auditory digit span was within the average range but mildly below expectation (WMS-R Digit Span). However, the backward span was high average and within expectation.

3. Executive function: On a test of problem solving and cognitive flexibility, performance was unimpaired (WCST). Ability to infer similarity between named items was in the very superior range (WAIS-R Similarities).

4. Verbal abilities: Naming of pictured items was almost error-free and within expectation (BNT). Letter fluency was in the very superior range, but category fluency was weaker and effortful, with some mild difficulty in switching between categories.

5. Visuospatial abilities: The patient's copies of simple designs from the DRS were distorted. His copy of the Rey-Osterreith Complex Figure was highly segmented and included misrepresentation of both the gestalt of the design and internal detail. When asked to draw a clock to command, he was unable to number the clock face. When asked to copy a drawing of a clock, he mispositioned the numbers on the face. Ability to configure block designs was impaired (WAIS-R Block Designs).

6. Memory: The patient was fully oriented. Both immediate and delayed structured verbal memory were within the average range although below expectation (WMS-R LM). Cumulative learning of unstructured verbal material was impaired, and there was further decline in recall after a time delay (CVLT). However, delayed recognition was within the average range, although below expectation. Reproduction of designs from immediate visual memory was impaired, although delayed memory was similar in quantity to immediate memory (WMS-R VR). Remote memory for academically based knowledge was high average, within expectation (WAIS-R Information).

7. Affect: Both the patient's clinical presentation and his responses to a questionnaire screening for depression (GDS) suggested that he was mildly depressed.

The evaluation report noted that the test findings together with the reported pattern of decline were consistent with a neurodegenerative disorder with prominent dysfunction of right hemisphere regions, possibly a visuospatial subtype of Alzheimer's disease.

The patient was reevaluated 1 year later. He reported that his general health had been stable and that he was not aware of decline in his cognitive abilities. The major findings of the reevaluation were as follows:

1. General intellectual function: The patient's DRS score was now 128/144.
2. Attention: Performance of mental control items continued to be largely accurate, with the exception of continued errors in reciting the months backward. The forward digit span continued to be average, and the backward span was high average.
3. Executive function: Performance on the WCST and ability to infer similarity between named items were unchanged and continued to be within expectation.
4. Verbal abilities: Naming of pictured items was unchanged and within expectation. Letter fluency continued to be in the very superior range, and category fluency continued to be below expectation, although unchanged.
5. Visuospatial abilities: The patient's copy of the Rey-Osterreith Complex Figure continued to be impaired. Clock drawing had deteriorated, with increased difficulty copying both the numbering on the clock face and the placement of the clock hands. Completion of block designs had declined.
6. Memory: The patient continued to be fully oriented. Immediate recall of structured verbal material remained within the average range, although below expectation. However, delayed recall had declined. Cumulative learning of unstructured verbal material had declined, and there continued to be impairment in delayed recall. Delayed recognition remained within the average range, although below expectation. Reproduction of designs from visual memory was similar in quality to that observed during the previous evaluation. Remote memory for academically based knowledge was now in the average range, mildly below expectation.
7. Affect: The patient no longer appeared to be depressed.

The patient was evaluated for a third time 1 year later. Although he reported only a mild decline in his abilities, his wife described his increasing confusion, including difficulty in reading an analogue wristwatch, occasional spatial disorientation even in his home, difficulty in recognizing common objects, and confusion about the duration of time.

The following test findings were obtained:

1. General intellectual function: His DRS score was now 122/144 points, representing a significant decline from that obtained 2 years before.
2. Attention: He had increased difficulty performing mental control items. He was unable to count forward by 3s and made more errors when reciting the months backward.
3. Executive function: He was no longer able to perform the WCST. Ability to infer similarity between named items had declined, although it remained in the superior range. In a variety of different tests, the patient had increased difficulty in establishing and maintaining task sets and exhibited perseverative responding.
4. Verbal abilities: Naming was now impaired, although it was facilitated by provision of phonemic cues. The patient exhibited perceptual confusion in recognizing the pictured objects. Performance on tests of letter fluency and category fluency remained consistent with that observed during previous evaluations.
5. Visuospatial and visuoconstructive abilities: Although visual acuity continued to be adequate (20/25), the patient showed further decline in copying simple designs, judgment of line orientation, and ability to configure block designs.
6. Memory: The patient was oriented in year, month, and date, although he was disoriented in day, location, and time. He was able to recall the names of the current and previous presidents without cuing. Immediate recall of structured verbal material was now at the lower end of the average range and had declined significantly since the previous evaluation. However, delayed recall was similar in quantity to immediate recall. Unstructured verbal memory continued to be impaired in conditions of both immediate and delayed recall. There was mild decline in delayed recognition. Reproduction of simple designs from either immediate or delayed visual memory continued to be impaired.
7. Affect: The patient's responses to the questionnaire screening for depression indicated a mild degree of depression.

The patient died 6 years after the initial evaluation. Autopsy of brain tissue revealed findings consistent with Alzheimer's disease. This patient's neuropsychological profile was consistent with a visuospatial subtype of Alzheimer's disease in which decline in visuospatial and visuoconstructive performance was initially most pronounced, followed by more widespread deficits.

CASE 3: EARLY-ONSET ALZHEIMER'S DISEASE WITH CORTICAL LEWY BODIES

The patient was a 50-year-old, right-handed man with a high school education, who had worked in a factory. He had experienced gradually increasing memory loss and confusion over the past year and had difficulty performing his work. His medical history was notable only for hypertension controlled by medication, a hearing loss in his left ear corrected with a hearing aid, and a heavy smoking habit. An MRI scan was unremarkable, and an EEG showed diffuse slowing. Other laboratory tests were normal. Family history was notable for dementia, presumed to be multi-infarct, in his mother.

The patient's behavioral presentation was unusual. Even though he appeared to be able to hear adequately, he often missed the point of questions that were addressed to him and gave partially unrelated responses. Even when he appreciated the meaning of a question, his responses often became disorganized and tangential. His affect was restrained and limited, and he did not appear to be concerned about the deficits that he exhibited. He often made defensive comments to explain these deficits. However, he was cooperative with formal testing and exerted effort to perform well.

Major neuropsychological findings included the following:

1. General intellectual function: Premorbid function was estimated to be average. The Verbal IQ, Performance IQ, and Full-Scale IQ were each in the borderline range, well below expectation, suggesting a significant decline in general intellectual function (WAIS-R).

2. Attention: These abilities were severely impaired. The only simple mental control task that the patient could perform was recitation of the alphabet. He was unable to count backward from 20, even when cued to start. When asked to count forward by 3s, he began correctly but became confused in the middle. He made an error in reciting the months forward. When next asked to recite the months backward, he made errors reflecting perseveration from a previous task set. The forward auditory digit span was within the average range, but he was unable to establish set to perform the backward span (WAIS-R Digit Span). Performance of mental arithmetic was severely impaired (WAIS-R Arithmetic).

3. Executive function: In a variety of different tests, the patient exhibited difficulty establishing, maintaining, and switching between response sets, with pronounced perseverative responding. Errors often reflected stimulus-boundedness. On a test requiring responses to questions requiring social knowledge and sensibility, performance was low average, mildly below expectation (WAIS-R Comprehension). Ability to infer similarity between named items was impaired (WAIS-R Similarities).

4. Verbal abilities: Spontanous expressive speech was impaired, as observed during the clinical interview. Although the patient had some difficulty in responding to questions during the clinical interview, this appeared to be more closely related to impaired ability to organize verbal responses (executive dysfunction) than to a verbal comprehension deficit. During formal testing, he appeared able to understand test instructions. Naming of pictured items was impaired, although the provision of phonemic cues mildly facilitated naming (BNT). Letter fluency was low

average, mildly below expectation, and category fluency was similar. Ability to define words was low average, mildly below expectation (WAIS-R Vocabulary).

5. Visuospatial and visuoconstructive abilities: When asked to draw a clock to command, the patient's numbering of the clock face was poorly positioned and he forgot task instructions. When reminded of the time he had been instructed to represent on the clock face, he was unable to do this, drawing only one clock hand. When asked to copy a drawing of a clock, he initially misnumbered the face. Analysis of visual detail in cartoon pictures, logical sequencing of cartoon pictures, and assembly of puzzles were each low average, mildly below expectation (WAIS-R Picture Completion, Picture Arrangement, Object Assembly). Configuration of block designs and performance of a visuospatial transcription task were each severely impaired (WAIS-R Block Design, Digit-Symbol).

6. Memory: The patient was oriented in year, month, day, and location but mildly disoriented in date and severely disoriented in time. He was able to recall the names of the current and previous presidents. Both immediate and delayed recall of structured verbal material were severely impaired and characterized by confabulation and disorganization (WMS-R LM). Although delayed memory was impaired, the patient did retain some of the distorted material he had initially recalled. In an unstructured verbal learning test, both learning and delayed memory were severely impaired and notable for multiple perseverative and intrusion errors (CVLT). Reproduction of designs from immediate or delayed visual memory was severely impaired, with segmentation of the designs' gestalt and rotation of design elements, as well as difficulty in remembering instructions (WMS-R VR). Remote memory for academically based knowledge was a relative strength, being only borderline impaired (WMS-R Information).

7. Motor abilities: Both the speed of finger tapping and performance of a visuomotor test of finger dexterity were impaired bilaterally (Finger Tapping, Grooved Pegboard). The patient had difficulty maintaining manual sequencing within each hand (Luria Motor Sequences).

The evaluation report noted that deficits in attention and in organizing and maintaining behavior, suggestive of severe frontal lobe dysfunction, seemed fundamental to other deficits, and that the test findings were not typical for Alzheimer's disease. However, it was noted that Alzheimer's disease often presents atypically in young-onset patients. It was recommended that the possibility of a frontotemporal lobar dementia might be considered.

The patient showed a rapidly progressive course and died 6 years later. A brain autopsy revealed pathology consistent with Alzheimer's disease but also cortical Lewy bodies. In retrospect, the cortical Lewy bodies, particularly in the frontal lobe, may have been the pathological basis for the patient's severe impairment in attention and executive function as well his relative lack of awareness of deficit. His memory deficit and impaired naming were more characteristic of Alzheimer's disease.

CASE 4: VASCULAR DEMENTIA

At the time of initial evaluation, the patient was a 65-year-old retired successful attorney. He had a history of alcohol abuse. Two years before, when he discontinued alcohol consumption prior to surgery, he had suffered severe symptoms of alcohol withdrawal, including delirium tremens. His memory had shown marked decline immediately following this episode and more gradual decline subsequently. He also has developed a progressive impairment in gait.

Medical history was notable for noncompliance with treatment for non-insulin-dependent diabetes over the past 8 years, diabetes-related peripheral neuropathy, including blind spots in his vision, and medically controlled hypertension. A recent MRI had revealed moderate volume loss and small infarcts in the thalamus and caudate nucleus.

The patient's family reported that he exhibited considerable cognitive impairment. He repeated questions and was disoriented in date, although he sometimes remembered appointments. He was no longer able to use the remote control for the television and had difficulty following his medication regimen, even when it was organized for him. He tended to sleep a lot during the day even when he slept well at night. The patient did not seem concerned about the changes that were described, and during formal testing, he had difficulty exerting effort on tasks of any difficulty.

Major neuropsychological findings included the following:

1. General intellectual function: Premorbid general intellectual function was estimated to be at least high average. The DRS score of 111/144 points was impaired.
2. Attention: The patient exhibited impairment on mental control items of any difficulty (WMS-R Mental Control). For example, he was able to count backward and recite the months forward, but could not recite the months backward or count forward by 3s. The forward auditory digit span was in the average range, and the backward span was in the low average range, each well below expectation (WMS-R Digit Span).
3. Executive function: Ability to infer similarity between named items was in the average range, below expectation. The patient exhibited motor persistence in following simple verbal commands (DRS).
4. Verbally based abilities: Speech comprehension was relatively preserved. Spontaneous expressive speech was halting and dysnomic. In formal testing, naming of pictured items was low average, below expectation, but the provision of phonemic cues facilitated naming (BNT). Performance on tests of letter or category fluency was severely impaired. Writing was notable for being imprecise and mildly micrographic.

5. Visuospatial and visuoconstructive abilities: The patient was able to match simple visual designs and to scan a page to detect target letters (DRS). When asked to draw a clock to command, his positioning of the numbers on the clock face was irregular. He was able to recall the time he'd been asked to represent but then did so in an incorrect, concrete fashion. He was able to copy a drawing of a clock, although the relative hand length was reversed. His drawing was mildly tremulous. Ability to configure block designs was impaired, in part owing to impaired motor control of the fingers (WAIS-R Block Design).

6. Memory: The patient was oriented in month, place, city, and time although disoriented in date and day. He was unable to recall the name of the current president, even when phonemically cued, although he could recall the name of the current vice president. He could recall the name of the previous president when cued. Immediate recall of structured verbal material was low average, well below expectation, and delayed recall was even more limited and impaired (WMS-R LM). However, his delayed recognition of content units from the material was relatively strong. Both immediate and delayed memory for unstructured verbal material was impaired (CVLT). However, the patient did not make any perseverative or intrusion errors, and his poor memory appeared, in part, to reflect a lack of effort. He was able to recall one out of two sentences after a short distractor task (DRS). Remote memory for academically based knowledge was in the high average range, mildly below expectation (WAIS-R Information).

7. Affect: Neither the patient's behavioral presentation nor his responses to a questionnaire screening for depression suggested that he was clinically depressed.

The evaluation report noted that the patient's medical history placed him at increased risk for alcoholic dementia or vascular dementia. His lack of concern about deficits, difficulty in maintaining task sets, and inertial behavior at home were suggestive of the frontal lobe dysfunction that is often associated with these disorders. In contrast, the findings of relatively preserved naming when cued, the absence of intrusion errors during memory recall, relatively strong delayed recognition memory, and possible remote memory loss were atypical of Alzheimer's disease.

The patient was seen 1 year later for reevaluation. His wife had perceived decline in his cognitive status over the past year. He had become dependent on others for help with bathing and dressing and recently had had difficulty recognizing her and his home.

The test findings were as follows:

1. General intellectual functions: The DRS score was now 102/144 points, representing a decline from the previous year.

2. Attention: Both performance of mental control items and the forward auditory digit span were similar in quality to those of the previous year, remaining below expectation. The backward digit span had become impaired.

3. Executive function: Ability to infer similarity between named items was within the average range, below expectation, and similar in quality to that of the previous year. The patient exhibited increased inability to establish and maintain task sets. He occasionally exhibited confusion in beginning tests, and in some cases he began tests correctly and then become confused and stopped.

4. Verbal abilities: Naming of pictured items continued to be low average, below expectation, and to benefit from phonemic cuing. The patient continued to exhibit impaired word fluency. Writing was irregular, with errors in spelling and capitalization.

5. Visuospatial and visuoconstructive abilities: The patient made errors in scanning a page to detect target letters. His clock drawing to command was similar in quality to that of the previous year, and he continued to be able to remember the time he was asked to represent but then to do so incorrectly. Configuration of block designs continued to be impaired.

6. Memory: The patient was oriented in place, city, day, and time, although not in date or month. He could spontaneously recall the names of the current and previous presidents, as well as the governor of his state and the mayor of his city. However, he could not recall his own age or date of birth. Immediate memory for structured verbal material was borderline impaired, and he was unable to recall any content units after a time delay. He continued to be able to accurately recognize content units from multiple choice alternatives. Immediate or delayed memory for unstructured verbal material continued to be severely impaired, although without notable occurrence of either perseverative or intrusion errors. Remote memory for academically based knowledge continued to be within the average range, below expectation.

7. Affect: The patient continued to appear relatively unconcerned and not depressed.

The report of the evaluation noted that the patient appeared to have a progressive disorder. Alzheimer's disease continued to be a less likely possibility because of the presence of features inconsistent with this disease, including his unimpaired naming, some preserved orientation, and relatively strong delayed memory recognition.

The patient died a year later. The autopsy of his brain was consistent with vascular dementia involving subcortical white matter disease, demyelination consistent with that of Binswanger's disease, and pathology in deep gray and brain stem structures. The autopsy report noted that the vascular disease may have been related to the clinical history of hypertension and diabetes.

Neuropsychological Evaluation of the Older Adult: A Clinician's Guidebook

CASE 5: PARKINSON'S DISEASE WITH MILD COGNITIVE DYSFUNCTION

The patient was a 63-year-old, right-handed man with a high school education, who worked as a salesman. He had a 15 year history of Parkinson's disease (PD). He reported that current PD symptoms included impaired balance, hypophonia, dysarthia, tremor, and dyskinesia. He had experienced nonthreatening visual hallucinations of people and animals in the past, which had been attributed to his Parkinson's medications. He described mild difficulty in concentrating when reading, but neither he nor family members reported major concern about his memory. The patient's medical history was notable for medically controlled hypertension, and family history was notable for PD in his father. He presented as a pleasant, alert man, whose verbal responses were slow and dysarthric. He was cooperative with the evaluation.

The patient was participating in a research protocol, from which the following findings were obtained:

1. General intellectual function: Premorbid general intellectual function was estimated to be average. On the DRS, the patient obtained 138/144 points, representing unimpaired performance.
2. Attention: Performance of mental control items was accurate and rapid, with the exception of two errors when counting forward by 3s. Both the forward and backward auditory digit spans were within the average range (WMS-R Digit Span).
3. Executive function: On an untimed test requiring problem solving and cognitive flexibility, performance was impaired (WCST). The patient had difficulty inferring rules for problem solving in response to feedback and in maintaining the task set.
4. Verbal abilities: Spontaneous expressive speech was dysarthric and hypophonic. Speech comprehension was unimpaired. Naming of pictured items was within the average range (BNT). Letter and category fluency were within the average range.
5. Visuospatial and visuoconstructive abilities – Judgment of line orientation was borderline impaired (JOLO).
6. Memory: On an unstructured verbal memory test, performance was impaired on measures of cumulative learning as well as on recall on the final learning trial (CVLT). However, delayed recall was in the low average range, and delayed recognition was within the average range.

Findings consistent with the mild cognitive dysfunction associated with PD included impairment in executive function, decline in visuospatial function, difficulty in acquiring new information in memory, particularly in unstructured conditions, and relatively preserved memory storage over time, especially in conditions involving recognition rather than recall.

CASE 6: PARKINSON'S DISEASE WITH ALZHEIMER'S PATHOLOGY

At the initial evaluation, the patient was a 50-year-old, right-handed woman, who had graduated from college and worked in a high-level management position in a large company. She had initially sought evaluation 3 years before when she developed difficulty using her right hand. Neurologic evaluation revealed an action and postural tremor and mild right arm and right toe dystonia. She was treated with dopaminergic medication and experienced some improvement in right body functioning. She was diagnosed with Parkinson's disease.

During the past year, she had experienced intellectual decline, including slowness in speech and reasoning, as well as difficulty in concentrating, organizing work, and completing tasks. Control of the right side of her body had become more impaired. She had also experienced considerable affective disorder, including anxiety, depression, and panic attacks and was being treated by a psychiatrist.

During the initial neuropsychological evaluation, the patient presented as an alert, pleasant, mildly anxious woman who was able to clearly describe her concerns in a well-organized, although slow, fashion. During formal testing, increased slowness and difficulty in organizing verbal responses were apparent.

Initial neuropsychological findings included the following:

1. General intellectual function: Premorbid general intellectual function was estimated to be high average. The Verbal IQ was within the average range, below expectation, and the Performance IQ was significantly lower, in the borderline range. The Full-scale IQ was low average (WAIS-R).

2. Attention: The patient made errors in performing mental control tasks, such as counting backward from 20 or counting forward by 3s (WMS-R Mental Control). The forward auditory digit span was within the average range, mildly below expectation, but the backward span was impaired (WMS-R Digit Span). Ability to perform mental arithmetic was impaired (WAIS-R Arithmetic).

3. Executive function: On a visuomotor test requiring mental tracking and cognitive flexibility, performance was impaired by slowness and errors (Trail-Making Test). Ability to infer similarity between named items was within the average range, mildly below expectation (WAIS-R Similarities). Responses to questions concerning social knowledge and sensibility were low average and below expectation (WAIS-R Comprehension).

4. Verbal abilities: The patient was slow in organizing verbal expression. Speech comprehension was preserved. Naming of pictured items was within the average range, mildly below expectation, although the provision of phonemic cues benefited naming. Both letter and category fluency were within expectation. Ability to define words was in the superior range.

5. Visuospatial and visuoconstructive abilities: These abilities were generally below expectation or impaired. Logical sequencing of cartoon pictures and ability to assemble puzzles were each low average, below expectation (WAIS-R Picture Arrangement, Object Assembly). Analysis of visual detail in cartoon pictures and ability to configure block designs were each borderline impaired (WAIS-R Picture Completion, Block Design). Performance of a visuomotor transcription task was impaired (WAIS-R Digit-Symbol).

6. Memory: The patient was fully oriented and could recall the name of the current president although not of the previous president. Immediate recall of structured verbal material was borderline impaired, although there was no significant memory loss over a time delay (WMS-R LM). On an unstructured verbal learning test, cumulative learning was impaired (CVLT). After a time delay, there was evidence of memory loss in conditions of recall or recognition. Delayed recognition was notable for a high false positive error rate. Reproduction of simple designs from immediate visual memory was borderline impaired, and there was no significant memory loss over a time delay (WMS-R VR). Remote memory for academically based knowledge was within the average range, below expectation (WAIS-R Information).
7. Motor abilities: Performance of a visuomotor task requiring finger dexterity was impaired bilaterally, worse for the right hand (Grooved Pegboard).
8. Affect: The patient's behavioral presentation as well as responses to a questionnaire screening for depression suggested that she was depressed (GDS).

The evaluation report noted that the most pronounced deficits occurred in attention, in ability to organize behavior, in visuospatial tasks, and in the acquisition of new material in memory. Storage of new information in memory was less problematic. The findings, together with the patient's history, were suggestive of dysfunction in frontal-subcortical brain systems, such as is associated with parkinsonian disorders. However, the severity of the neuropsychological deficits that the patient exhibited was somewhat uncharacteristic of the mild cognitive change associated with Parkinson's disease, particularly in a relatively younger, premorbidly high-functioning patient with recently diagnosed disease. The patient had never experienced the visual hallucinations that are associated with Lewy body dementia.

The patient showed a rapidly progressive course. Two years later her DRS score was 95/144, representing severely impaired performance. She exhibited more widespread deficits, with impairment in attention, executive function, verbal abilities, and visuospatial abilities. Relative strengths were the forward digit span and memory retention of structured verbal material, each of which remained low average. One year later, the DRS score had declined to 49/144 points, and the following year the patient was totally dysfunctional and near death. A biopsy of brain tissue showed evidence of pathology consistent with both Parkinson's disease and Alzheimer's disease. The rapid progression of neuropsychological decline was highly uncharacteristic of the cognitive change associated with Parkinson's disease alone.

CASE 7: PARKINSON'S DISEASE WITH CORTICAL LEWY BODIES AND HIPPOCAMPAL GLIOSIS

The patient was a 66-year-old, right-handed man who had been diagnosed with Parkinson's disease (PD) 1 year prior to the neuropsychological evaluation.

Initial motor symptoms included a shuffling gait, and had appeared 2 to 3 years before the PD was diagnosed. In the past year, the patient had experienced hallucinations, which were reduced when his antiparkinson's medication was adjusted. He had a master's degree in mathematics and had taught in the third grade through college. He had been asked to retire 3 years prior to the neuropsychological evaluation, in part because of difficulty in writing, speaking, and problem solving.

During the clinical interview, it was reported that the patient had shown personality change, becoming easily and suddenly belligerent toward others. The patient himself reported being unaware of this behavior until after it occurred. He had shown poor judgment in caring for himself, an impaired sense of direction, and mild dysnomia. Memory problems were not described as a major concern. His appetite was described as poor, with a tendency to desire sweet foods, but he reported sleeping fairly well and being in good spirits most of the time.

Major neuropsychological findings included the following:

1. General intellectual function: Premorbid general intellectual function was estimated to be high average. The DRS score of 100/144 was impaired.
2. Attention: The patient had difficulty in completing more challenging mental control items (WMS-R Mental Control). For example, he was able to recite the alphabet but required a second attempt in order to recite numbers backward from 20. When asked to recite the months backward, he became confused in the middle and perseverated in a previous task set. The forward auditory digit span was high average, within expectation, but the backward span was low average, below expectation (WMS-R Digit Span).
3. Executive function: Ability to infer similarity between named items was borderline impaired, well below expectation (WAIS-R Similarities). He exhibited difficulty in establishing, switching, and maintaining task sets.
4. Verbal abilities: Naming of pictured items was impaired but benefited from phonemic cuing (BNT). Both letter and category fluency were impaired. Writing was micrographic.
5. Visuospatial and visuoconstructive abilities: The patient had difficulty in copying simple designs. When asked to copy a simple alternating design, he began correctly but then became gradually more micrographic and perseverated in copying a single design (DRS). He was able to copy a simple embedded design on a second attempt. Both judgment of line orientation and configuration of block designs were impaired (JOLO, WAIS-R Block Design).
6. Memory: The patient was oriented in month, day, city, and time but disoriented in year, date, and location. Immediate recall of structured verbal material was impaired, although delayed recall was borderline impaired (WMS-R LM). On a unstructured verbal memory test, both immediate and delayed memory were impaired, even in conditions of recognition

(CVLT). Ability to reproduce simple designs from immediate visual memory was low average, and delayed memory was impaired (WMS-R VR). Remote memory for academically based knowledge was low average and below expectation (WAIS-R Information).

7. Affect: The patient did not appear to be depressed.

The report of the neuropsychological evaluation noted that the severity and rapid progression of the patient's cognitive change was not highly characteristic of PD alone and raised the possibility that he might have another neurodegenerative disorder in addition to PD.

The patient died 4 years after the neuropsychological evaluation was conducted. Neuropathological analysis of brain tissue was interpreted as evidencing idiopathic PD with associated cortical Lewy bodies as well as gliosis in the hippocampus and amygdala. In retrospect, the pronounced deficits in attention and executive function may have reflected the presence of cortical Lewy bodies, which exacerbated subcortical-cortical dysfunction directly related to PD. The hippocampal gliosis may have contributed to the severity of the patient's memory deficit.

CASE 8: MULTIPLE SYSTEM ATROPHY (OLIVOPONTOCEREBELLAR DEGENERATION)

The patient was a 48-year-old right-handed woman with a college education, who had worked as a teacher. Three years before, she had developed motor symptoms including decline in motor dexterity, motor rigidity and stiffness, balance problems, and severe fatigue. The symptoms were worse on the left side of her body.

Neuropsychological data were collected during her participation in a research study, and the major findings were as follows:

1. General intellectual function: Her Verbal IQ was in the very superior range (WAIS-R).

2. Attention: The auditory digit spans were in the very superior range (WAIS-R Digit Span). Ability to perform mental arithmetic was in the very superior range (WAIS-R Mental Arithmetic).

3. Executive function: On a test of problem solving and cognitive flexibility, performance was unimpaired and within expectation (WCST). Responses to questions requiring social knowledge and sensibility were in the very superior range (WAIS-R Comprehension). Ability to infer similarity between named items was in the very superior range (WAIS-R Similarities). On a timed visuomotor test requiring mental tracking and cognitive flexibility, performance was high average, although below expectation (Trail-Making Test), possibly owing to motor impairment.

4. Verbal abilities: Spontaneous expressive speech and speech comprehension were unimpaired. Naming of pictured items was in the very superior range (BNT). Letter fluency was in the average range, below expectation.

5. Visuospatial and visuoconstructive abilities: The patient was able to discriminate between visual forms without error (Benton Visual Form Discrimination). Ability to configure block designs was in the very superior range (WAIS-R Block Design).

6. Memory: Immediate and delayed recall of structured verbal material were each within the average range, well below expectation (WMS-R LM). On an unstructured verbal learning test, cumulative learning as well as final trial recall were in the low average range, well below expectation (CVLT). Delayed free recall was impaired, although delayed recognition was within the average range, still below expectation. Remote memory for academically based knowledge was in the high average range, mildly below expectation (WAIS-R Information).

7. Affect: The patient did not appear to be depressed on the basis of her behavioral presentation or a questionnaire inventory.

The patient died 3 years later of causes unrelated to her movement disorder. The brain autopsy was interpreted as evidencing olivopontocerebellar degeneration. Her neuropsychological profile, particularly evidence of mild decline in word fluency and in memory acquisition and recall although not in memory recognition, was consistent with a parkinsonian syndrome. However, the absence of executive dysfunction was somewhat atypical of idiopathic Parkinson's disease.

CASE 9: DEMENTIA WITH LEWY BODIES

At the initial evaluation, the patient was a 71-year-old, right-handed man with a 6-year history of progressive cognitive change and pronounced decline over the past 2 years. He had had difficulty keeping his car on the road and remembering the names of familiar individuals and recent events. Over the past year, he had exhibited distinct episodes of increased confusion, including visual hallucinations and excessive sleeping. His writing had become micrographic and his speech slurred, and he was often disoriented even when at home. The patient had a college degree and had worked as a salesman.

His medical history was notable for medically controlled hypertension and hypercholesterolemia. Recent brain scans were interpreted as showing old bilateral lacunar basal ganglia infarcts and periventricular white matter disease.

The patient's behavior was notable for slow, effortful speech, masked facies, and bilateral tremor of the hands.

The major neuropsychological test findings were as follows:

1. General intellectual function: Premorbid general intellectual function was estimated as high average. The patient's DRS score of 121/144 points was interpreted as impaired performance.

2. Attention: The patient had great difficulty in performing simple mental control tasks (WMS-R Mental Control). For example, he became confused in the middle of counting backward from 20 and made four errors

of omission near the end of reciting the alphabet. The forward auditory digit span was low average and below expectation, while the backward span was average, mildly below expectation (WMS-R Digit Span).

3. Executive function: Ability to infer similarity between named items was average, mildly below expectation (WAIS-R Similarities). The patient exhibited variable difficulty in establishing, maintaining, and switching between task sets.

4. Verbal abilities: Spontaneous speech was slow and effortful, although speech comprehension was preserved. Naming of pictured items was unimpaired (BNT). Letter fluency was impaired, although category fluency was relatively stronger. Writing of simple sentences was unremarkable.

5. Visuospatial and visuoconstructive abilities: The patient obtained 20/30 on a screening of visual acuity. He was able to copy a simple embedded design, but could not maintain the alternation of a simple alternating design (DRS). When asked to draw a clock to command, he was unable to number the clock face or to represent a specified time. When asked to copy a clock drawing, his positioning of the numbers on the clock face was distorted, although he could copy the clock hands in a grossly correct fashion. Judgment of line orientation was within the average range although mildly below expectation (JOLO). Ability to configure block designs was impaired (WAIS-R Block Design).

6. Memory: The patient was oriented in year, month, date, day, time, and city, although not in exact location. He was able to recall the names of the current and previous president. Immediate recall of structured verbal material was low average, and delayed recall was borderline impaired (WMS-R LM). Errors reflected poor retention of the structure of the material. Cumulative immediate memory of unstructured verbal material was impaired, although delayed recall was similar in quantity to immediate memory, suggesting some preserved ability to store new information (CVLT). Reproduction of simple designs from immediate visual memory was low average and notable for micrographia and distortion of the gestalt (WMS-R VR). Delayed reproduction was also low average. Remote memory for academically based knowledge was within the average range, mildly below expectation (WAIS-R Information).

7. Affect: The patient did not appear to be depressed.

The patient was reevaluated 1 year later. His wife reported that he continued to have visual hallucinations, largely of other people in his home. His confusion had increased, including loss of behavioral initiative, spatial disorientation at home, suspiciousness concerning his wife's behavior, and difficulty maintaining a train of thought.

Major neuropsychological findings included the following:

1. General intellectual function: He obtained 97/144 points on the DRS, representing impaired performance and a significant decline from the previous year.

2. Attention: These abilities continued to be impaired and were similar in quality to those of the previous evaluation.
3. Executive function: He exhibited decreased ability to establish, maintain, and switch between task sets, with marked perseverative responding. Ability to infer similarity between named items had declined.
4. Verbal abilities: Spontaneous expressive speech and speech comprehension were unchanged. Naming of pictured items continued to be unimpaired. Category fluency had declined dramatically and was impaired.
5. Visuospatial and visuoconstructive abilities: These abilities had deteriorated. He was no longer able to copy a simple embedded design or perform a test involving judgment of line orientation.
6. Memory: He was fully oriented and able to recall the names of the current and previous presidents. However, his performance on formal tests of memory, either visual or verbal, was now impaired in conditions of either immediate or delayed memory. However, remote memory for academically based knowledge continued to be in the average range and represented a relative strength.

The patient died 2 years later. The brain autopsy revealed multiple Lewy bodies at cortical and subcortical sites; parkinsonian changes, including degeneration within the substantia nigra; mild changes consistent with Alzheimer's disease; and atherosclerotic changes, including an old left basal ganglia infarct. In retrospect, the presence of a fluctuating state of arousal, visual hallucinations, pronounced impairment in attention and executive function, and extrapyramidal motor symptoms were consistent with the diagnosis of dementia with Lewy bodies. It seems likely that vascular disease exacerbated the neuropsychological change associated with Lewy body disease.

CASE 10: FRONTOTEMPORAL DEMENTIA (PICK'S DISEASE)

At initial evaluation, the patient was a 56-year-old, formerly high-functioning executive, who had 23 years of education. He had first seen a psychiatrist 2 years earlier after exhibiting personality changes. These included excessive alcohol consumption, offensive comments to others, obsessive behavior, questionable judgment, and reduced interest in formerly enjoyable activities. An MRI revealed frontal lobe atrophy. A position emission tomography (PET) scan revealed hypometabolism in the bilateral medial frontal, left inferior and superior frontal, and bitemporal brain regions.

The patient's behavioral presentation was notable for a lack of concern about the changes that his wife described. During formal testing, he exerted effort to perform well, but his affect was flat and he continued to appear unconcerned. It was difficult to establish rapport with him, and throughout the evaluation, he exhibited laughter at inappropriate times.

Major neuropsychological findings included the following:

1. General intellectual function: Premorbid function was estimated to be in the superior range. The patient's Verbal, Performance, and Full-Scale IQ

scores were each within the average range, well below expectation (WAIS-R).

2. Attention: Performance of mental control items was unimpaired (WMS-R Mental Control). The auditory digit span was in the superior range, within expectation (WMS-R Digit Span). Ability to perform mental arithmetic was in the high average range, mildly below expectation (WMS-R Mental Arithmetic).

3. Executive function: Performance was impaired on a test of problem solving and cognitive flexibility (WCST). Ability to infer similarity between named items was impaired (WAIS-R Similarities). The patient's general response style was impulsive and inattentive to detail.

4. Verbal abilities: Spontaneous expressive speech and speech comprehension were unimpaired. Naming of pictured items was low average, well below expectation, and the provision of phonemic cues did not facilitate naming (BNT). Letter fluency was also low average, below expectation. However, category fluency was stronger than letter fluency. Ability to define words was within the average range, below expectation (WAIS-R Vocabulary).

5. Visuospatial and visuoconstructive abilities: The patient's drawing of a clock to command was notable only for one self-corrected error. Abilities to analyze visual detail in cartoon pictures, to logically sequence cartoon pictures, or to configure block designs were each within the average range, below expectation (WAIS-R Picture Completion, Picture Arrangement, Block Design). Performance of a visuomotor transcription task was in the superior range, representing a relative strength (WAIS-R Digit-Symbol).

6. Memory: The patient was fully oriented and able to recall the names of the current and previous presidents. Immediate recall of structured verbal material was in the average range, below expectation, and delayed recall was in the low average range, well below expectation (WMS-R LM). The presence of confabulatory content was notable. Performance was weaker in a less structured verbal memory test (CVLT). Cumulative immediate learning was borderline impaired. Both long-delay free recall and long-delay recognition were impaired. Visual memory was a relative strength (WMS-R VR). Reproduction of designs from immediate visual memory was high average, mildly below expectation, and delayed reproduction was in the superior range. Remote memory for academically based knowledge was in the average range, well below expectation (WAIS-R Information).

The patient was seen for a brief reevaluation 6 months later. He continued to appear cooperative but unconcerned. Letter fluency was adequate in the number of words generated, but with a great increase in perseverative errors. The patient was unable to interpret common proverbs. He continued to be largely oriented, although he was now inaccurate in recalling the name of the previous president. Immediate recall of structured verbal material continued to be in the average

Neuropsychological Evaluation of the Older Adult: A Clinician's Guidebook
Copyright © 2000 by Academic Press. All rights of reproduction in any form reserved.

range, although well below expectation, but there had been a decline in delayed recall, which was now in the borderline impaired range. Visual memory continued to be a relative strength, in the very superior range.

Biopsy of brain tissue revealed findings consistent with frontotemporal dementia. Characteristic of this disease were the patient's early change in personality, including inappropriate, impulsive behavior accompanied by a lack of concern about change. Although below expectation for many measures, his performance on formal neuropsychological tests was not dramatically impaired. Visuospatial performance and visual memory were relatively preserved. The most pronounced weaknesses were observed on tests sensitive to frontal lobe function. Confabulation was present in verbal memory recall, and verbal memory was weaker in unstructured conditions.

CASE 11: DEPRESSION WITHOUT DEMENTIA

The patient was a 69-year-old, right-handed man with a 10th-grade education who had a history of depression since his teenage years. He had been treated with medication and also with electroconvulsive therapy (ECT), most recently about 3 months before the neuropsychological evaluation. He was referred because he had expressed concerns about increased forgetfulness even before his recent ECT. He reported that when he felt lonely, he became inactive and forgot to take his antidepressant medication, resulting in increased depression and forgetfulness. His sister had plans for him to move into her home in the near future. His medical history was otherwise notable only for phlebitis, which was being medically treated. He had worked on an assembly line and had never married.

The patient appeared alert, but sad, and he rarely smiled. He exhibited extrapyramial motor symptoms, including tremor of his lip, a short gait, stooped posture, and mildly dysarthric speech. He had difficulty exerting effort on some tests.

Major neuropsychological findings included the following:

1. General intellectual function: Premorbid general intellectual function was estimated to be average. On the DRS, the patient obtained 113/144 points, which was interpreted as impaired performance.
2. Attention: Performance of simple mental control tasks was borderline impaired and well below expectation (WMS-III Mental Control). The forward auditory digit span was low average and mildly below expectation, but the backward span was within the average range and within expectation (WMS-III Digit Span).
3. Executive function: On a timed test requiring concentration and cognitive flexibility, performance was impaired (Trail-Making Test). The patient exhibited motor persistence in following simple verbal commands.
4. Verbal Ability: Naming of pictured items was within the average range (BNT). Ability to generate words either beginning with specified letters or representing specified categories was low average and mildly below expectation (Word Fluency).

5. Visuospatial and visuoconstructive ability: The patient was able to match simple visual designs, although he missed a letter when scanning the page to detect target letters. He made perseverative errors in copying a simple alternating design but was able to copy a simple embedded design, as well as more complex designs. However, his drawing was notable for being tremulous and micrographic. In drawing a clock to command, he was able to remember the time that he had been asked to represent, but then set the time in an incorrect, concrete fashion. Judgment of line orientation was impaired (JOLO). However, ability to configure block designs was low average, only mildly below expectation (WAIS-III Block Design).

6. Memory and learning: The patient was able to spontaneously recall his age, his date of birth, and the name of the current president. He required a phonemic cue to recall the name of the previous president. He was oriented in year, month, date, place, city, and day, although mildly disoriented in time. Remote memory for academically based knowledge was within the average range (WAIS-III Information). Immediate recall of structured verbal material was borderline impaired (WMS-III LM). The percent retained after a 30-minute delay was also borderline impaired. However, on an unstructured verbal learning test (WMS-III Words), cumulative immediate memory was within the average range, and delayed recall was also within the average range. Ability to reproduce simple designs from immediate or delayed visual memory was within the average range (WMS-III VR).

7. Affect: The patient's behavior and his responses to a questionnaire screening for depression (BDI) suggested that he was significantly depressed.

The neuropsychological report noted that the patient's performance was mildly below expectation in each of the neuropsychological domains that was examined, largely because of inconsistency. On tests of memory, his performance was inconsistent but was unimpaired on an unstructured verbal memory test and also on a visual memory test. Although his score on the DRS indicated significant impairment, this was largely due to variability, and his performance within specific neuropsychological domains did not suggest that he had a significant degree of dementia. There was some tendency for performance to be stronger in more demanding conditions, a pattern that is often associated with mild depression. The presence of tremulousness, micrographia, and a relative weakness in executive function raised the possibility of extrapyramidal motor symptoms, possibly related to his medication regimen or to subcortical vascular disease. It was concluded that the overall pattern of findings was largely consistent with the mild cognitive dysfunction associated with depression.

BASIC BRAIN NEUROANATOMY

Lateral View of the Brain

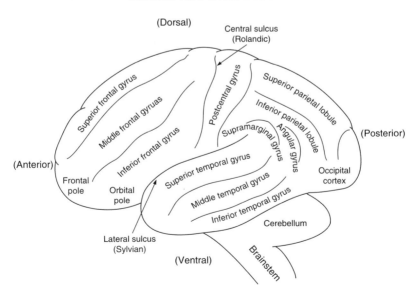

(Dorsal)

Central sulcus
(Rolandic)

Superior frontal gyrus

Middle frontal gyruas

Inferior frontal gyrus

Postcentral gyrus

Superior parietal lobule

Inferior parietal lobule

Supramarginal gyrus

Angular gyrus

(Posterior)

(Anterior)

Frontal
pole

Orbital
pole

Superior temporal gyrus

Middle temporal gyrus

Inferior temporal gyrus

Occipital
cortex

Cerebellum

Lateral sulcus
(Sylvian)

(Ventral)

Brainstem

Horizontial View of the Brain through the Basal Ganglia
(gray areas indicate gray matter)

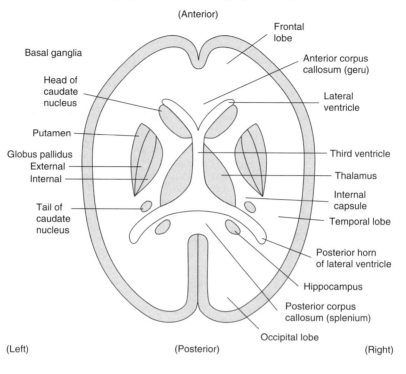

(Anterior)

Frontal lobe

Basal ganglia

Anterior corpus callosum (geru)

Head of caudate nucleus

Lateral ventricle

Putamen

Globus pallidus
External
Internal

Third ventricle

Thalamus

Internal capsule

Tail of caudate nucleus

Temporal lobe

Posterior horn of lateral ventricle

Hippocampus

Posterior corpus callosum (splenium)

Occipital lobe

(Left)   (Posterior)   (Right)

Major Arteries of the Brain (inferior view)

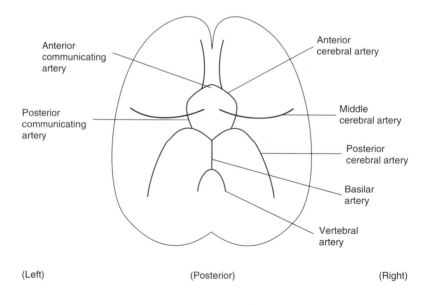

(Anterior)

Anterior communicating artery

Anterior cerebral artery

Posterior communicating artery

Middle cerebral artery

Posterior cerebral artery

Basilar artery

Vertebral artery

(Left)   (Posterior)   (Right)

LIST OF ABBREVIATIONS

ACA = anterior cerebral artery
AcoA = anterior communicating artery
AD = Alzheimer's disease
ADRDA = Alzheimer's Disease and Related Disorders Association
AK = alcoholic Korsakoff's syndrome
AMNART = American New Adult Reading Test
ApoE = apolipoprotein E
AVM = arteriovenous malformation
BDI = Beck Depression Inventory
BNT = Boston Naming Test
CABG = coronary artery bypass graft
CADASIL = cerebral autosomal dominant arteriopathy with subcortical infarcts
    and leukoencephalopathy
CBD = corticobasal degeneration
COWA = Controlled Oral Word Association
CSF = cerebrospinal fluid
CT = computed tomography
CVLT = California Verbal Learning Test
DRS = Dementia Rating Scale

ECT = electroconvulsive therapy
EPS = extrapyramidal motor symptoms
DLB = dementia with Lewy bodies
DSM = Diagnostic and Statistical Manual of Mental Disorders
FTLD = frontotemporal lobar degeneration
FTD = frontotemporal dementia
FSIQ = Full-Scale Intelligence Quotient
GCS = Glasgow Coma Scale
HD = Huntington's disease
I-O = Information and Orientation
IQ = Intelligence Quotient
JOLO = Judgment of Line Orientation
LM = Logical Memory
MAST = Michigan Alcohol Screening Test
MCA = middle cerebral artery
MOANS = Mayo's Older Americans Normative Study
MRI = magnetic resonance imaging
MSA = multiple system atrophy
NART = National Adult Reading Test
NINCDS = National Institute of Neurologic and Communicative Disorders and
    Stroke
NPH = normal pressure hydrocephalus
PD = Parkinson's disease
PSP = progressive supranuclear palsy
PIQ = Performance Intelligence Quotient
PCA = posterior cerebral artery
PcoA = posterior communicating artery
SD = standard deviation
SEM = standard error of measurement
SSRI = selective serotonin reuptake inhibitors
TBI = traumatic brain injury
TCA = tricyclic antidepressant medication
TIA = transient ischemic attack
VaD = vascular dementia
VIQ = Verbal Intelligence Quotient
VR = Visual Reproduction
WMS = Wechsler Memory Scale
WMS–R = Wechsler Memory Scale, Revised
WMS–III = Wechsler Memory Scale, Third Edition
WAIS = Wechsler Adult Intelligence Scale
WAIS–R = Wechsler Adult Intelligence Scale, Revised
WAIS–R NI = WAIS–R as a Neuropsychological Instrument
WAIS–III = Wechsler Adult Intelligence Scale, Third Edition
WCST = Wisconsin Card Sorting Test
WL = Word Lists

Neuropsychological Evaluation of the Older Adult: A Clinician's Guidebook
Copyright © 2000 by Academic Press. All rights of reproduction in any form reserved.

REFERENCES

Aarsland, D., Tandberg, E., Larsen, J., & Cummings, J. (1996). Frequency of dementia in Parkinson disease. *Archives of Neurology, 53,* 538–542.

Abrams, R. (1992). *Electroconvulsive therapy.* New York: Oxford University Press.

Abrams, R., Swartz, C., & Vedak, C. (1991). Antidepressant effects of high-dose right unilateral electroconvulsive therapy. *Archives of General Psychiatry, 48,* 746–748.

Ackeman, H., & Hertrick, I. (1997). Voice onset time in ataxic dysarthria. *Brain and Language, 156,* 321–333.

Adams, R., Fisher, C., Hakim, S., Ojemann, R., & Sweet, W. (1965). Symptomatic occult hydrocephalus with "normal" cerebrospinal fluid pressure. *New England Journal of Medicine, 273,* 117–126.

Agid, Y. (1998). Levodopa: Is toxicity a myth? *Neurology, 50,* 858–863.

Aharon-Peretz, J., Kliot, D., Amyel-Zvi, E., Tomer, R., Rakier, A., & Feinsod, M. (1997). Neurobehavioral consequences of closed head injury in the elderly. *Brain Injury, 11,* 871–875.

Ainslie, N., & Murden, R.A. (1993). Effect of education on the clock-drawing dementia screen in non-demented elderly persons. *Journal of the American Geriatrics Society, 41,* 249–252.

Akshoomoff, N., Delis, D., & Kiefner, M. (1989). Block constructions of chronic alcoholic and unilateral brain-damaged patients: A test of the right hemisphere vulnerability hypothesis of alcoholism. *Archives of Clinical Neuropsychology, 4,* 275–281.

Alberico, A., Ward, J., Choi, S., Marmarou, A., & Young, H. (1987). Outcome after severe head injury; relationship to mass lesions, diffuse injury and ICP course in pediatric and adult patients. *Journal of Neurosurgery, 67,* 648–656.

Albert, M. (1996). Cognitive and neurobiologic markers of early Alzheimer's disease. *Proceedings of the National Academy of Sciences, 93,* 13547–13551.

Albert, M., Butters, N., & Brandt, J. (1980). Memory for remote events in alcoholics. *Journal of Studies on Alcohol, 41,* 1071–1081.

Albert, M., Butters, N., & Brandt, J. (1981). Development of remote memory loss in patients with Huntington's disease. *Journal of Clinical Neuropsychology, 3,* 1–12.

Albert, M., Butters, N., & Levin, J. (1979). Temporal gradients in the retrograde amnesia of patients with alcoholic Korsakoff disease. *Archives of Neurology, 36,* 211–216.

Albert, M., Feldman, R., & Willis, A. (1974). The subcortical dementia of progressive supranuclear palsy. *Journal of Neurology, Neurosurgery and Psychiatry, 37,* 121–130.

Alexander, G., DeLong, M., & Strick, P. (1986). Parallel organization of functionally segregated circuits linking basal ganglia and cortex. *Annual Review of Neuroscience, 9,* 357–381.

Alexander, G., Furey, M., Grady, C., Pietrini, P., Brady, D., Mentis, M., & Schapiro, M. (1997). Association of premorbid intellectual function with cerebral metabolism in Alzheimer's disease: Implications for the cognitive reserve hypothesis. *American Journal of Psychiatry, 154,* 165–172.

Alexander, G.E., Crutcher, M.D., & DeLong, M.R. (1990). Basal ganglia-thalamocortical circuits: Parallel substrates for motor, oculomotor, "prefrontal" and "limbic" functions. In H.B.M. Uylings, C.G. Van Eden, J.P.C. De Bruin, M.A. Corner, & M.G.P. Feenstra (Eds.), *Progress in Brain Research.* New York: Elsevier Science Publishers.

Alexopoulos, G., Meyers, B., Young, R., Mattis, S., & Kakuma, T. (1993a). The course of geriatric depression with "reversible dementia": A controlled study. *American Journal of Psychiatry, 150,* 1693–1699.

Alexopoulos, G., Young, R., & Meyers, B. (1993b). Geriatric depression: Age of onset and dementia. *Biological Psychiatry, 34,* 141–145.

Allegri, R., Mangone, C., Villavicencio, A., Rymberg, S., Taragano, F., & Baumann, D. (1997). Spanish Boston Naming Test norms. *Clinical Neuropsychologist, 11,* 416–420.

Alzheimer's Disease and Related Dementias Guideline Panel. (1996). *Recognition and Initial Assessment of Alzheimer's Disease and Related Dementias.* (Vol. 19). Rockville, MD: U.S. Department of Health and Human Services. AHCPR Publication No. 97–0702.

Amaducci, L., Fratiglioni, L., Rocca, W., Fieschi, C., Livrea, P., Pedone, D., Bracco, L., Lippi, A., Gandolfo, C., & Bino, G. (1986). Risk factors for clinically diagnosed Alzheimer's disease: A case-control study of an Italian population. *Neurology, 36,* 922–931.

American Psychiatric Association. (1990). *Benzodiazepine Dependence, Toxicity and Abuse. A Task Force Report of the American Psychiatric Association.* Washington, DC: American Psychiatric Association.

American Psychiatric Association. (1994). *Diagnostic Criteria from DSM-IV.* Washington, D.C.: American Psychiatric Association.

American Psychological Association. (1989). Guidelines regarding the use of nondoctoral personnel in clinical neuropsychological assessment. *The Clinical Neuropsychologist, 3,* 23–24.

American Psychological Association. (1991). Recommendations for education and training of nondoctoral personnel in clinical neuropsychology. *The Clinical Neuropsychologist, 5,* 20–23.

American Psychological Association. (1992). Ethical principles of psychologist and code of conduct. *American Psychologist, 47,* 1597–1611.

Anastasi, A., & Urbina, S. (1997). *Psychological Testing* (7th ed.). Upper Saddle River, NJ: Prentice-Hall.

Anderson, S., Damasio, H., Jones, R., & Tranel, D. (1991). Wisconsin Card Sorting Test Performance as a measure of frontal lobe damage. *Journal of Clinical and Experimental Neuropsychology, 13,* 909–922.

Appelbaum, P., & Grisso, T. (1988). Assessing patients' capacities to consent to treatment. *New England Journal of Medicine, 319,* 1635–1638.

Army Individual Test Battery. (1944). Washington, DC: War Department, Adjutant General's Office.

Artiola i Fortuny, L., & Heaton, R.K. (1996). Standard versus computerized version of the Wisconsin Card Sorting Test. *The Clinical Neuropsychologist, 10,* 419–424.

Artman, H., Gall, M., Hacker, H., & Herrlich, J. (1981). Reverible enlargement of cerebral spinal fluid spaces in chronic alcoholics. *American Journal of Neuroradiology, 2,* 23–27.

Atkinson, R., & Shiffrin, R. (1968). Human memory: A proposed system and its control processes. In K. Spence & J. Spence (Eds.), *The Psychology of Learning and Motivation (Vol. 2)* (pp. 89–195). Orlando: Academic Press.

Atkinson, R., & Shiffrin, R. (1971). The control of short-term memory. *Scientific American, 225,* 82–90.

Atkinson, R., Tolson, R., & Truner, J. (1990). Late versus early onset problem drinking in older men. *Alcoholism: Clinical and Experimental Research, 14,* 574–579.

Auchus, A.P., Goldstein, F.C., Green, J., & Green, R.C. (1994). Unawareness of cognitive impairments in Alzheimer's disease. *Neuropsychiatry, Neuropsychology, and Behavioral Neurology, 7,* 25–29.

Auchus, A.P., Goldstein, F.C., & Green, R.C. (1992). Unawareness of cognitive impairments in Alzheimer's disease. *Neurology, 42*(Suppl 3), 224.

Auriacombe, S., Grossman, M., Carvell, S., Gollomp, S., Stern, M., & Hurtig, H. (1993). Verbal fluency deficits in PD. *Neuropsychology, 2,* 182–192.

Avery, D., & Silverman, J. (1984). Psychomotor retardation and agitation in depression: relationship to age, sex and response to treatment. *Journal of Affective Disorders, 7,* 67–76.

Axelrod, B., Henry, R., & Woodard, J. (1992). Analysis of the abbreviated form of the Wisconsin Card Sorting Test. *The Clinical Neuropsychologist, 6,* 27–31.

Axelrod, B., Jiron, C., & Henry, R. (1993). Performance of adults ages 20 to 90 on the abbreviated Wisconsin Card Sorting Test. *The Clinical Neuropsychologist, 7,* 205–209.

Babikian, V., & Ropper, A. (1987). Binswanger's disease: A review. *Stroke, 18,* 2–12.

Baddeley, A. (1986). *Working Memory.* Oxford: Oxford University Press.

Baddeley, A., & Hitch, G. (1974). Working memory. In G. Bower (Ed.), *The Psychology of Learning and Motivation* (Vol. 8, pp. 47–90). San Diego: Academic Press.

Baddeley, A., & Weiskrantz, L. (Eds.). (1993). *Attention: Selection, Awareness and Arousal: A Tribute to Donald Broadbent.* New York: Oxford University Press.

Baldini, I., Vita, A., Mauri, M., Amodei, V., Carrisi, M., Bravin, S., & Cantalamessa, L. (1997). Psychopathological and cognitive features in subclinical hypothyroidism. *Progress in Neuro-Psychopharmacology and Biological Psychiatry, 21,* 925–935.

Barbarotto, R., DeSantis, A., Laiacona, M., Basso, A., Spagnoli, D., & Capitani, E. (1989). Neuropsychological follow-up of patients operated for aneurysms of the middle cerebral artery and posterior communicating artery. *Cortex, 25,* 275–288.

Barona, A., Reynolds, C., & Chastain, R. (1984). A demographically-based index of premorbid intelligence for the WAIS-R. *Journal of Consulting and Clinical Psychology, 52,* 885–887.

Barr, A., Benedict, R., Tune, L., & Brandt, J. (1992). Neuropsychological differentiation of Alzheimer's disease from vascular dementia. *International Journal of Geriatric Psychiatry, 7,* 621–627.

Barr, A., & Brandt, J. (1996). Word-list generation deficits in dementia. *Journal of Clinical and Experimental Neuropsychology, 18,* 810–822.

Baum, C., Kennedy, P., & Forbes, M. (1984). Drug use in the United States in 1981. *Journal of the American Medical Association, 241,* 1293.

Baxter, L.J., Schwartz, J., Phelps, M., Mazziota, J., Guze, B., Selin, C., Gerner, R., & Sumida, R. (1989). Reduction of prefrontal cortex glucose metabolism common to three types of depression. *Archives of General Psychiatry, 46,* 243–250.

Bayles, K. (1991). Age at onset of Alzheimer's disease: Relation to language dysfunction. *Archives of Neurology, 48,* 155–159.

Bayles, K., Trosset, M., Tomoeda, C., Montgomery, E., Jr, & Wilson, J. (1993). Generative naming in Parkinson disease patients. *Journal of Clinical and Experimental Neuropsychology, 15,* 547–562.

Beatty, W., Salmon, D., Butters, N., Heindel, W., & Granholm, E. (1988). Retrograde amnesia in patients with Alzheimer's disease or Huntington's disease. *Neurobiology of Aging, 9,* 181–186.

Beatty, W., Staton, R., Weir, W., Monson, N., & Whitaker, H. (1989). Cognitive disturbances in Parkinson's disease. *Journal of Geriatric Psychiatry and Neurology, 2,* 22–33.

Beck, A., & Steer, R. (1990). *Beck Anxiety Inventory.* San Antonio, Texas: The Psychological Corporation.

Beck, A., Ward, C., Mendelson, M., Mock, J., & Erbaugh, J. (1961). An inventory for measuring depression. *Archives of General Psychiatry, 4,* 561–571.

Becker, J., Hubb, F., Nebes, R., Holland, A., & Boller, F. (1988). Neuropsychological function in Alzheimer's disease: Pattern of impairment and rates of progression. *Archives of Neurology, 45,* 263–268.

Benson, D., & Cummings, J. (1982). Angular gyrus syndrome simulating Alzheimer's disease. *Archives of Neurology, 39,* 616–620.

Benton, A. (1992). Gerstmann's syndrome. *Archives of Neurology, 49,* 445–447.

Benton, A., & Hamsher, K. (1989). *Multilingual Aphasia Examination.* Iowa City, Iowa: AJA Associates.

Benton, A., Hamsher, K., Varney, N., & Spreen, O. (1983). *Contributions to Neuropsychological Assessment.* New York: Oxford University Press.

Benton, A., & Tranel, D. (1993). Visuoperceptual, visuospatial and visuoconstructive disorders. In K. Heilman & E. Valenstein (Eds.), *Clinical Neuropsychology* (3rd ed., pp. 168–214). New York: Oxford University Press.

Ben-Yishay, Y., Diller, L., Mandleberg, I., Gordon, W., & Gerstman, L. (1971). Similarities and differences in block design performance between older normal and brain-injured persons: A task analysis. *Journal of Abnormal Psychology, 78,* 17–25.

Berent, S., Giordani, B., Gilman, S., Junck, L., Lehtinen, S., Markel, D., Boivin, M., Kluin, K., Parks, R., & Koeppe, R. (1990). Neuropsychological changes in olivopontocerebellar atrophy. *Archives of Neurology, 47,* 997–1001.

Berg, E. (1948). A simple objective technique for measuring flexibility in thinking. *Journal of General Psychology, 39,* 15–22.

Berg, L., Danziger, W., Storandt, M., Coben, L., Gado, M., Hughes, C., Knesevich, J., & Botwinick, J. (1984). Predictive features in mild senile dementia of the Alzheimer type. *Neurology, 34,* 563–569.

Bergman, H., Borg, S., Hindmarsh, T., Idestrom, C., & Mutzell, S. (1980). Computed tomography of the brain and neuropsychological assessment of male alcoholic patients and a random sample from the general male population. *Acta Psychiatrica Scandinavica, 286 (Suppl.),* 77–88.

Berman, K., Ostrem, J., Randolph, C., Gold, J., Goldberg, T., Coppola, R., Carson, R., Herscovitch, P., & Weinberger, D. (1995). Physiological activation of a cortical network during performance of the Wisconsin Card Sorting Test: A positron emission study. *Neuropsychologia, 33,* 1027–1046.

Bieliauskas, L. (1993). Depressed or not depressed? That is the question. *Journal of Clinical and Experimental Neuropsychology, 15,* 119–134.

Biggens, C., Boyd, J., Harrop, F., Madeley, P., Mindham, R., Randall, J., & Spokes, E. (1992). A controlled, longitudinal study of dementia in Parkinson's disease. *Journal of Neurology, Neurosurgery, and Psychiatry, 55,* 566–571.

Bigler, E. (1988). Frontal lobe damage and neuropsychological assessment. *Archives of Clinical Neuropsychology, 3,* 279–297.

Black, F. (1986). Digit repetition in brain-damaged adults: Clinical and theoretical implications. *Journal of Clinical Psychology, 42,* 770–782.

Black, F., & Strub, R. (1976). Constructional apraxia in patients with discrete missile wounds. *Cortex, 12,* 212–220.

Black, P. (1980). Idiopathic normal-pressure hydrocephalus. Results of shunting in 62 patients. *Journal of Neurosurgery, 52,* 371–377.

Black, P., Ojemann, R., & Tzouras, A. (1985). CSF shunts for dementia, incontinence, and gait disturbance. *Clinical Neurosurgery, 32,* 632–656.

Blacker, D., Haines, J., Rodes, L., Terwedow, H., Go, R., Harrell, L., Perry, R., Bassett, S., Chase, G., Meyers, D., Albert, M., & Ranzi, R. (1997). ApoE-4 and age at onset of Alzheimer's disease: The NIMH genetics initiative. *Neurology, 48,* 139–147.

Blair, J., & Spreen, O. (1989). Predicting premorbid IQ: A revision of the National Adult Reading Test. *The Clinical Neuropsychologist, 3,* 129–136.

Blansjaar, B., & van Dijk, J. (1992). Korsakoff minus Wernicke syndrome. *Alcohol and Alcoholism, 27,* 435–437.

Blazer, D. (1993). *Depression in Late Life.* (2nd ed.). St. Louis: CV Mosby.

Block, R., DeVoe, M., Stanley, B., Staley, M., & Pomara, N. (1985). Memory performance in individuals with primary degenerative dementia: Its similarity to diazepam-induced impairments. *Experimental Aging Research, 11,* 151–155.

Blonder, L., Gur, R., Gur, R., Saykin, A., & Hurtig, H. (1989). Neuropsychological functioning in hemiparkinsonism. *Brain and Cognition, 9,* 244–257.

Bodis-Wollner, I., Marx, M., Mitra, M., Bobak, P., Mylin, L., & Yahr, M. (1987). Visual dysfunction in Parkinson's disease. *Brain, 110,* 1675–1698.

Bogen, J. (1993). The callosal syndrome. In K. Heilman & C. Valenstein (Eds.), *Clinical Neuropsychology.* New York: Oxford University Press.

Bokura, H., & Robinson, R. (1997). Long-term cognitive impairment associated with caudate stroke. *Stroke, 28,* 970–975.

Bolla, K., Lindgren, K., Bonaccorsy, C., & Bleecker, M. (1990). Predictions of verbal fluency (FAS) in the healthy elderly. *Journal of Clinical Psychology, 46,* 623–628.

Bolla-Wilson, K., Robinson, R., Starkstein, S., Boston, J., & Price, T. (1989). Lateralization of dementia of depression in stroke patients. *American Journal of Psychiatry, 146,* 627–634.

Boller, F., Mizutani, T., Roessmann, U., & Gambetti, P. (1980). Parkinson's disease, dementia and Alzheimer's disease: Clinicopathologic correlations. *Annals of Neurology, 7,* 329–335.

Bondareff, W., Mountjoy, C., & Roth, M. (1982). Loss of neurons of origin of the adrenergic projection to cerebral cortex (nucleus locus ceruleus) in senile dementia. *Neurology, 32,* 164–167.

Bondi, M., & Kaszniak, A. (1991). Implicit and explicit memory in Alzheimer's disease and Parkinson's disease. *Journal of Clinical and Experimental Neuropsychology, 13,* 339–358.

Bondi, M., Kaszniak, A., Bayles, K., & Vance, K. (1993). Contributions of frontal system dysfunction to memory and perceptual abilities in Parkinson's disease. *Neuropsychology, 7,* 89–102.

Bondi, M., Salmon, D., Monsch, A., Galasko, D., Butters, N., Klauber, M., Thal, L., & Saitoh, T. (1995). Episodic memory changes are associated with the ApoE-e4 allele in nondemented older adults. *Neurology, 45,* 2203–2206.

Boone, K., Lesser, I., Miller, B., Wohl, M., Berman, N., Lee, A., Palmer, B., & Black, D. (1995). Cognitive functioning in older depressed outpatients: Relationship of presence and severity of depression to neuropsychological test scores. *Neuropsychology, 9,* 390–398.

Boone, K., Miller, B., Lesser, I., Mehringer, C., Hill-Gutierrez, E., Goldberg, M., & Berman, N. (1992). Neuropsychological correlates of white-matter lesions in healthy, elderly subjects. A threshold effect. *Archives of Neurology, 49,* 549–554.

Bornstein, R. (1986). Contributions of various neuropsychological measures to detection of frontal lobe impairment. *International Journal of Clinical Neuropsychology, 8,* 18–22.

Bornstein, R., & Suga, L. (1988). Educational level and neuropsychological performance in healthy elderly subjects. *Developmental Neuropsychology, 4,* 17–22.

Bornstein, R., Weir, B., Petruk, K., & Disney, L. (1987). Neuropsychological function in patients after subarachnoid hemorrhage. *Neurosurgery, 21,* 651–654.

Bowden, S. (1990). Separating cognitive impairment in neurologically asymptomatic alcoholism from Wernicke-Korsakoff syndrome: Is the neuropsychological distinction justified? *Psychological Bulletin, 107,* 355–366.

Bradshaw, J., & Nettleton, N. (1983). *Human Cerebral Asymmetry.* Englewood Cliffs, NJ: Prentice-Hall, Inc.

Brandt, J. (1985). Access to knowledge in the dementia of Huntington's disease. *Developmental Neuropsychology, 1,* 335–348.

Brandt, J., & Butters, N. (1996). Neuropsychological characteristics of Huntington's disease. In I. Grant & K. Adams (Eds.), *Neuropsychological Assessment of Neuropsychiatric Disorders* (pp. 312–341). New York: Oxford University Press.

Brandt, J., Butters, N., Ryan, C., & Bayog, R. (1983). Cognitive loss and recovery in long-term alcohol abusers. *Archives of General Psychiatry, 40,* 435–442.

Brandt, J., Bylsma, F., Gross, R., Stine, O., Ranen, N., & Ross, C. (1996). Trinucleotide repeat length and clinical progression in Huntington's disease. *Neurology, 46,* 527–531.

Breen, E. (1993). Recall and recognition in Parkinson's disease. *Cortex, 29,* 91–102.

Breitner, J.C.S., Silverman, J.M., Mohs, R.C., & Davis, K.L. (1988). Familial aggregation in Alzheimer's disease: Comparison of risk among relatives of early- and late-onset cases and among male and female relatives in successive generations. *Neurology, 38,* 207–212.

Bremer, B., Wert, K., Durica, A., & Weaver, A. (1997). Neuropsychological, physical and psychosocial functioning of individuals with end-stage renal disease. *Annals of Behavioral Medicine, 19,* 348–352.

Breteler, M., Van Amerongen, N., Van Swieten, J., Claus, J., Grobbee, D., Van Gijn, J., Hofman, A., & Van Harskamp, F. (1994). Cognitive correlates of ventricular enlargement and cerebral white matter lesions on magnetic resonance imaging: The Rotterdam study. *Stroke, 25,* 1109–1115.

Brodaty, H., & Moore, C. (1997). The Clock Drawing Test for dementia of the Alzheimer's type: A comparison of three scoring methods in a memory disorders clinic. *International Journal of Geriatric Psychiatry, 12,* 619–627.

Brouwers, P., Cox, C., Marin, A., Chase, T., & Fedio, T. (1984). Differential perceptual-spatial impairment in Huntington's and Alzheimer's dementia. *Archives of Neurology, 41,* 1073–1076.

Brower, K., Mudd, S., Blow, F., Young, J., & Hill, E. (1994). Severity and treatment of alcohol withdrawal in elderly individuals versus younger patients. *Alcoholism: Clinical and Experimental Research, 18,* 196–201.

Brown, G., & Bornstein, R. (1991). Anatomic imaging methods for neurobehavioral studies. In R. Bornstein & G. Brown (Eds.), *Neurobehavioral Aspects of Cerebrovascular Disease* (pp. 83–108). New York: Oxford University Press.

Brown, G., Spicer, K., Robertson, W., Baird, A., & Malik, G. (1989). Neuropsychological signs of lateralized arteriovenous malformations: Comparison with ischemic stroke. *The Clinical Neuropsychologist, 3,* 340–352.

Brown, R., Crane, A., & Goldman, P. (1979). Regional distribution of monoamines in the cerebral cortex and subcortical structures of the rhesus monkey: concentrations and in vitro synthesis rates. *Brain, 168,* 133–150.

Brown, R., & Marsden, C. (1991). Dual task performance and processing resources in normal subjects and patients with Parkinson's disease. *Brain, 114,* 215–231.

Brun, A. (1987). Frontal lobe degeneration of the non-Alzheimer type. I., Neuropathology. *Archives of Gerontology and Geriatrics, 6,* 193–208.

Brun, A., Englund, B., Gustafson, L., Passant, U., Mann, D., Neary, D., & Snowden, J: (1994). Clinical and neuropathological criteria for frontotemporal dementia. *Journal of Neurology, Neurosurgery, and Psychiatry, 57,* 416–418.

Buffett-Jerrott, S., Stewart, S., & Teehan, M. (1998). A further examination of the time-dependent effects of oxazepam and lorazepam on implicit and explicit memory. *Psychopharmacology, 138,* 344–353.

Burke, W., Roccaforte, W., Wengel, S., McArthur-Miller, D., Folks, D., & Potter, J. (1998). Disagreement in the reporting of depressive symptoms between patients with dementia of the Alzheimer type and their collateral sources. *American Journal of Geriatric Psychiatry, 6,* 308–319.

Burt, D., Zembar, M., & Niederehe, G. (1995). Depression and memory impairment: A meta-analysis of the association, its pattern and specificity. *Psychological Bulletin, 117,* 285–305.

Butters, M., Lopez, O., & Becker, J. (1996). Focal temporal lobe dysfunction in probable Alzheimer's disease predicts a slow rate of cognitive decline. *Neurology, 46,* 687–692.

Butters, N., & Cermak, L. (1980). *Alcoholic Korsakoff's Syndrome.* New York: Academic Press.

Butters, N., Granholm, E., Salmon, D., Grant, I., & Wolfe, J. (1987). Episodic and semantic memory: A comparison of amnesic and demented patients. *Journal of Clinical and Experimental Neuropsychology, 9,* 479–497.

Butters, N., Sax, D., Montgomery, K., & Tarlow, S. (1978). Comparison of the neuropsychological deficits associated with early and advanced Huntington's disease. *Archives of Neurology, 35,* 585–589.

Butters, N., Wolfe, J., Granholm, E., & Martone, M. (1986). An assessment of verbal recall, recognition and fluency abilities in patients with Huntington's disease. *Cortex, 22,* 11–32.

Butters, N., Wolfe, J., Marone, M., Granholm, E., & Cermak, L. (1985). Memory disorders associated with Huntington's disease: Verbal recall, verbal recognition, and procedural memory. *Neuropsychologia, 23,* 729–743.

Buytenhuijs, E., Berger, H., Van Spaendonck, K., Horstink, M., Borm, G., & Cools, A. (1994). Memory and learning strategies in patients with Parkinson's disease. *Neuropsychologia, 32,* 335–342.

Bylsma, F. (1997). Huntington's disease. In P. Nussbaum (Ed.), *Handbook of Neuropsychology and Aging* (pp. 246–259). New York: Plenum Press.

Bylsma, F., Brandt, J., & Strauss, M. (1990). Aspects of procedural memory are differentially impaired in Huntington's disease. *Archives of Clinical Neuropsychology, 5,* 287–297.

Cahn, D., & Kaplan, E. (1997). Clock drawing in the oldest old. *The Clinical Neuropsychologist, 11,* 96–100.

Cahn, D., Salmon, D., Butters, N., Wiederholt, W., Corey-Bloom, J., Edelstein, S., & Barrett-Connor, E. (1995). Detection of dementia of the Alzheimer type in a population-based sample: Neuropsychological test performance. *Journal of the International Neuropsychological Society, 1,* 252–260.

Cahn, D., Salmon, D., Monsch, A., Butters, N., Wiederholt, W., Corey-Bloom, J., & Barrett-Conner, E. (1996). Screening for dementia of the Alzheimer type in the community: The utility of the Clock Drawing Test. *Archives of Clinical Neuropsychology, 11,* 529–539.

Caine, E., Lyness, J., & King, D. (1993). Reconsidering depression in the elderly. *The American Journal of Geriatric Psychiatry, 1,* 4–20.

Calev, A., Nigal, D., Shapira, B., Tubi, N., Chazan, S., Ben-Yehuda, Y., Kugelmass, S., & Lerer, B. (1991). Early and long-term effects of electroconvulsive therapy on memory and other cognitive functions. *Journal of Nervous and Mental Disease, 179,* 526–533.

Caltagirone, C., Carlesimo, A., Nocentini, U., & Vicari, S. (1989). Defective concept formation in parkinsonians is independent from mental deterioration. *Journal of Neurology, Neurosurgery and Psychiatry, 52,* 334–337.

Caltagirone, C., Gainotti, G., Masullo, C., & Villa, E. (1982). Neurophysiological study of normal pressure hydrocephalus. *Acta Psychiatrica Scandinavica, 63,* 93–100.

Canavan, A., Passingham, R., Marsden, C., Quinn, N., Wyke, M., & Polkey, C. (1989). The performance on learning tasks of patients in the early stages of Parkinson's disease. *Neuropsychologia, 27,* 141–156.

Caparros-Lefebvre, D., Pecheux, N., Petit, V., Duharnel, A., & Petit, H. (1995). Which factors predict cognitive decline in Parkinson's disease. *Journal of Neurology, Neurosurgery, and Psychiatry, 58,* 51–55.

Caplan, B. (1985). Stimulus effects in unilateral neglect. *Cortex, 21,* 69–80.

Caplan, L., Schmahmann, J., Kase, C., Feldmann, E., Baquis, G., Greenberg, J., Gorelick, P., Helgason, C., & Hier, D. (1990). Caudate infarcts. *Archives of Neurology, 47,* 133–143.

Carlen, P., Wortzman, G., Holgate, R., Wilkinson, D., & Rankin, J. (1978). Reversible cerebral atrophy in recently abstinent chronic alcoholics measured by computed tomography scans. *Science, 200,* 1076–1078.

Castillo, C., Starkstein, S., Fedoroff, J., Price, T., & Robinson, R. (1993). Generalized anxiety disorder following stroke. *Journal of Nervous and Mental Disorders, 181,* 100–106.

Cercy, S., & Bylsma, F. (1997). Lewy bodies and progressive dementia: A critical review and meta-analysis. *Journal of the International Neuropsychological Society, 3,* 179–194.

Chan, A., Salmon, D., Butters, N., & Johnson, S. (1995). Semantic network abnormality predicts rate of cognitive decline in patients with probable Alzheimer's disease. *Journal of the International Neuropsychological Society, 1,* 297–303.

Chan, W., Pristach, E., Welte, J., & Russell, M. (1993). Use of the TWEAK test in screening for heavy drinking in three populations. *Alcoholism: Clinical and Experimental Research, 17,* 1188–1192.

Chase, T., Fedio, P., Foster, N., Brooks, R., DiChiro, G., & Mansi, L. (1984). Wechsler Adult Intelligence Scale performance. Cortical localization by fluorodeoxyglucose F18–positron emission tomography. *Archives of Neurology, 41,* 1244–1247.

Chawluk, J., Mesulam, M.-M., Hurtig, H., Kushner, M., Weintraub, S., Saykin, A., Rubin, N., Alavi, A., & Reivich, M. (1986). Slowly progressive aphasia without generalized dementia: Studies with positron emission tomography. *Annals of Neurology, 19,* 68–74.

Chelune, G., & Bornstein, R. (1988). WMS-R patterns among patients with unilateral brain lesions. *The Clinical Neuropsychologist, 2,* 121–132.

Chui, H., Lyness, S., Sobel, E., & Schneider, L. (1994). Extrapyramidal signs and psychiatric symptoms predict faster cognitive decline in Alzheimer's disease. *Archives of Neurology, 51,* 676–681.

Chui, H., Teng, E., Henderson, V., & Moy, A. (1985). Clinical subtypes of dementia of the Alzheimer type. *Neurology, 35,* 1544–1550.

Chui, H., Victoroff, J., Margolin, D., Jagust, W., Shankle, R., & Katzman, R. (1992). Criteria for the diagnosis of ischemic vascular dementia proposed by the State of California Alzheimer's Disease Diagnostic and Treatment Centers. *Neurology, 42,* 473–480.

Clarfield, A. (1989). Normal pressure hydrocephalus: Saga or swamp? *Journal of the American Medical Association, 262,* 2592–2593.

Coblentz, J., Mattis, S., Zingesser, L., Kasoff, S., Wisniewski, H., & Katzman, R. (1973). Presenile dementia: Clinical aspects and evaluation of cerebrospinal fluid dynamics. *Archives of Neurology, 29,* 299–308.

Codori, A., & Brandt, J. (1994). Psychological costs and benefits of predictive testing for Huntington's disease. *American Journal of Medical Genetics (Neuropsychiatric Genetics), 54,* 174–184.

Coffey, C., Figiel, G., Djang, W., & Weiner, R. (1990). Subcortical hyperintensity on magnetic resonance imaging: A comparison of normal and depressed elderly subjects. *American Journal of Psychiatry, 147,* 187–189.

Cole, A. (1992). A survey of frontal lobe dementia in a psychogeriatric day unit population. *International Journal of Geriatric Psychiatry, 7,* 731–738.

Coleman, E., Sackheim, H., Prudic, J., Devanand, D., McElhiney, M., & Moody, B. (1996). Subjective memory complaints prior to and following electroconvulsive therapy. *Biological Psychiatry, 39,* 346–356.

Colombo, A., Sorgato, P., & Scarpa, M. (1989). Language disturbances following vascular lesions restricted to the left basal ganglia, thalamus and white matter. *Neuropsychology, 3,* 75–80.

Colwell, J., Lopes-Virella, M., & Halushka, P. (1981). Pathogenesis of atherosclerosis in diabetes mellitus. *Diabetes Care, 4,* 121–129.

Conneally, P. (1984). Huntington's disease: genetics and epidemiology. *American Journal of Human Genetics, 36,* 506–526.

Connors, G. (1995). Screening for alcohol problems. In J. Allen & M. Columbus (Eds.), *Assessing Alcohol Problems: A Guide for Clinicians and Researchers* (pp. 17–29). Bethesda, MD: National Institute on Alcohol Abuse and Alcoholism. NIH publication 95–3745.

Cooper, J., & Sagar, H. (1993a). Encoding deficits in untreated Parkinson's disease. *Cortex, 1993,* 251–265.

Cooper, J., & Sagar, H. (1993b). Incidental and intentional recall in Parkinson's disease: An account based on diminished attentional resources. *Journal of Experimental and Clinical Neuropsychology, 15,* 713–731.

Cooper, J., Sagar, H., Doherty, S., Jordan, N., Tidswell, P., & Sullivan, E. (1992). Different effects of dopaminergic and anticholinergic therapies on cognitive and motor function in Parkinson's disease: A follow-up study of untreated patients. *Brain, 115,* 1701–1725.

Cooper, J., Sagar, H., Jordan, N., Harvey, N., & Sullivan, E. (1991). Cognitive impairment in early, untreated Parkinson's disease and its relationship to motor disability. *Brain, 114,* 2095–2122.

Cooper, J., Sagar, H., Tidswell, P., & Jordan, N. (1994). Slowed central processing in simple and go/no-go reaction time tasks in Parkinson's disease. *Brain, 117,* 517–529.

Corder, E.H., Saunders, A.M., Strittmatter, W.J., Schmechel, D.E., Gaskell, P.C., Small, G.W., Roses, A.D., Haines, J.L., & Pericak-Vance, M.A. (1993). Gene dose of apolipoprotein E type 4 allele and the risk of Alzheimer's disease in late onset families. *Science, 261,* 921–923.

Corkin, S. (1984). Last consequences of medial temporal lobectomy: Clinical cause and experimental findings in H.M. *Seminars in Neurology, 4,* 249–259.

Cornford, M., Chang, L., & Miller, B. (1995). The neuropathology of parkinsonism: An overview. *Brain and Cognition, 28,* 321–341.

Costa, L. (1975). The relationship of visuospatial dysfunction to digit span performance in patients with cerebral lesions. *Cortex, 11,* 31–36.

Costa, L. (1988). Clinical neuropsychology: prospects and problems. *The Clinical Neuropsychologist, 2,* 3–11.

Costa, P.J., Williams, T., Albert, M., Butters, N., Folstein, M., Gilman, S., Gurland, B., Gwyther, L., Heyman, A., Kaszniak, A., Katz, I., Levy, L., Lombardo, N., Orr-Rainey, N., Phillips, L., Storandt, M., Tangalos, E., & Wykle, M. (1996). *Recognition and Initial Assessment of Alzheimer's Disease and Related Dementias. Clinical Practice Guideline No. 19.* Rockville, MD. US Department of Health and Human Services, Public Health Service, Agency for Health Care Policy and Research. AHCPR Publication No. 97–0702.

Costello, A.D.L., & Warrington, E. (1989). Dynamic aphasia: The selective impairment of verbal planning. *Cortex, 25,* 103–114.

Coyle, J., Price, D., & DeLong, M. (1983). Alzheimer's disease: A disorder of cortical cholinergic innervation. *Science, 219,* 1184–1190.

Craft, S., Teri, L., Edland, S., Kukull, W., Schellenberg, G., McCormick, W., Bowen, J., & Larson, E. (1998). Accelerated decline in apoliprotein E-e4 homozygotes with Alzheimer's disease. *Neurology, 51,* 149–153.

Craik, F., & Jennings, J. (1992). Human memory. In F. Craik & T. Salthouse (Eds.), *The Handbook of Aging and Cognition* (pp. 51–110). Hillsdale, NJ: Lawrence Erlbaum Associates.

Craik, F., & Lockhart, R. (1972). Levels of processing: A framework for memory research. *Journal of Verbal Learning and Verbal Behavior, 11,* 671–684.

Crawford, J., Moore, J., & Cameron, I. (1992). Verbal fluency: A NART-based equation for estimation of premorbid performance. *British Journal of Clinical Psychology, 31,* 327–329.

Crawford, J., Parker, D., Stewart, L., Besson, J., & DeLacey, G. (1989). Prediction of WAIS IQ with the National Adult Reading Test: Cross-validation and extension. *British Journal of Clinical Psychology, 28,* 267–273.

Cummings, J. (1990a). Introduction. In J. Cummings (Ed.), *Subcortical Dementia* (pp. 3–16). New York: Oxford University Press.

Cummings, J. (1990b). *Subcortical Dementia.* New York: Oxford University Press.

Cummings, J. (1992a). Depression and Parkinson's disease: A review. *American Journal of Psychiatry, 149,* 443–454.

Cummings, J. (1992b). Neuropsychiatric complications of drug treatment in Parkinson's disease. In S. Huber & J. Cummings (Eds.), *Parkinson's disease: Neurobehavioral aspects* (pp. 313–327). New York: Oxford University Press.

Cummings, J., & Benson, D. (1992a). *Dementia: A Clinical Approach.* Boston: Butterworth-Heinemann.

Cummings, J., & Benson, D. (1992b). Laboratory aids in the diagnosis of dementia. In J. Cummings & D. Benson (Eds.), *Dementia: A Clinical Approach* (2nd ed., pp. 345–364). Boston: Butterworth-Heinemann.

Cummings, J., & Benson, F. (1984). Subcortical dementia: Review of an emerging concept. *Archives of Neurology, 41,* 874–879.

Cummings, J., & Duchen, L. (1981). The Kluver-Bucy syndrome in Pick disease. *Neurology, 31,* 1415–1422.

Cummings, J., & Huber, S. (1992). Visuospatial abnormalities in Parkinson's disease. In S. Huber & J. Cummings (Eds.), *Parkinson's Disease: Neurobehavioral Aspects* (pp. 59–73). New York: Oxford University Press.

Cummings, J., Mega, M., Gray, K., Rosenberg-Thompson, S., Carusi, D., & Gornbein, J. (1994). The Neuropsychiatric Inventory: Comprehensive assessment of psychopathology in dementia. *Neurology, 44,* 2308–2314.

Cummings, J., Miller, B., Hill, M., & Neshkes, R. (1987). Neuropsychiatric aspects of multiinfarct dementia and dementia of the Alzheimer type. *Archives of Neurology, 44,* 389–393.

Cummings, J., & Victoroff, J. (1990). Noncognitive neuropsychiatric syndromes in Alzheimer's disease. *Neuropsychiatry, Neuropsychology and Behavioral Neurology, 3,* 140–158.

Cummings, J., Vinters, H., Cole, G., & Khachaturian, Z. (1998). Alzheimer's disease: Etiologies, pathophysiology, cognitive reserve, and treatment opportunities. *Neurology, 51 (Suppl.1),* S2–S17.

Curran, H. (1991). Benzodiazepines, memory and mood: A review. *Psychopharmacology, 105,* 1–8.

Curran, H., Pooviboonsuk, P., Dalton, J., & Lader, M. (1998). Differentiating the effects of centrally acting drugs on arousal and memory: An event-related potential study of scopolamine, lorazepam and diphenhydramine. *Psychopharmacology, 135,* 27–36.

Curran, H., Sakulsripring, M., & Lader, M. (1998). Antidepressants and human memory: An investigation of four drugs with different sedative and anticholinergic profiles. *Psychopharmacology, 95,* 520–527.

Cutting, J. (1978). The relationship between Korsakoff's syndrome and alcoholic dementia. *British Journal of Psychiatry, 132,* 240–251.

Damasio, A. (1995). The frontal lobes. In K. Heilman & E. Valenstein (Eds.), *Clinical Neuropsychology* (2nd ed., pp. 409–460). New York: Oxford University Press.

Damasio, A., Graff-Radford, N., Eslinger, P., & Damasio, H. (1985). Amnesia following basal forebrain lesions. *Archives of Neurology, 42,* 263–271.

Daniel, W., & Crovitz, H. (1986). Disorientation during electroconvulsive therapy: Technical, theoretical and neuropsychological issues. *Annals of the New York Academy of Science, 482,* 293–306.

Danielczyk, W. (1983). Various mental behavioral disorders in Parkinson's disease, primary degenerative senile dementia, and multiple infarction dementias. *Journal of Neural Transmission, 56,* 161–176.

Danion, J.-M., Zimmermann, M.-A., Willard-Schroeder, D., Grange, D., Welsch, M., Imbs, J., & Singer, L. (1990). Effects of scopolamine, trimipramine, diazepam on explicit memory and repetition priming in healthy volunteers. *Psychopharmacology, 102,* 422–424.

Dannenbaum, S., Parkinson, S., & Inman, V. (1988). Short-term forgetting: Comparison between patients with dementia of the Alzheimer type, depressed and normal elderly. *Cognitive Neuropsychology, 5,* 213–233.

Dejerine, J., & Thomas, A. (1900). L'atrophie olivo-ponto-cerebelleuse. *Novelle Iconographie Salpetriere, 13,* 330–370.

DeLacoste, M., & White, C., III (1993). The role of cortical connectivity in Alzheimer's disease pathogenesis: A review and model system. *Neurobiology of Aging, 14,* 1–16.

Delis, D., & Massman, P. (1992). The effects of dopamine fluctuation on cognition and affect. In S. Huber & J. Cummings (Eds.), *Parkinson's Disease: Neurobehavioral Aspects* (pp. 288–302). New York: Oxford University Press.

Delis, D., Massman, P., Butters, N., Salmon, D., Cermak, L., & Kramer, J. (1991). Profiles of demented and amnestic patients on the California Verbal Learning Test: Implications for assessment of memory disorders. *Psychological Assessment: A Journal of Consulting and Clinical Psychology, 3,* 19–26.

Della Sala, S., & Logie, R. (1993). When working memory does not work: The role of working memory in neuropsychology. In F. Boller & J. Grafman (Eds.), *Handbook of Neuropsychology* (Vol. 8, pp. 1–62). Amsterdam: Elsevier.

DeLuca, J. (1992). Cognitive dysfunction after aneurysm of the anterior communicating artery. *Journal of Clinical and Experimental Neuropsychology, 14,* 924–934.

Derogatis, L., & Spencer, P. (1982). *Administration and Procedures: Brief Symptom Checklist.* Baltimore: Johns Hopkins University Press.

DesRosiers, G., Hodges, J., & Berrios, B. (1995). The neuropsychological differentiation of patients with very mild Alzheimer's disease and/or major depression. *Journal of the American Geriatrics Society, 43,* 1256–1263.

Deutsch, G., Bourbon, W., Papanicolaou, A., & Eisenberg, H. (1988). Visuospatial tasks compared via activation of regional cerebral blood flow. *Neuropsychologia, 26,* 445–452.

Devanand, D., Sano, M., Tang, M.-X., Taylor, S., Gurland, B., Wilder, D., Stern, S., & Mayeux, R. (1996). Depressed mood and the incidence of Alzheimer's disease in the elderly living in the community. *Archives of General Psychiatry, 53,* 175–182.

Devanand, D., Verma, A., Tirumalasetti, F., & Sackheim, H. (1991). Absence of cognitive impairment after more than 100 lifetime ECT treatments. *American Journal of Psychiatry, 148,* 929–932.

Diaz, J., Merskey, H., Hachinski, V., Lee, D., Boniferro, M., Wong, C., Mirsen, R., & Fox, H. (1991). Improved recognition of leukoaraisosis and cognitive impairment in Alzheimer's disease. *Archives of Neurology, 48,* 1022–1025.

Ditter, S., & Mirra, S. (1987). Neuropathologic and clinical features of Parkinson's disease in Alzheimer's disease patients. *Neurology, 37,* 754–760.

Dom, R., Malfroid, M., & Baro, F. (1976). Neuropathology of Huntington's disease. *Neurology, 26,* 64–68.

Donaldson, A. (1979). CT scan in Alzheimer disease. In A. Glen & L. Whalley (Eds.), *Alzheimer's disease. Early recognition of potentially reversible deficits* (pp. 97–101). New York: Churchill Livingstone.

Doody, R., & Jankovic, J. (1992). The alien hand syndrome and related signs. *Journal of Neurology, Neurosurgery, and Psychiatry, 55,* 806–810.

Drachman, D., & Leavitt, J. (1974). Human memory and the cholinergic system. *Archives of Neurology, 30,* 113–124.

Draelos, M., Jacobson, A., Weinger, K., Widom, B., Ryan, C., Finkelstein, D., & Simonson, D. (1995). Cognitive function in patients with insulin-dependent diabetes mellitus during hyperglycemia and hypoglycemia. *American Journal of Medicine, 98,* 135–144.

Drewe, E. (1974). The effect of type and area of brain lesion on Wisconsin Card Sorting Test performance. *Cortex, 10,* 159–170.

Dubois, B., Pillon, B., Lhermitte, F., & Agid, Y. (1990a). Cholinergic deficiency and frontal dysfunction in Parkinson's disease. *Annals of Neurology, 28,* 117–121.

Dubois, B., Pillon, B., Sternic, N., Lhermitte, F., & Agid, Y. (1990b). Age-induced cognitive disturbances in Parkinson's disease. *Neurology, 40,* 38–41.

Dubois, B., Ruberg, M., Javoy-Agid, F., Ploska, A., & Agid, Y. (1983). A subcortical-cortical cholinergic system is affected in Parkinson's disease. *Brain Research, 288,* 213–221.

Dugbartey, A. (1998). Neurocognitive aspects of hypothyroidism. *Archives of Internal Medicine, 158,* 1413–1418.

Dunn, E., Searight, H., Grisso, T., Margolis, R., & Gibbons, J. (1990). The relation of the Halstead-Reitan Neuropsychological Battery to functional daily living skills in geriatric patients. *Archives of Clinical Neuropsychology, 5,* 103–117.

Duvoisin, R. (1986). Genetics of Parkinson's disease, *Advances in Neurology* (Vol. 45, pp. 307–312). New York: Raven Press.

Duyao, M., Ambrose, C., Myers, R., Novelletto, A., Persichetti, F., Frontali, M., Folstein, S., Ross, C., Franz, M., Abbott, M., Gray, J., Conneally, P., Young, A., Penney, J., Hollingsworth, Z., Shoulson, I., Lazzarinia, A., Falek, A., Koroshetz, W., Sax, D., Bird, E., Vonsattel, J., Bonilla, E., Alvir, J., Bickham Conde, J., Cha, J.-H., Dure, L., Gomez, F., Ramos, M., Sanchez-Ramos, J., Snodgrass, S., de Young, M., Wexler, N., Moscowitz, C., Penchaszadeh, G., MacFarlane, H., Anderson, M., Jenkins, B., Srinidhi, J., Barnes, G., Gusella, J., & MacDonald, M. (1993). Trinucleotide repeat length instability and age of onset in Huntington's disease. *Nature Genetics, 4,* 387–392.

Eckardt, M., & Martin, P. (1986). Clinical assessment of cognition in alcoholism. *Alcoholism: Clinical and Experimental Research, 10,* 123–127.

Eckardt, M., Stapleton, J., Rawlings, R., Davis, E., & Grodin, D. (1995). Neuropsychological functioning in detoxified alcoholics between 18 and 35. *American Journal of Psychiatry, 152,* 45–52.

Egelko, S., Gordon, W., Hibbard, M., Diller, L., Lieberman, A., Holliday, R., Ragnarsson, K., Shaver, M., & Orazem, J. (1988). Relationship between CT scans, neurological exam, and neuropsychological test performance in right brain-damaged stroke patients. *Journal of Clinical and Experimental Neuropsychology, 10,* 539–564.

Ellor, J., & Kurz, D. (1982). Misuse and abuse of prescription and nonprescription drugs by the elderly. *Nursing Clinics of North America, 17,* 319–330.

Erickson, R., Eimon, P., & Hebben, N. (1994). A bibliography of normative articles on cognitive tests for older adults. In M. Storandt & G. Vandenbos (Eds.), *Neuropsychological Assessment of Dementia and Depression in Older Adults: A Clinician's Guide.* Washington, DC: American Psychological Association.

Erkinjuntti, T., Sipponen, J., Iavanainen, M., Kotenen, L., Sulkava, R., & Sepponen, R. (1984). Cerebral NMR and CT imaging in dementia. *Journal of Computer Assisted Tomography, 8,* 614–618.

Erkinjuntti, T., Sulkava, R., Kovanen, J., & Palo, J. (1987). Suspected dementia: Evaluation of 323 consecutive referrals. *Acta Neurologica Scandanavia, 76,* 359–364.

Evans, D., Beckett, L., Field, T., Feng, L., Albert, M., Bennett, D., Tycko, B., & Mayeux, R. (1997). Apolipoprotein E epsilon 4 and incidence of Alzheimer's disease in a community population of older adults. *Journal of the American Medical Association, 277,* 822–824.

Evans, D., Funkenstein, H., Albert, M., Scherr, P., Cook, N., Chown, M., Hebert, L., Hennedens, C., & Taylor, J. (1989). Prevalence of Alzheimer's disease in a community population of older persons. Higher than previously reported. *Journal of the American Medical Association, 262,* 2551–2556.

Ewing, J. (1984). Detecting alcoholism: The CAGE questionnaire. *Journal of the American Medical Association, 252,* 1905–1907.

Eysenck, M. (1982). *Attention and Arousal.* New York: Springer-Verlag.

Faber, R., & Trimble, M. (1991). Electroconvulsive therapy in Parkinson's disease and other movement disorders. *Movement Disorders, 6,* 293–303.

Faber-Langendoen, K., Morris, J., Knesevich, J., LaBarge, E., Miller, J., & Berg, L. (1988). Aphasia in senile dementia of the Alzheimer type. *Annals of Neurology, 23,* 365–370.

Fabian, M., & Parsons, O. (1983). Differential improvement of cognitive functions in recovering alcoholic women. *Journal of Abnormal Psychology, 92,* 87–95.

Fahn, S. (1996). Is levodopa toxic? *Neurology, 47 (Suppl.),* S184–S195.

Fahn, S., & Elton, R., Members of the UPDRS Development Committee. (1987). Unified Parkinson's disease rating scale. In S. Fahn, C. Marsden, D. Calne, & M. Goldstein (Eds.), *Recent Developments in Parkinson's Disease* (Vol. 2, pp. 153–164). Florham Park, NJ: Macmillan Healthcare Information.

Farrer, L. (1986). Suicide and attempted suicide in Huntington's disease: Implications for preclinical testing of persons at risk. *American Journal of Medical Genetics, 24,* 305–311.

Farrer, L., Cupples, L., van Duijn, C., Kurz, A., Zimmer, R., Uller, U., Green, R., Clarke, V., Shoffner, J., Wallace, D., Chui, H., Flanagan, S., Duara, R., St.George-Hyslop, P., Auerback, S., Volicer, L., Wells, J., van Broeckhoven, C., Growdon, J., & Haines, J. (1995). Apolipoprotein E genotype in patients with Alzheimer's disease: Implications for the risk of dementia among relatives. *Annals of Neurology, 38,* 797–808.

Feher, E., Larrabee, G., & Crook, T.R. (1992). Factors attenuating the validity of the Geriatric Depression Scale in a dementia population. *Journal of the American Geriatrics Society, 40,* 906–909.

Feher, E.P., Mahurin, R.K., Inbody, S.B., Crook, T.H., & Pirozzolo, F.J. (1991). Anosognosia in Alzheimer's disease. *Neuropsychiatry, Neuropsychology, and Behavioral Neurology, 4*(2), 136–146.

Ferraro, F., & Bercier, B. (1996). Boston Naming Test performance in a sample of native American elderly adults. *Clinical Gerontologist, 17,* 58–60.

Ferrucci, L., Cecchi, F., Guralnik, J., Giampaoli, S., Lo Noce, C., Salani, B., Bandinelli, S., & Baroni, A. (1996). Does the Clock Drawing Test predict cognitive decline in older persons independent of the Mini-Mental State Examination? The FINE (Finland, Italy, the Netherlands Elderly) Study Group. *Journal of the American Geriatrics Society, 44,* 1326–1331.

Fields, R. (1994). *Traumatic brain injury in the elderly.* Paper presented at the National Academy of Neuropsychology, Dallas, Texas.

Fields, R. (1997). Geriatric head injury. In P. Nussbaum (Ed.), *Handbook of Neuropsychology and Aging* (pp. 280–297). New York: Plenum Press.

Figiel, G., Krishnan, K., Doraiswamy, P., Rao, V., Nemeroff, C., & Boyko, O. (1991). Subcortical hypointensities on brain magnetic resonance imaging: A comparison between late age onset and early onset elderly depressed subjects. *Neurobiology of Aging, 12,* 245–247.

Fillenbaum, G., Huber, M., & Taussig, I. (1997). Performance of elderly white and African-American community residents on the abbreviated CERAD Boston Naming Test. *Journal of Clinical and Experimental Neuropsychology, 19,* 204–210.

Fillenbaum, G., & Smyer, M. (1981). The development, validity, and reliability of the OARS Multidimensional Functional Assessment Questionnaire. *Journal of Gerontology, 36,* 428–434.

Filley, C., Kelly, J., & Heaton, R. (1986). Neuropsychologic features of early- and late-onset Alzheimer's disease. *Archives of Neurology, 43,* 574–576.

Fischer, P., Jellinger, K., Gatterbi, G., & Danielcyzk, W. (1991). Prospective neuropathological validation of Hachinski's Ischemia Score in dementias. *Journal of Neurology, Neurosurgery, and Psychiatry, 54,* 580–583.

Fisher, C. (1977). The clinical picture of occult hydrocephalus. *Clinical Neurosurgery, 24,* 270–284.

Fisher, C. (1982). Hydrocephalus as a cause of disturbances of gait in the elderly. *Neurology, 32,* 1358–1363.

Fisher, N., Rourke, B., Bieliauskas, L., Giordani, B., Berent, S., & Foster, N. (1996). Neuropsychological subgroups of Alzheimer's disease. *Journal of Clinical and Experimental Neuropsychology, 18,* 349–370.

Flashman, L., Horner, M., & Freides, D. (1991). Note on scoring perseveration on the Wisconsin Card Sorting Test. *The Clinical Neuropsychologist, 5,* 190–194.

Foelker, G., Jr., Schewchuk, R., & Niederehe, G. (1987). Confirmatory factor analysis of the short form Beck Depression Inventory in elderly community samples. *Journal of Clinical Psychology, 43,* 111–118.

Fogel, B., & Duffy, J. (1994). Elderly patients. In J. Silver, S. Yudofsky, & R. Hales (Eds.), *Neuropsychiatry of Traumatic Brain Injury* (pp. 412–441). Washington, DC: American Psychiatric Press.

Folstein, M., & McHugh, P. (1978). Dementia syndrome of depression. In R. Katzman, R. Terry, & K. Bick (Eds.), *Alzheimer's Disease, Senile Dementia and Related Disorders* (pp. 281–289). New York: Raven Press.

Folstein, S., Brandt, J., & Folstein, M. (1991). Huntington's disease. In J. Cummings (Ed.), *Subcortical Dementia* (pp. 87–107). New York: Oxford University Press.

Fontenot, D., & Benton, A. (1970). Perception of direction in the right and left visual fields. *Neuropsychologia, 10,* 447–452.

Fox, G., Bowden, S., Bashford, G., & Smith, D. (1997). Alzheimer's disease and driving: Prediction and assessment of driving performance. *Journal of the American Geriatrics Society, 45,* 949–953.

Franceschi, M., Cecchetto, R., Minicucci, F., Smirne, S., Baio, G., & Canal, N. (1984). Cognitive processes in insulin-dependent diabetes. *Diabetes Care, 7,* 228–231.

Frankowski, R. (1986). Descriptive epidemiologic studies of head injury in the United States: 1974–1984. *Advances in Psychosomatic Medicine, 16,* 153–172.

Franzen, M., Haut, M., Rankin, E., & Keefover, R. (1995). Empirical comparisons of alternate forms of the Boston Naming Test. *The Clinical Neuropsychologist, 9,* 225–229.

Freedman, M., Leach, L., Kaplan, E., Winocur, G., Shulman, K., & Delis, D. (1994). *Clock Drawing A Neuropsychological Analysis.* New York: Oxford University Press.

Freedman, M., Rivoira, P., Butters, N., Sax, D., & Feldman, R. (1984). Retrograde amnesia in Parkinson's disease. *Canadian Journal of Neurological Science, 11,* 297–301.

Freeman, C., Weeks, D., & Kendell R. (1980). ECT II: Patients who complain. *British Journal of Psychiatry, 137,* 17–25.

Freund, G., & Ballinger, W. (1991). Loss of synaptic receptors can precede morphological changes induced by alcoholism. *Alcohol and Alcoholism (Suppl), 1,* 385–391.

Friedland, R., Koss, E., Kumar, A., Gaine, S., Metzler, D., Haxby, J., & Moore, A. (1988). Motor vehicle crashes in dementia of the Alzheimer type. *Annals of Neurology, 24,* 782–786.

Frith, C., Friston, K., Liddle, P., & Frackowiak, R. (1991). A PET study of word finding. *Neuropsychologia, 29,* 1137–1148.

Fuld, P. (1984). Test profile of cholinergic dysfunction and of Alzheimer-type dementia. *Journal of Clinical Neuropsychology, 6,* 380–392.

Funkenstein, H., Albert, M., Cook, N., West, C., Scherr, P., Chown, M., Pilgrim, D., & Evans, D. (1993). Extrapyramidal signs and other neurologic findings in clinically diagnosed Alzheimer's disease. *Archives of Neurology, 50,* 51–56.

Fuster, J. (1997). *The Prefrontal Cortex: Anatomy, Physiology, and Neuropsychology of the Frontal Lobe.* Philadelphia: Lippincott-Raven.

Gabrieli, J., Singh, J., Stebbins, G., & Goetz, C. (1996). Reduced working memory span in Parkinson's disease: Evidence for the role of a frontostriatal system in working and strategic memory. *Neuropsychology, 3,* 322–332.

Gainotti, G., Parloato, E., Monteleone, D., & Carlomagno, S. (1989). Verbal memory disorders in Alzheimer's disease and multi-infarct dementia. *Journal of Neurolinguistics, 4,* 327–345.

Galasko, D., Hansen, L., Katzman, R., Wiederholt, W., Masliah, E., Terry, R., Hill, L., Lessin, P., & Thal, L. (1994). Clinical-neuropathological correlations in Alzheimer's disease and related disorders. *Archives of Neurology, 51,* 888–895.

Galasko, D., Katzman, R., Salmon, D., & Hansen, L. (1997). Clinical and neuropathological findings in Lewy body dementias. *Brain and Cognition, 31,* 166–175.

Galasko, D., Saitoh, T., Xia, Y., Thal, L., Katzman, R., Hill, L., & Hansen, L. (1995). The apolipoprotein E allele e4 is over-represented in patients with Lewy body variant of Alzheimer's disease. *Neurology, 44,* 1950–1951.

Gallo, J., Royall, D., & Anthony, J. (1993). Risk factors for the onset of depression in middle-age and later life. *Social Psychiatry and Psychiatric Epidemiology, 28,* 101–108.

Gathercole, S. (1994). Neuropsychology and working memory: A review. *Neuropsychology, 8,* 494–505.

Gearing, M., Mirra, S., Sumi, S., Hansen, L., Hedreen, J., & Heyman, A. (1995). The Consortium to Establish a Registry for Alzheimer's Disease (CERAD) Part X: Neuropathology confirmation of the clinical diagnosis of Alzheimer's disease. *Neurology, 45,* 461–466.

Ghoneim, M., & Hinrichs, J. (1997). Drugs, memory and sedation: Specificity of effects. *Anesthesiology, 87,* 734–736.

Ghoneim, M., Mewaldt, S., Berie, J., & Hinrichs, J. (1981). Memory and performance effects of single and 3-week administration of diazepam. *Psychopharmacology, 73,* 147–151.

Gibb, W., & Lees, A. (1988). The relevance of the Lewy body to the pathogenesis of idiopathic Parkinson's disease. *Journal of Neurology, Neurosurgery and Psychiatry, 51,* 745–752.

Gibb, W., Luther, P., & Marsden, C. (1989). Corticobasal degeneration. *Brain, 112,* 1171–1192.

Gilley, D., & Wilson, R. (1997). Criterion-related validity of the Geriatric Depression Scale in Alzheimer's disease. *Journal of Clinical and Experimental Neuropsychology, 19,* 489–499.

Gilman, S., Adams, K., Koeppe, R., Brunberg, J., Kluin, K., Berent, S., & Kroll, P. (1990). Cerebellar and frontal hypometabolism in alcohol cerebellar degeneration studied with positron emission tomography. *Annals of Neurology, 28,* 775–785.

Glass, R., Uhlenhuth, E., Hartel, F., Matuzas, W., & Fischman, M. (1981). Cognitive dysfunction and imipramine in outpatient depressives. *Archives of General Psychiatry, 38,* 1048–1051.

Glatt, S., & Koller, W. (1992). Effect of antiparkinsonian drugs on memory. In S. Huber & J. Cummings (Eds.), *Parkinson's disease: Neurobehavioral aspects* (pp. 303–312). New York: Oxford University Press.

Glenn, S., Parsons, O., & Sinha, R. (1994). Assessment of recovery of electrophysiological and neuropsychological functions in chronic alcoholics. *Biological Psychiatry, 36,* 443–452.

Goate, A., Chatier-Harlin, M., Mullan, M., Brown, J., Crawford, F., Fidani, L., Giuffra, L., Haynes, A., Irving, N., James, L., Mant, R., Newton, P., Rooke, K., Roques, P., Talbot, C., Pericakvance, M., Roses, A., Williamson, R., Rossor, M., Owen, M., & Hardy, J. (1991). Segregation of a missense mutation in the amyloid precursor protein gene with familial Alzheimer's disease. *Nature, 349,* 704–706.

Golbe, L. (1991). Young onset PD (YOPD): A clinical review. *Neurology, 41,* 168–173.

Golbe, L. (1997). Progressive supranuclear palsy. In R. Watts & W. Koller (Eds.), *Movement Disorders: Neurologic Principles and Practice* (pp. 277–295). New York: McGraw-Hill.

Golbe, L., Davis, P., Schoenberg, B., & Duvoisin, R. (1988). Prevalence and natural history of progressive supranuclear palsy. *Neurology, 38,* 1031–1034.

Golbe, L., Di Iorio, G., Bonavita, V., Miller, D., & Duvoisin, R. (1990). A large kindred with autosomal dominant Parkinson's disease. *Annals of Neurology, 27,* 276–282.

Goldberg, E., & Barr, W. (1991). Three possible mechanisms of unawareness of deficit. In G. Prigatano & D. Schacter (Eds.), *Awareness of Deficit after Brain Injury* (pp. 152–175). New York: Oxford University Press.

Goldberg, T., Weinberger, D., Berman, K., Pliskin, N., & Podd, M. (1987). Further evidence for dementia of the prefrontal type in schizophrenia? A controlled study of teaching the Wisconsin Card Sorting Test. *Archives of General Psychiatry, 44,* 1008–1014.

Goldman, W., Baty, J., Buckles, V., Sahrmann, S., & Morris, J. (1998). Cognitive and motor functioning in Parkinson disease: Subjects with and without questionable dementia. *Archives of Neurology, 55,* 674–680.

Goldstein, F., Levin, H., Goldman, W., Kalechstein, W., Clark, A., & Kenehan-Altonen, T. (1999). Cognitive and behavioral sequelae of closed head injury in older adults according to their significant others. *Journal of Neuropsychiatry and Clinical Neuroscience, 11,* 38–44.

Goldstein, F., Levin, H., Presley, R., Searcy, J., Colohan, A., Eisenberg, H., Jann, B., & Bertolino-Kusnerik, L. (1994). Neurobehavioral consequences of closed head injury in older adults. *Journal of Neurology, Neurosurgery and Psychiatry, 57,* 961–966.

Goldstein, F., Levin, H., Roberts, V., Goldman, W., Kalechstein, A., Winslow, M., & Goldstein, S. (1996). Neuropsychological effects of closed head injury in older adults: A comparison with Alzheimer's disease. *Neuropsychology, 10,* 147–154.

Goldstein, G. (1985). Dementia associated with alcoholism. In R. Tarter & D. VanThiel (Eds.), *Alcohol and the Brain: Chronic Effects* (pp. 283–294). New York: Plenum Press.

Goldstein, K. (1939). *The Organism: A Holistic Approach to Biology Derived From Pathological Data in Man.* New York: American Press.

Gomberg, E. (1995). Older women and alcohol: Use and abuse. *Recent Developments in Alcoholism, 12,* 61–79.

Goodglass, H., & Kaplan, E. (1983). *The Assessment of Aphasia and Related Disorders.* (2nd ed.). Philadelphia: Lea and Febiger.

Goodwin, F. (1971). Psychiatric side effects of levodopa in man. *Journal of the American Medical Association, 218,* 1915–1920.

Gorell, J., Johnson, C., Rybicki, B., Peterson, E., & Richardson, R. (1998). The risk of Parkinson's disease with exposure to pesticides, farming, well water and rural living. *Neurology, 50,* 1346–1350.

Gotham, A., Brown, R., & Marsden, C. (1986). Depression in Parkinson's disease: A quantitative and qualitative analysis. *Journal of Neurology, Neurosurgery, and Psychiatry, 49,* 381–389.

Gotham, A., Brown, R., & Marsden, C. (1988). "Frontal" cognitive function in patients with Parkinson's disease "ON" and "OFF" levodopa. *Brain, 111,* 299–321.

Graff-Radford, N., Eslinger, P., Damasio, A., & Yamada, T. (1984). Nonhemorrhagic infarction of the thalamus: Behavioral, anatomic and physiologic correlates. *Neurology, 34,* 14–23.

Grafman, J., Jonas, B., & Salazar, A. (1990a). Wisconsin Card Sorting Test performance based on location and size of neuroanatomical lesion in Vietnam veterans with penetrating head injury. *Perceptual and Motor Skills, 71,* 1120–1122.

Grafman, J., Litvan, I., Gomez, C., & Chase, T. (1990b). Frontal lobe function in progressive supranuclear palsy. *Archives of Neurology, 47,* 553–558.

Grafman, J., Litvan, I., & Stark, M. (1995). Neuropsychological features of progressive supranuclear palsy. *Brain and Cognition, 28,* 311–320.

Grahama, J., & Oppenheimer, D. (1969). Orthostatic hypotension and nicotine sensitivity in a case of multiple system atrophy. *Journal of Neurology, Neurosurgery, and Psychiatry, 32,* 28–34.

Grant, A., & Berg, A. (1948). A behavioral analysis of degree of reinforcement and ease of shifting to new responses in a Weigl-type card-sorting problem. *Journal of Experimental Psychology, 38,* 404–411.

Grant, I. (1987). Alcohol and the brain: Neuropsychological correlates. *Journal of Consulting and Clinical Psychology, 55,* 310–324.

Grant, I., Adams, K., & Reed, R. (1984). Aging, abstinence and medical risk factors in the prediction of neuropsychological deficit amongst chronic alcoholics. *Archives of General Psychiatry, 41,* 710–718.

Grant, I., Prigatano, G., Heaton, R., McSweeny, A., Wright, E., & Adams, K. (1987a). Progressive neuropsychologic impairment and hypoxemia. *Archives of General Psychiatry, 44,* 999–1006.

Grant, I., Reed, R., & Adams, K. (1987b). Diagnosis of intermediate-duration and sub-acute organic mental disorders in abstinent alcoholics. *Journal of Clinical Psychiatry, 48,* 319–323.

Green, J., Goldstein, F.C., Sirockman, B.E., & Green, R.C. (1993). Variable awareness of deficits in Alzheimer's disease. *Neuropsychiatry, Neuropsychology and Behavioral Neurology, 6,* 159–165.

Green, R.C., Woodard, J.L., & Green, J. (1995). Validity of the Mattis Dementia Rating Scale for detection of cognitive impairment in the elderly. *Journal of Neuropsychiatry, 7,* 357–360.

Greenlief, C., Margolis, R., & Erker, G. (1985). Application of the Trail-Making Test in differentiating neuropsychological impairment of elderly persons. *Perceptual and Motor Skills, 61,* 1283–1289.

Gregory, C., & Hodges, J. (1996). Frontotemporal dementia: Use of consensus criteria and prevalence of psychiatric features. *Neuropsychiatry, Neuropsychology and Behavioral Neurology, 9,* 145–153.

Grisso, T. (1994). Clinical assessments for legal competence of older adults. In M. Storandt & G. VandenBos (Eds.), *Neuropsychological Assessment of Dementia and Depression in Older Adults: A Clinician's Guide* (pp. 119–140). Washington, DC: American Psychological Association.

Grober, E., & Sliwinski, M. (1991). Development and validation of a model for estimating premorbid verbal intelligence in the elderly. *Journal of Clinical and Experimental Neuropsychology, 13,* 933–949.

Growdon, J., Kieburtz, K., McDermott, M., Panisset, M., & Friedman, J. (1998). Levodopa improves motor function without impairing cognition in mild non-demented Parkinson's disease patients. *Neurology, 50,* 1327–1331.

Growdon, J., Locascio, J., Corkin, S., Gomez-Isla, T., & Hyman, B. (1996). Apolipoprotein E genotype does not influence rates of cognitive decline in Alzheimer's disease. *Neurology, 47,* 444–448.

Gupta, S., Naheedy, M., Young, J., Ghobrial, M., Rubino, F., & Hindo, W. (1988). Periventricular white matter changes and dementia. Clinical, neuropsychological, radiological and pathological correlation. *Archives of Neurology, 45,* 637–641.

Gusella, J., Wexler, N., Conneally, P., Naylor, S., Anderson, M., Tanzi, B., Shoulson, I., Bonilla, E., & Martin, J. (1983). A polymorphic DNA marker genetically linked to Huntington's disease. *Nature, 306,* 234–238.

Gustafson, L. (1987). Frontal lobe degeneration of the non-Alzheimer type. II. Clinical picture and differential diagnosis. *Archives of Gerontology and Geriatrics, 6,* 209–233.

Gustafson, L. (1993). Clinical picture of frontal lobe degeneration of non-Alzheimer type. *Dementia, 4*, 143–148.

Hachinski, V., Iliff, L., Zilhka, E., Du Boulay, G., McAllister, V., Marshall, J., Russell, R., & Symon, L. (1975). Cerebral blood flow in dementia. *Archives of Neurology, 32*, 632–637.

Hachinski, V., & Norris, J. (1985). *The Acute Stroke*. Philadelphia: FA Davis.

Hachinski, V., Potter, P., & Merskey, H. (1987). Leuko-araiosis. *Archives of Neurology, 44*, 21–23.

Halstead, W. (1947). *Brain and Intelligence: A Quantitative Study of the Frontal Lobes*. Chicago: University of Chicago Press.

Hamilton, M. (1967). Development of a rating scale for primary depressive illness. *British Journal of Social and Clinical Psychology, 6*, 278–296.

Hannay, H., Falgout, J., Leli, D., Katholi, C., Halsey, J., & Wills, E. (1987). Focal right temporo-occipital blood flow changes associated with judgment of line orientation. *Neuropsychologia, 25*, 755–763.

Hanninen, T., Hallikainen, M., Koivisto, K., Partanen, K., Laakso, M., Riekkinen, P., & Soininen, H. (1997). Decline of frontal lobe functions in subjects with age-associated memory impairment. *Neurology, 48*, 148–153.

Hansen, L., Salmon, D., Galasko, D., Masliah, E., Katzman, R., DeTersa, R., Thal, L., Pay, M., Hofstetter, R., Klauber, M., Rice, V., Butters, N., & Alford, M. (1990). The Lewy body variant of Alzheimer's disease: A clinical and pathological entity. *Neurology, 40*, 1–8.

Harris, M. (1999). *Wisconsin Card Sorting Test: Scoring Program*. Odessa, FL: Psychological Assessment Resources.

Hart, R., Kwentus, J., Hamer, R., & Taylor, J. (1987). Selective reminding procedure in depression and dementia. *Psychology and Aging, 2*, 111–115.

Hata, T., Meyer, J., Tanahashi, N., Ishikawa, Y., Imai, A., Shinohara, T., Velez, M., Fann, W., Kandul, P., & Sakai, F. (1987a). Three-dimensional mapping of local cerebral perfusion in alcholic encephalopathy with and without Wernicke-Korsakoff syndrome. *Journal of Cerebral Blood Flow and Metabolism, 7*, 35–44.

Hata, T., Meyer, J., Tanahashi, N., Ishikawa, Y., Imai, A., Shinohara, T., Velez, M., Fann, W., Kandula, P., & Sakai, F. (1987b). Three-dimensional mapping of local cerebral perfusion in alcoholic encephalopathy with and without Wernicke-Korsakoff syndrome. *Journal of Cerebral Blood Flow and Metabolism, 7*, 35–44.

Hawkins, K., Sledge, W., Orleans, J., Quinlan, D., Rakfeldt, J., & Hoffman, R. (1993). Normative implications of the relationship between reading vocabulary and Boston Naming Test performance. *Archives of Clinical Neuropsychology, 8*, 525–537.

Haxby, J., Grady, C., Duara, R., Schlageter, N., Berg, G., & Rapoport, S. (1986). Neocortical metabolic abnormalities precede nonmemory cognitive deficits in early Alzheimer's-type dementia. *Archives of Neurology, 43*, 882–885.

Haxby, J., Grady, C., Koss, E., Horwitz, B., Heston, L., Schapiro, M., Friedland, R., & Rapoport, S. (1990). Longitudinal study of cerebral metabolic asymmetries and associated neuropsychological patterns in early dementia of the Alzheimer's type. *Archives of Neurology, 47*, 753–760.

Haxby, J., Grady, C., Koss, E., Horwitz, B., Schapiro, M., Friedland, R., & Rapoport, S. (1988). Heterogeneous anterior-posterior metabolic patterns in dementia of the Alzheimer type. *Neurology, 38*, 1853–1863.

Haxby, J., Juara, R., Grady, C., Cutler, N., & Rapoport, S. (1985). Relations between neuropsychological and cerebral metabolic abnormalities in early Alzheimer's disease. *Journal of Cerebral Blood Flow and Metabolism, 5*, 193–200.

Heaton, R., Chelune, G., Talley, J., Kay, G., & Curtiss, G. (1993). *Wisconsin Card Sorting Test Manual*. Odessa, Florida: Psychological Assessment Resources.

Heaton, R., Grant, I., & Matthews, C. (1991). *Comprehensive Norms for an Expanded Halstead-Reitan Battery: Demographic Corrections, Research Findings and Clinical Applications*. Odessa, Florida: Psychological Assessment Resources.

Heaton, R., & Pendleton, M. (1981). Use of neuropsychological tests to predict adult patients' everyday functioning. *Journal of Consulting and Clinical Psychology, 49*, 807–821.

Heaton, R., & Psychological Assessment Resources staff. (1999). *WCST: Computer Version-3 Research Edition.* Odessa, FL: Psychological Assessment Resources, Inc.

Heikkila, V., Turkka, J., Korpelainen, J., Kallanranta, T., & Summala, H. (1998). Decreased driving ability in people with Parkinson's disease. *Journal of Neurology, Neurosurgery and Psychiatry, 64,* 325–330.

Heilbronner, R., Henry, G., Buck, P., Adams, R., & Fogle, L. (1991). Lateralized brain damage and performance on Trail Making A and B, Digit Span forward and backward, TPT memory and location. *Archives of Clinical Neuropsychology, 6,* 251–258.

Heilman, K., Bowers, D., & Valenstein, E. (1993a). Emotional disorders associated with neurological diseases. In K. Heilman & E. Valenstein (Eds.), *Clinical Neuropsychology* (3rd ed., pp. 461–498). New York: Oxford University Press.

Heilman, K., & Valenstein, E. (1993). *Clinical Neuropsychology.* (3rd ed.). New York: Oxford University Press.

Heilman, K., Watson, R., & Valenstein, E. (1993b). Neglect and related disorders. In K. Heilman & E. Valenstein (Eds.), *Clinical Neuropsychology* (3rd ed.). New York: Oxford University Press.

Heindel, W., Butters, N., & Salmon, D. (1988). Impaired learning of a motor skill in patients with Huntington's disease. *Behavioral Neuroscience, 102,* 141–147.

Heindel, W., Salmon, D., & Butters, N. (1991). The biasing of weight judgments in Alzheimer's and Huntington's disease: A priming or programming phenomenon. *Journal of Clinical and Experimental Neuropsychology, 13,* 189–203.

Heindel, W., Salmon, D., Shults, C., Walicke, P., & Butters, N. (1989). Neuropsychological evidence for multiple implicit memory systems: a comparison of Alzheimer's, Huntington's and Parkinson's disease patients. *The Journal of Neuroscience, 9,* 582–587.

Helmes, E. (1996). Use of the Barona method to predict premorbid intelligence in the elderly. *The Clinical Neuropsychologist, 10,* 255–261.

Helzer, J., Burnam, A., & McEvoy, L. (1991). Alcoholic abuse and dependence. In L. Robins & D. Regier (Eds.), *Psychiatric Disorders in America: The Epidemiologic Catchment Area Study* (pp. 81–115). New York: Free Press.

Henderson, A., Easteal, S., Jorm, A., Mackinnon, A., Korten, A., Christensen, H., Croft, L., & Jacomb, P. (1995). Apolipoprotein E allele e4, dementia and cognitive decline in a population sample. *Lancet, 346,* 1387–1390.

Henderson, V., Paganini-Hill, A., Emanuel, C., Dunn, M., & Buckwalter, J. (1994). Estrogren replacement therapy in older women. *Archives of Neurology, 51,* 896–900.

Hersch, S., Jones, R., Koroshetz, W., & Quaid, K. (1994). The neurogenetics genie: Testing for the Huntington's disease mutation. *Neurology, 44,* 1369–1373.

Heyman, A., Fillenbaum, G., Welsh-Bohmer, K., Gearing, M., Mirra, S., Mohs, R., Peterson, B., & Pieper, C. (1998). Cerebral infarcts in patients with autopsy-proven Alzheimer's disease. *Neurology,* 159–162.

Hietanen, M., & Teravainen, H. (1988). The effect of age of disease onset on neuropsychological performance in Parkinson's disease. *Journal of Neurology, Neurosurgery and Psychiatry, 51,* 244–249.

Hill, C., Stoudemire, A., Morris, R., Martino-Saltzman, D., & Markwalter, H. (1993). Similarities and differences in memory deficits in patients with primary dementia and depression-related cognitive dysfunction. *Journal of Neuropsychiatry and Clinical Neurosciences, 5,* 277–282.

Hill, C., Stoudemire, A., Morris, R., Martino-Saltzman, D., Markwalter, H., & Lewison, B. (1992). Dysnomia in the differential diagnosis of major depression, depression-related cognitive dysfunction, and dementia. *Journal of Neuropsychiatry and Clinical Neurosciences, 4,* 64–69.

Hinrichs, J., & Ghoneim, M. (1987). Diazepam, behavior, and aging: Increased sensitivity or lower baseline performance? *Psychopharmacology, 92,* 100–105.

Hinrichs, J., Mewaldt, S., Ghoneim, M., & Berie, J. (1982). Diazepam and learning: Assessment of acquisition deficits. *Pharmacology, Biochemistry and Behavior, 17,* 165–170.

Hodges, J., & Patterson, K. (1996). Nonfluent progressive aphasia and semantic dementia: A comparative neuropsychological study. *Journal of the International Neuropsychological Society, 6,* 511–524.

Hodges, J., Patterson, K., Ward, R., Garrard, P., Bak, T., Perry, R., & Gregory, C. (1999). The differentiation of semantic dementia and frontal lobe dementia (temporal and frontal variants of frontotemporal dementia) from early Alzheimer's disease: A comparative neuropsychological study. *Neuropsychology, 13,* 31–40.

Hodges, J., Patterson, S., Oxbury, S., & Funnell, E. (1992a). Semantic dementia: Progressive fluent aphasia with temporal lobe atrophy. *Brain, 115,* 1783–1806.

Hodges, J., Salmon, D., & Butters, N. (1990). Differential impairment of semantic and episodic memory in Alzheimer's disease and Huntington's disease: A controlled prospective study. *Journal of Neurology, Neurosurgery and Psychiatry, 53,* 1089–1095.

Hodges, J., Salmon, D., & Butters, N. (1991). The nature of the naming deficits in Alzheimer's and Huntington's disease. *Brain, 114,* 1547–1558.

Hodges, J., Salmon, D., & Butters, N. (1992b). Semantic memory impairment in Alzheimer's disease: Failure of access or degraded knowledge? *Neuropsychologia, 30,* 301–314.

Hoehn, M., & Yahr, M. (1967). Parkinsonism: Onset progression and mortality. *Neurology, 17,* 427–442.

Hom, J., Turner, M.B., Risser, R., Bonte, F.J., & Tintner, R. (1994). Cognitive deficits in asymptomatic first-degree relatives of Alzheimer's disease patients. *Journal of Clinical and Experimental Neuropsychology, 16,* 568–675.

Hommer, D. (1991). Benzodiazepines: Cognitive and psychomotor effects. In P. Roy-Byrne & D. Cowley (Eds.), *Benzodiazepines in Clinical Practice: Risks and Benefits* (pp. 113–129). Washington, DC: American Psychiatric Press.

Hua, M.-S., & Lu, C.-S. (1994). Multiple system atrophy and visuospatial function. *Neuropsychology, 1,* 91–94.

Huber, S., Christy, J., & Paulson, G. (1991). Cognitive heterogeneity associated with clinical subtypes of PD. *Neuropsychiatry, Neurology and Behavioral Neurology, 4,* 147–157.

Huber, S., Freidenberg, D., Paulson, G., Shuttleworth, E., & Christy, J. (1990). The pattern of depressive symptoms varies with the progression of Parkinson's disease. *Journal of Neurology, Neurosurgery, and Psychiatry, 53,* 275–278.

Huber, S., Freidenberg, D., Shuttleworth, E., Paulson, G., & Christy, J. (1989a). Neuropsychological impairment associated with severity of Parkinson's disease. *Journal of Neuropsychiatry and Clinical Neurosciences, 1,* 154–158.

Huber, S., Paulson, G., & Shuttleworth, E. (1988). Depression in Parkinson's disease. *Neuropsychiatry, Neuropsychology and Behavioral Neurology, 1,* 47–51.

Huber, S., Shuttleworth, E., & Freidenberg, D. (1989b). Neuropsychological differences between the dementias of Alzheimer's and Parkinson's disease. *Archives of Neurology, 46,* 1287–1291.

Huber, S., Shuttleworth, E., & Paulson, G. (1986a). Dementia in Parkinson's disease. *Archives of Neurology, 43,* 987–990.

Huber, S., Shuttleworth, E., Paulson, G., Bellchambers, M., & Clapp, L. (1986b). Cortical vs subcortical dementia: Neuropsychological differences. *Archives of Neurology, 43,* 392–394.

Huff, F.J., Auerbach, J., Chakravarti, A., & Boller, F. (1988). Risk of dementia in relatives of patients with Alzheimer's disease. *Neurology, 38,* 786–790.

Hughes, A., Daniel, S., Blankson, S., & Lees, A. (1993). A clinicopathologic study of 100 cases of Parkinson's disease. *Archives of Neurology, 50,* 140–148.

Hunt, A., Orrison, W., Yeo, R., Haaland, K., Rhyne, R., Garry, P., & Rosenberg, G. (1989). Clinical significance of MRI white matter lesions in the elderly. *Neurology, 39,* 1470–1474.

Hunt, L., Morris, J., Edwards, D., & Wilson, B. (1993). Driving performance in persons with senile dementia of the Alzheimer type. *Journal of the American Geriatrics Society, 41,* 747–752.

Hunt, L., Murphy, C., Carr, D., Duchek, J., Buckles, V., & Morris, J. (1997). Reliability of the Washington University Road Test. A performance-based assessment for drivers with dementia of the Alzheimer type. *Archives of Neurology, 54,* 707–712.

Huntington, G. (1972). On chorea. *Advances in Neurology, 1,* 33–35.

Huntington's Disease Collaborative Research Group. (1993) A novel gene containing a trinucleotide repeat that is expanded and unstable on Huntington's disease chromosomes. *Cell, 72,* 971–983.

Hyman, B. (1998). New neuropathological criteria for Alzheimer disease. *Archives of Neurology, 55,* 1174–1176.

Hyman, B., Van Horsen, G., Damasio, A., & Barnes, C. (1984). Alzheimer's disease: Cell-specific pathology isolates the hippocampal formation. *Science, 225,* 1168–1170.

Ineichen, B. (1987). Measuring the rising tide. How many dementia cases will there be by 2001? *British Journal of Psychiatry, 150,* 193–200.

Ishii, N., Nishihara, Y., & Imamura, T. (1986). Why do frontal lobe syndromes predominate in vascular dementia with lacunes? *Neurology, 36,* 340–345.

Ivnik, R., Malec, J., Smith, G., Tangalos, E., & Peterson, R. (1996). Neuropsychological test norms above age 55: COWAT, BNT, MAE Token, WRAT-R Reading, AMNART, Stroop, TMT, JLO. *The Clinical Neuropsychologist, 10,* 1–111.

Ivnik, R., Malec, J., Smith, G., Tangalos, E., Peterson, R., Kokmen, E., & Kurland, L. (1992a). Mayo's older Americans normative studies: WAIS-R norms for ages 56 to 97. *The Clinical Neuropsychologist, 6,* 1–30.

Ivnik, R., Malec, J., Smith, G., Tangalos, E., Peterson, R., Kokmen, E., & Kurland, L. (1992b). Mayo's older Americans normative studies: WMS-R norms for ages 56 to 94. *The Clinical Neuropsychologist, 6,* 49–82.

Ivnik, R., Malec, J., Smith, G., Tangalos, E., Peterson, R., Kokmen, E., & Kurland, L. (1992c). Mayo's older Americans normative studies: Updated AVLT norms for ages 56 to 97. *The Clinical Neuropsychologist, 6,* 83–104.

Jacobs, D., Marder, K., Cote, L., Sano, M., Stern, Y., & Mayeux, R. (1995a). Neuropsychological characteristics of preclinical dementia in Parkinson's disease. *Neurology, 45,* 1691–1696.

Jacobs, D., Sano, M., Dooneief, G., Marder, K., Bell, K., & Stern, Y. (1995b). Neuropsychological detection and characterization of preclinical Alzheimer's disease. *Neurology, 45,* 957–62.

Jacobs, D., Sano, M., Marder, K., Bell, K., Bylsma, F., Lafleche, G., Albert, M., Brandt, J., & Stern, Y. (1994). Age at onset of Alzheimer's disease: Relationship to pattern of cognitive dysfunction and rate of decline. *Neurology, 44,* 1215–1220.

Jarvik, L., & Perl, M. (1981). Overview of physiologic dysfunctions related to psychiatric problems in the elderly. In A. Levenson & R. Hall (Eds.), *Neuropsychiatric Manifestations of Physical Disease in the Elderly* (pp. 1–15). New York: Raven Press.

Jeffreys, R. (1987). Hydrocephalus. In J. Millder (Ed.), *Northfield's Surgery of the Central Nervous System* (pp. 543–573). Edinburgh: Blackwell.

Jernigan, R., Schafer, K., Butters, N., & Cermak, L. (1991a). Magnetic resonance imaging of alcoholic Korsakoff's patients. *Neuropsychopharmacology, 4,* 175–186.

Jernigan, T., Butters, N., DiTraglia, G., Schafer, K., Smith, T., Irwin, M., Grant, I., Schuckit, M., & Cermak, L. (1991b). Reduced cerebral gray matter observed in alcoholics using magnetic resonance imaging. *Alcoholism: Clinical and Experimental Research, 15,* 418–427.

Jernigan, T., Schafer, K., Butters, N., & Cermak, L. (1991c). Magnetic resonance imaging of alcoholic Korsakoff patients. *Neuropsychopharmacology, 4,* 175–186.

Jetter, W., Poser, U., Freeman, R., & Markowitsch, J. (1986). A verbal long term memory deficit in frontal lobe damaged patients. *Cortex, 22,* 229–242.

Jinks, M., & Raschko, R. (1990). A profile of alcohol and prescription drug abuse in a high-risk community-based elderly population. *Drug Intelligence and Clinical Pharmacy, 24,* 971–975.

Johansson, K., & Lundberg, C. (1997). The 1994 International Consensus Conference on Dementia and Driving: A brief report. Swedish National Road. *Alzheimer's Disease and Related Disorders, 11 Suppl 1,* 62–69.

Johnson, J.R., Litvan, I., & Grafman, J. (1991). Progressive supranuclear palsy: Altered sensory processing leads to degraded cognition. *Neurology, 41,* 1257–1262.

Johnson, W. (1991). Genetic susceptibility to Parkinson's disease. *Neurology, 41,* 82–87.

Johnstone, P., Rundell, J., & Esposito, M. (1990). Mental status changes of Addison's disease. *Psychosomatics, 31,* 103–106.

Jones, B., & Parsons, O. (1971). Impaired abstracting ability in chronic alcoholics. *Archives of General Psychiatry, 24,* 71–75.

Jones, R. (1996). *Walking the Tightrope: Living at Risk for Huntington's disease.* Huntington's Disease Society of America.

Jonides, J., Smith, E., Koeppe, R., Awh, E., Minoshima, S., & Mintun, M. (1993). Spatial working memory in humans as revealed by PET. *Nature, 363,* 623–626.

Jorm, A. (1990). *The Epidemiology of Alzheimer's Disease and Related Disorders.* London: Chapman and Hall.

Jorm, A., Korten, A., & Henderson, A. (1987). The prevalence of dementia: A quantitative integration of the literature. *Acta Psychiatrica Scandinavica, 76,* 465–479.

Josiassen, R., Curry, L., & Mancall, E. (1983). Development of neuropsychological deficits in Huntington's disease. *Archives of Neurology, 40,* 791–796.

Joutel, A., Vahedi, K., Corpechot, C., Troesch, A., Chabriat, H., Vayssiere, C., Cruaud, C., Maciazek, J., Weissenbach, J., Bousser, M., Back, J., & TournierLasserve, E. (1997). Strong clustering and stereotyped nature of Notch3 mutations in CADASIL patients. *Lancet, 350,* 1511–1515.

Junque, C., Pujol, J., Vendrell, P., Bruna, O., Jodar, M., Ribas, J., Vinas, J., Capdevila, A., & Marti-Vilalta, J. (1990). Leuko-araiosis on magnetic resonance imaging and speed of mental processing. *Archives of Neurology, 47,* 151–156.

Kahn, R., Zarit, S., Hilbert, N., & Niederehe, G. (1975). Memory complaint and impairment in the aged: The effect of depression and altered brain function. *Archives of General Psychiatry, 32,* 1569–1573.

Kahneman, D. (1973). *Attention and Effort.* Englewood Cliffs, NJ: Prentice-Hall, Inc.

Kanne, S., Balota, D., Storandt, M., McKeel, D., & Morris, J. (1998). Relating anatomy to function in Alzheimer's disease: Neuropsychological profiles predict regional neuropathology 5 years later. *Neurology, 50,* 979–985.

Kaplan, D., Goodglass, H., & Weintraub, S. (1983). *Boston Naming Test.* Philadelphia: Lea & Febiger.

Kaplan, E. (1983). Process and achievement revisited. In S. Wapner & B. Kaplan (Eds.), *Toward a Holistic Developmental Psychology* (pp. 143–156). Hillsdale, NJ: Lawrence Erlbaum Publishers.

Kaplan, E. (1988). A process approach to neuropsychological assessment. In T. Boll & B. Bryant (Eds.), *Clinical Neuropsychology and Brain Function: Research, Measurement and Practice* (pp. 129–167). Washington, DC: American Psychological Association.

Kaplan, E., Fein, D., Morris, R., & Delis, D. (1991). *WAIS-R as a Neuropsychological Instrument.* San Antonio: The Psychological Corporation.

Kapust, L., & Weintraub, S. (1992). To drive or not to drive: Preliminary results from road testing of patients with dementia. *Journal of Geriatric Psychiatry and Neurology, 5,* 210–216.

Kaszniak, A. (1987). Neuropsychological consultation to geriatricians: Issues in the assessment of memory complaints. *The Clinical Neuropsychologist, 1,* 35–46.

Katz, D., Alexander, M., & Mandell, A. (1987). Dementia following strokes in the mesencephalon and diencephalon. *Archives of Neurology, 44,* 1127–1133.

Katz, S., Ford, A., Moskowitz, R., Jackson, B., & Jaffee, M. (1963). Studies of illness in the aged: The Index of ADL, a standardized measure of biological and psychosocial function. *Journal of the American Medical Association, 185,* 94–99.

Katzen, H., Levin, B., & Llabre, M. (1998). Age of disease onset influences cognition in Parkinson's disease. *Journal of the International Neuropsychological Society, 4,* 285–290.

Katzman, R. (1993). Education and the prevalence of dementia and Alzheimer's disease. *Neurology, 43,* 13–20.

Katzman, R., & Kawas, C. (1994). The epidemiology of dementia and Alzheimer disease. In R. Terry, R. Katzman, & K. Bick (Eds.), *Alzheimer Disease.* New York: Raven Press.

Katzman, R., & Rowe, J. (Eds.). (1992). *Principles of Geriatric Neurology.* Philadelphia: FA Davis.

Kaufman, A., McLean, J., & Reynolds, C. (1988). Sex, race, residence, region and education differences on 11 WAIS-R subtests. *Journal of Clinical Psychology, 44,* 231–248.

Kaufman, A., McLean, J., & Reynolds, C. (1991). Analysis of WAIS-R factor patterns by sex and race. *Journal of Clinical Psychology, 47,* 548–557.

Kawas, C. (1990). Early clinical diagnosis: Status of the NINCDS-ADRDA criteria. In R.E. Becker & E. Giacobini (Eds.), *Alzheimer Disease: Current Research in Early Diagnosis* (pp. 9–18). New York: Taylor and Francis.

Kawas, C., Resnick, S., Morrison, A., Brookmeyer, R., Corrada, M., Zonderman, A., Bacal, C., Lingle, D., & Metter, E. (1997). A prospective study of estrogen replacement therapy and the risk of developing Alzheimer's disease. *Neurology, 48,* 1517–1521.

Kay, T., Harrington, D., Adams, R., Anderson, T., Berrol, S., Cicerone, K., Dahlberg, C., Gerber, D., Goka, R., Harley, P., Hilt, J., Horn, L., Lehmkuhl, D., & Malec, J. (1993). Definition of mild traumatic brain injury. *Journal of Head Trauma Rehabilitation, 8,* 86–87.

Keane, M., Gabrieli, J., Fennema, A., Growdon, J., & Corkin, S. (1991). Evidence for a dissociation between perceptual and conceptual priming in Alzheimer's disease. *Behavioral Neuroscience, 105,* 326–342.

Kemper, T. (1994). Neuroanatomical and neuropathological changes during aging and dementia. In M. Albert & J. Knoefel (Eds.), *Clinical Neurology of Aging,* (2nd ed., pp. 3–67). New York: Oxford University Press.

Kertesz, A., & Clydesdale, S. (1994). Neuropsychological deficits in vascular dementia vs Alzheimer's disease: Frontal lobe deficits prominent in vascular dementia. *Archives of Neurology, 51,* 1226–1231.

Kiloh, L. (1961). Pseudodementia. *Acta Psychiatrica Scandinavica, 37,* 336–351.

King, D., & Caine, E. (1995). Cognitive impairment and major depression: Beyond the pseudodementia syndrome. In I. Grant & D. Adams (Eds.), *Neuropsychological Assessment of Neuropsychiatric Disorders* (pp. 200–217). New York: Oxford University Press.

King, D., Caine, E., Conwell, Y., & Cox, C. (1991a). The neuropsychology of depression in the elderly: A comparative study of normal aging and Alzheimer's disease. *Journal of Neuropsychiatry and Clinical Neurosciences, 3,* 163–168.

King, D., Cox, D., Lyness, J., & Caine, E. (1995). Neuropsychological effects of depression and age in an elderly sample: A confirmatory study. *Neuropsychology, 9,* 399–408.

King, E., Caine, E., Conwell, Y., & Cox, C. (1991b). Predicting severity of depression in the elderly at six-months follow-up: A neuropsychological study. *Journal of Neuropsychiatry and Clinical Neuroscience, 3,* 64–66.

Kish, S., El-Awar, M., Shut, L., Oscar-Berman, M., & Freedman, M. (1988). Cognitive deficit in olivopontocerebellar atrophy: Implications for the cholinergic hypothesis of Alzheimer's dementia. *Annals of Neurology, 24,* 200–206.

Kitagaki, H., Mori, E., Yamaji, S., Ishii, K., Hirono, N., Kobashi, S., & Hata, Y. (1998). Frontotemporal dementia and Alzheimer disease: Evaluation of cortical atrophy with automated hemispheric surface display generated with MR images. *Radiology, 208,* 431–439.

Kline, D., & Scialfa, C. (1996). Visual and auditory aging. In J. Birren & K. Schaie (Eds.), *Handbook of the Psychology of Aging,* (4th ed., pp. 181–203). San Diego: Academic Press.

Knight, B. (1994). Providing clinical interpretations to older clients and their families. In M. Storandt & G. VandenBos (Eds.), *Neuropsychological Assessment of Dementia and Depression in Older Adults: A Clinician's Guide* (pp. 141–154). Washington, DC: American Psychological Association.

Knight, B. (1996). *Psychotherapy With Older Adults (2nd ed.).* Thousand Oaks, CA: Sage Publications.

Knopman, D., Mastri, A., Frey, W., Sung, J., & Rustan, T. (1990). Dementia lacking distinctive histologic features: A common non-Alzheimer degenerative dementia. *Neurology, 40,* 251–256.

Koller, W., Veter-Overfield, B., Gray, C., Alexander, C., Chin, R., Colezal, J., Hassanein, R., & Tanner, C. (1990). Environmental risk factors in Parkinson's disease. *Neurology, 40,* 1218–1221.

Kosaka, K. (1990). Diffuse Lewy Body disease in Japan. *Journal of Neurology, 237,* 197–204.

Koss, E., Edland, S., Fillenbaum, G., Mohs, R., Clark, C., Galasko, D., & Morris, J. (1996). Clinical and neuropsychological differences between patients with earlier and later onset of Alzheimer's disease: A CERAD analysis, part XII. *Neurology, 46,* 136–141.

Kozora, E., & Cullum, C. (1995). Generative naming in normal aging: Total output and qualitative changes using phonemic and semantic constraints. *The Clinical Neuropsychologist, 9,* 313–320.

Kraus, J. (1987). Epidemiology of head injury. In P. Cooper (Ed.), *Head Injury* (pp. 1–19). Baltimore: Williams & Wilkins.

Krull, K., Scott, J., & Sherer, M. (1995). Estimation of premorbid intelligence from combined performance and demographic variables. *The Clinical Neuropsychologist, 9,* 83–88.

Kulisevsky, J., Avila, A., Barnaboj, M., Antonijoan, R., Berthier, M., & Gironell, A. (1996). Acute effects of levodopa on neuropsychological performance in stable and fluctuating Parkinson's disease patients at different levodopa plasma levels. *Brain, 119,* 2121–2132.

Kuzis, G., Sabe, L., Tiberti, C., Leiguarda, R., & Starkstein, S. (1997). Cognitive functions in major depression and disease. *Archives of Neurology, 54,* 982–986.

LaBerge, E., Balota, D., Storandt, M., & Smith, D. (1992). An analysis of confrontation naming errors in senile dementia of the Alzheimer's type. *Neuropsychology, 6,* 77–95.

Lacey, M., Gore, P., Pliskin, N., Henry, G., Helibronner, R., & Hamer, D. (1996). Verbal fluency task equivalence. *The Clinical Neuropsychologist, 10,* 305–308.

Lafleche, G., & Albert, M. (1995). Executive function deficits in mild Alzheimer's disease. *Neuropsychology, 9,* 313–320.

Lamping, D., Spring, B., & Gelenberg, A. (1984). Effects of two antidepressants on memory performance in depressed outpatients: A double-blind study. *Psychopharmacology, 84,* 254–261.

Larrabee, G., Largen, J., & Levin, H. (1985). Sensitivity of age-decline resistant ("Hold") WAIS subtests to Alzheimer's disease. *Journal of Clinical and Experimental Neuropsychology, 7,* 497–504.

Larrabee, G., & Levin, H. (1986). Memory self-ratings and objective test performance in a normal elderly sample. *Journal of Experimental and Clinical Neuropsychology, 8,* 275–284.

LaRue, A., & Jarvik, L. (1987). Cognitive function and prediction of dementia in old age. *International Journal of Aging and Human Development, 25,* 79–89.

Lawson, J., Erdahl, D., Monga, T., Bird, C., Donald, M., Surridge, D., & Letemendia, F. (1984). Neuropsychological function in diabetic patients with neuropathy. *British Journal of Psychiatry, 145,* 263–268.

Lawton, M. (1971). The functional assessment of elderly people. *Journal of the American Geriatrics Society, 19,* 465–481.

Lawton, M., Moss, M., Fulcomer, M., & Kleban, M. (1982). A research and service oriented multilevel assessment instrument. *Journal of Gerontology, 37,* 91–99.

Learoyd, B. (1972). Psychotropic drugs and the elderly patients. *Medical Journal of Australia, 1,* 1131–1133.

Lechtenberg, R., & Gilman, S. (1978). Speech disorders in cerebellar disease. *Annals of Neurology, 3,* 285–290.

Lee, G., & Loring, D. (1993). Acute confusional states in toxic and metabolic disorders. In R. Parks, R. Zec, & R. Wilson (Eds.), *Neuropsychology of Alzheimer's Disease and Other Dementias* (pp. 375–415). New York: Oxford University Press.

Lee, H., & Lawlor, B. (1995). State-dependent nature of the clock drawing task in geriatric depression. *Journal of the American Geriatrics Society, 43*(7), 796–8.

Lee, H., Swanwick, G., Coen, R., & Lawlor, B. (1996). Use of the clock drawing task in the diagnosis of mild and very mild Alzheimer's disease. *International Psychogeriatrics, 8,* 469–476.

Lees, A., & Smith, E. (1983). Cognitive deficits in the early stages of Parkinson's disease. *Brain, 106,* 257–270.

Legrand, F., Vidailhet, P., Danion, J., Grange, D., Giersch, A., Van der Linden, M., & Imbs, J. (1995). Time course of the effects of diazepam and lorazepam on perceptual priming and explicit memory. *Psychopharmacology, 118,* 475–479.

Lehtovirta, M., Soininen, H., Helisalmi, A., Mannermaa, M., Helkala, E.-L., Hartikainen, P., Hanninen, T., Ryynanen, M., & Riekkinen, P. (1996). Clinical and neuropsychological characteristics in familial and sporadic Alzheimer's disease: Relationship to apolipoprotein E polymorphism. *Neurology, 46,* 413–419.

Leiguarda, R., Lees, A., Merello, M., Starkstein, S., & Marsden, C. (1994). The nature of apraxia in corticobasal degeneration. *Journal of Neurology, Neurosurgery and Psychiatry, 57,* 455–459.

Leininger, B., Gramling, S., Farrell, A., Kreutzer, J., & Peck, E. (1990). Neuropsychological deficits in symptomatic minor head injury patients after concussion and mild concussion. *Journal of Neurology, Neurosurgery and Psychiatry, 53,* 293–296.

Lerer, B., Shapira, B., Calev, A., Tubi, N., Drexler, H., Kindler, S., Lidsky, D., & Schwartz, J. (1995). Antidepressant and cognitive effects of twice- versus three-times-weekly ECT. *American Journal of Psychiatry, 152,* 564–570.

Lerner, A., Friedland, R., Riley, D., Whitehouse, P., Lanska, D., Vick, N., Cochran, E., Tresser, N., Cohen, M., & Gambetti, P. (1992). Dementia with pathological findings of corticobasal ganglionic degeneration. *Annals of Neurology, 32,* 271.

Lesser, I., Boone, K., Mehringer, C., Wohl, M., Miller, B., & Berman, N. (1996). Cognition and white matter hyperintensities in older depressed patients. *American Journal of Psychiatry, 153,* 1280–1287.

Levenson, A., & Hall, R. (1981). Preface: A statement of the problem. In A. Levenson & R. Hall (Eds.), *Neuropsychiatric Manifestations of Physical Disease in the Elderly* (pp. v–vi). New York: Raven Press.

Leverenz, J., & Sumi, M. (1986). Parkinson's disease in patients with Alzheimer's disease. *Archives of Neurology, 43,* 662–664.

Levin, B., Llabre, M., Reisman, S., Weiner, W., Sanchez-Ramos, J., Singer, C., & Brown, M. (1991). Visuospatial impairment in Parkinson's disease. *Neurology, 41,* 365–369.

Levin, B., Llabre, M., & Weiner, W. (1988). Parkinson's disease and depression: Psychometric properties of the Beck Depression Inventory. *Journal of Neurology, Neurosurgery and Psychiatry, 51,* 1401–1404.

Levin, B., Llabre, M., & Weiner, W. (1989). Cognitive impairments associated with early Parkinson's disease. *Neurology, 39,* 557–561.

Levin, B., Tomer, R., & Rey, G. (1992). Clinical correlates of cognitive impairment in Parkinson's disease. In S. Huber & J. Cummings (Eds.), *Parkinson's Disease: Neurobehavioral Aspects.* New York: Oxford University Press.

Levin, D., & Finklestein, S. (1982). Delayed psychosis after right temporoparietal stroke or trauma: Relation to epilepsy. *Neurology, 32,* 267–273.

Levy, M., Miller, B., Cummings, J., Fairbanks, L., & Craig, A. (1997). Alzheimer disease and frontotemporal dementias. Behavioral distinctions. *Archives of Neurology, 53,* 687–690.

Levy-Lahad, E., Wasco, W., Poorkaj, P., Romano, D., Oshima, J., Pettingell, W., Yu, C., Jondro, P., Schmidt, S., Wang, K., Crowley, A., Fu, Y., Guenette, S., Galas, D., Nemens, E., Wijsman, E., Bird, T., Schellenberg, G., & Tanzi, R. (1995). Candidate gene for the chromosome 1 familial Alzheimer disease. *Science, 269,* 973–977.

Lewin, R. (1985). Parkinson's disease: An environmental cause? *Science, 229,* 257–258.

Lezak, M. (1995). *Neuropsychological Assessment, Third Edition.* New York: Oxford University Press.

L'Hermitte, F. (1986). Human anatomy and the frontal lobes: Part II: Patient behavior in complex and social situations: The "environmental dependency syndrome." *Annals of Neurology, 19,* 335–343.

Li, G., Shen, Y., Chen, C., Zhao, C., & Li, S. (1989). An epidemiological survey of age-related dementia in an urban area of Beijing. *Acta Psychiatrica Scandinavica, 79,* 557–563.

Liberto, J., Oslin, D., & Ruskin, P. (1992). Alcoholism in older persons: A review of the literature. *Hospital and Community Psychiatry, 43,* 975–984.

Libon, D., Malamut, B., Swenson, R., Sands, L., & Cloud, B. (1996). Further analyses of clock drawings among demented and nondemented older subjects. *Archives of Clinical Neuropsychology, 11,* 193–205.

Libon, D., Scanlon, M., Swenson, R., & Coslet, H. (1990). Binswanger's disease: Some neuropsychological considerations. *Journal of Geriatric Psychiatry and Neurology, 3,* 31–40.

Libon, D., Swenson, R., Barnoski, E., & Sands, L. (1993). Clock drawing as an assessment tool for dementia. *Archives of Clinical Neuropsychology, 8,* 405–415.

Lieberman, A. (1998). Managing the neuropsychiatric symptoms of Parkinson's disease. *Neurology, 50 (Suppl 6),* S33–S38.

Lieberman, A., Dziatolowski, M., Duupersmith, M., Serby, M., Goodgold, A., Korein, J., & Goldstein, M. (1979). Dementia in Parkinson disease. *Annals of Neurology, 6,* 355–359.

Lishman, W. (1986). Alcoholic dementia: A hypothesis. *Lancet, 1,* 1184–1185.

Lister, R., Weingartner, H., Eckardt, M., & Linnoila, M. (1988). Clinical relevance of effects of benzodiazepines on learning and memory. *Psychopharmacology Series, 6,* 117–127.

Litvan, I., Grafman, J., Gomez, C., & Chase, T. (1989). Memory impairment in patients with progressive supranuclear palsy. *Archives of Neurology, 46,* 765–767.

Loeb, C., Gandolfo, C., Croce, R., & Conti, M. (1992). Dementia associated with lacunar infarction. *Stroke, 23,* 1225–1229.

Loewenstein, D., Amigo, E., Duara, R., Guterman, A., Hurwitz, D., Berkowitz, N., Wilkie, F., Weinberg, G., Black, B., Gittleman, B., & Eisdorfer, C. (1981). A new scale for the assessment of functional status in Alzheimer's disease and related disorders. *Journal of Gerontology: Psychological Sciences, 44,* 114–121.

Logsdon, R., Teri, L., & Larson, E. (1992). Driving and Alzheimer's disease. *Journal of General Internal Medicine, 7,* 583–588.

Loke, W., Hinrichs, J., & Ghoneim, M. (1985). Caffeine and diazepam: Separate and combined effects on mood, memory, and psychomotor performance. *Psychopharmacology, 87,* 344–350.

Lopez, O., Becker, J., Brenner, R., Rosen, J., Bajulaiye, O., & Reynolds III, C. (1991). Alzheimer's disease with delusions and hallucinations: Neuropsychological and electroencephalographic correlates. *Neurology, 41,* 906–912.

Lopez, O., Boller, F., Becker, J., Miller, M., & Reynolds, C. (1990). Alzheimer's disease and depression: Neuropsychological impairment and progression of the illness. *American Journal of Psychiatry, 147,* 855–860.

Lopez, O., Gonzalez, M., Becker, J., Reynolds III, D., Sudilovksy, A., & DeKosky, S. (1996). Symptoms of depression and psychosis in Alzheimer's disease and frontotemporal dementia. Exploration of underlying mechanisms. *Neuropsychiatry, Neuropsychology and Behavioral Neurology, 9,* 154–161.

Loring, D. (Ed.). (1999). *INS Dictionary of Neuropsychology.* New York: Oxford University Press.

Loring, D., & Largen, J. (1985). Neuropsychological patterns of presenile and senile dementia of the Alzheimer type. *Neuropsychologia, 23,* 351–357.

Lorusso, S., Poli, V., & Casmiro, M. (1994). Cognitive improvement following treatment in a case of idiopathic hypoparathyroidism. *European Neurology, 34,* 292–294.

Lucas, J., Ivnik, R., Smith, G., Bohac, D., Tangalos, E., Graff-Radford, N., & Peterson, R. (1998). Mayo's Older Americans Normative Studies: Category Fluency Norms. *Journal of Clinical and Experimental Neuropsychology, 20,* 194–200.

Lucas-Blaustein, M., Filipp, L., Dungan, C., & Tune, L. (1988). Driving in patients with dementia. *Journal of the American Geriatric Society, 36,* 1087–1091.

Luerssen, T., Klauber, M., & Marshall, L. (1988). Outcome from head injury related to patient's age: A longitudinal prospective study of adult and pediatric head injury. *Journal of Neurosurgery, 68,* 409–416.

Lundberg, C., Hakamies-Blomqvist, L., Almkvist, O., & Johansson, K. (1998). Impairments of some cognitive functions are common in crash-involved older drivers. *Accident Analysis and Prevention, 30,* 371–377.

Lyketsos, G., Tune, L., Pearlson, G., & Steele, C. (1996). Major depression in Alzheimer's disease: An interaction between gender and family history. *Psychosomatics, 37,* 380–384.

Lynch, T., Sano, M., Marder, K., Bell, K., Foster, N., Defendini, R., Sima, A., Keohane, C., Nygaard, T., Fahn, S., Mayeux, R., Rowland, L., & Wilhelmsen, K. (1994). Clinical characteristics of a family with chromosome 17-linked disinhibition-dementia-parkinsonism-amyotrophy complex. *Neurology, 44,* 1878–1844.

Lyness, S., Eaton, E., & Schneider, L. (1994). Cognitive performance in older and middle-aged depressed outpatients and controls. *Journal of Gerontology: Psychological Sciences, 49,* P129–P136.

Mack, W., Freed, D., Williams, B., & Henderson, V. (1992). Boston Naming Test: Shortened version for Alzheimer's disease. *Journal of Gerontology, 47,* 164–168.

Mackenzie, T., Robiner, W., & Knopman, D. (1989). Differences between patient and family assessments of depression in Alzheimer's disease. *American Journal of Psychiatry, 146,* 1174–1178.

Maddrey, A., Cullum, C., Weiner, M., & Filley, C. (1996). Premorbid intelligence and level of dementia in Alzheimer's disease. *Journal of the International Neuropsychological Society, 2,* 551–555.

Mahalik, D., Ruff, R., & U, H. (1991). Neuropsychological sequelae of arteriovenous malformations. *Neurosurgery, 29,* 351–357.

Mahendra, B. (1987). *Dementia: A Survey of the Syndrome of Dementia (2nd edition).* Lancaster, UK: MTP Press.

Maier, W., Lichtermann, D., Minges, J., Heun, R., Hallmayer, J., & Klingler, T. (1991). Unipolar depression in the aged: Determinants of family aggregation. *Journal of Affective Disorder, 23,* 53–61.

Mair, W., Warrington, E., & Weiskrantz, L. (1979). Memory disorder in Korsakoff psychosis: A neuropathological and neuropsychological investigation of two cases. *Brain, 102,* 749–783.

Malec, J., Ivnik, R., Smith, G., Tangalos, E., Peterson, R., Kokmen, E., & Kurland, L. (1992). Mayo's Older Americans Normative Studies: Utility of corrections for age and education for the WAIS-R. *The Clinical Neuropsychologist, 6,* 31–48.

Manly, J., Jacobs, D., Sano, M., Bell, K., Merchant, C., Small, S., & Stern, Y. (1998). Cognitive test performance among nondemented African Americans and whites. *Neurology, 50,* 1238–1245.

Marcopulus, B., & Graves, R. (1990). Antidepressant effect on memory in depressed older persons. *Journal of Clinical Experimental Neuropsychology, 12,* 655–663.

Marder, K., Tang, M., Alfaro, B., Mejia, H., Cote, L., Jacobs, D., Stern, Y., Sano, M., & Mayeux, R. (1998). Postmenopausal estrogen use and Parkinson's disease with and without dementia. *Neurology, 50,* 1141–1143.

Marder, K., Tang, M.-X., Cote, L., Stern, Y., & Mayeux, R. (1995). The frequency and associated risk factors for dementia in patients with Parkinson's disease. *Archives of Neurology, 52,* 695–701.

Markowitsch, H. (1982). Thalamic mediodorsal nucleus and memory: A critical evaluation of studies in animals and in man. *Neuroscience Biobehavioral Review, 6,* 351–380.

Marson, D., Dymek, M., Duke, L., & Harrell, L. (1997). Subscale validity of the Mattis Dementia Rating Scale. *Archives of Clinical Neuropsychology, 12,* 269–275.

Martin, A., Brouwers, P., Lalonde, F., Cox, C., Teleska, P., Fedio, P., Foster, N., & Chase, T. (1986). Towards a behavioral typology of Alzheimer's patients. *Journal of Clinical and Experimental Neuropsychology, 8,* 594–610.

Martin, A., & Fedio, P. (1983). Word production and comprehension in Alzheimer's disease: The breakdown of semantic knowledge. *Brain and Language, 19,* 124–141.

Martin, W., Young, W., & Anderson, V. (1973). Parkinson's disease: A genetic study. *Brain, 96,* 495–506.

Massman, P., Delis, D., Butters, N., Dupont, R., & Gillin, J. (1992). The subcortical dysfunction hypothesis of deficits in depression: Neuropsychological validation in a subgroup of patients. *Journal of Clinical and Experimental Neuropsychology, 14,* 687–706.

Massman, P., Kreiter, K., Jankovic, J., & Doody, R. (1996). Neuropsychological functioning in cortical-basal ganglionic degeneration: Differentiation from Alzheimer's disease. *Neurology, 46,* 720–726.

Masur, D., Sliwinski, M., Lipton, R., Blau, A., & Crystal, H. (1994). Neuropsychological prediction of dementia and the absence of dementia in healthy elderly persons. *Neurology, 44,* 1427–1432.

Matison, R., Mayeux, R., Rosen, J., & Fahn, S. (1982). "Tip-of-the-tongue" phenomenon in Parkinson's disease. *Neurology, 29,* 951–956.

Mattis, S. (1988). *Dementia rating scale.* Odessa, FL: Psychological Assessment Resources, Inc.

Mayberg, H., Starkstein, S., Sadzot, B., Preziosis, T., Andrezejewski, P., Dannals, R., Wagner, H.J., & Robinson, R. (1990). Selective hypometabolism in the inferior frontal lobe in depressed patients with Parkinson's disease. *Annals of Neurology, 28,* 57–64.

Mayeux, R., Chen, J., Mirabello, E., Marder, K., Bell, K., Dooneief, G., Cote, L., & Stern, Y. (1990). An estimate of the incidence of dementia in idiopathic Parkinson's disease. *Neurology, 40,* 1513–1517.

Mayeux, R., Denaro, J., Hemenegildo, N., Marder, K., Tang, M., Cote, L., & Stern, Y. (1992). A population-based investigation of Parkinson's disease with and without dementia: Relationships to age and gender. *Archives of Neurology, 42,* 492–497.

Mayeux, R., Ottman, R., Maestre, G., Ngai, C., Tang, M.-X., Ginsberg, H., Chun, M., Tycko, B., & Shelanski, M. (1995). Synergistic effects of traumatic head injury and apolipoprotein e4 in patients with Alzheimer's disease. *Neurology, 45,* 555–557.

Mayeux, R., Sano, M., Chen, J., Tatemichi, T., & Stern, Y. (1991). Risk of dementia in first-degree relatives of patients with Alzheimer's disease and related disorders. *Archives of Neurology, 48,* 269–273.

Mayeux, R., Saunders, A., Shea, S., Mirra, S., Evans, D., Roses, A., Hyman, B., Crain, B., Tang, M.-X., & Phelps, C. (1998). Utility of the apolipoprotein e genotype in the diagnosis of Alzheimer's disease. *New England Journal of Medicine, 338,* 506–511.

Mayeux, R., Stern, Y., Cote, L., & Williams, J. (1984). Altered serotonin metabolism in depressed patients with Parkinson's disease. *Neurology, 34,* 642–646.

Mayeux, R., Stern, Y., Ottman, R., Tatemichi, T., Tang, M.-X., Maestre, G., Ngai, C., Tycko, B., & Ginsberg, H. (1993). The apolipoprotein e4 allele in patients with Alzheimer's disease. *Annals of Neurology, 34,* 752–754.

Mayeux, R., Stern, Y., Rosen, J., & Benson, D. (1983). Is subcortical dementia a recognizable clinical entity? *Annals of Neurology, 14,* 278–283.

Mayeux, R., Stern, Y., Sano, M., Williams, J., & Cote, I. (1988). The relationship of serotonin to depression in Parkinson's disease. *Movement Disorders, 3,* 237–244.

Mayeux, R., Stern, Y., & Spanton, S. (1985). Heterogeneity in dementia of the Alzheimer type. *Neurology, 35,* 453–461.

Mayeux, R., Stern, Y., Williams, J., Cote, L., Frantz, A., & Dyrenfurth, I. (1986). Clinical and biochemical features of depression in Parkinson's disease. *American Journal of Psychiatry, 143,* 756–759.

Mayfield, D., McLeod, G., & Hall, P. (1974). The CAGE questionnaire: Validation of a new alcoholism screening instrument. *American Journal of Psychiatry, 131,* 1121–1123.

McFie, J. (1975). *Assessment of Organic Intellectual Function.* London: Academic Press.

McGlynn, S.M., & Kaszniak, A.W. (1991). When metacognition fails: Impaired awareness of deficit in Alzheimer's disease. *Journal of Cognitive Neuroscience, 3,* 183–189.

McHugh, P., & Folstein, M. (1975). Psychiatric syndromes in Huntington's disease. In D. Benson & D. Blumer (Eds.), *Psychiatric Aspects of Neurologic Disease* (pp. 267–285). New York: Grune & Stratton.

McKeith, I., Galasko, D., Kosak, K., Perry, E., Dickson, D., Hansen, L., Salmon, D., Lowe, J., Mirra, S., Byrne, E., Lennos, G., Quinn, N., Edwardson, J., Ince, P., Bergeron, C., Burns, A., Miller, B., Lovestone, S., Collerton, D., Jansen, E., Ballard, C., de Vos, R., Wilcock, G., Jellinger, K., & Perry, R. (1996). Consensus guidelines for the clinical and pathologic diagnosis of dementia with Lewy bodies (DLB): Report of the consortium on DLB international workshop. *Neurology, 47,* 1113–1124.

McKhann, G., Drachman, D., Folstein, M., Katzman, R., Price, D., & Stadlan, E. (1984). Clinical diagnosis of Alzheimer's disease: Report of the NINCDS-ADRDA Work Group, Department of Health and Human Services Task Force on Alzheimer's Disease. *Neurology, 34,* 939–944.

Meador, K., Loring, D., Davis, H., Sethi, K., Patel, B., Adams, R., & Hammond, E. (1987). Cholinergic and serotonergic effects on the P3 potential and memory. *Journal of Clinical and Experimental Neuropsychology, 11,* 252–260.

Mega, M., Cummings, J., Fiorello, T., & Gornbein, J. (1996). The spectrum of behavioral changes in Alzheimer's disease. *Neurology, 46,* 130–135.

Mendez, M., Adams, N., & Leewandowksi, K. (1989). Neurobehavioral changes associated with caudate lesions. *Neurology, 39,* 349–354.

Mendez, M., & Ashla-Mendez, M. (1991). Differences between multi-infarct dementia and Alzheimer's disease on unstructured neuropsychological tasks. *Journal of Clinical and Experimental Neuropsychology, 13,* 923–932.

Mendez, M., Cherrier, M., Perryman, K., Nachana, N., Miller, B., & Cummings, J. (1996). Frontotemporal dementia versus Alzheimer's disease. *Neurology, 47,* 1189–1194.

Mendez, M., Underwood, K., Zander, B., Mastri, A., Sung, J., & Frey, W., II. (1992a). Risk factors in Alzheimer's disease: A clinicopathologic study. *Neurology, 42,* 770–775.

Mendez, M.F., Ala, T., & Underwood, K.L. (1992b). Development of scoring criteria for the clock drawing task in Alzheimer's disease. *Journal of the American Geriatrics Society, 40,* 1095–1099.

Mendlewicz, J., & Baron, M. (1991). Morbidity risks in subtypes of unipolar depressive illness. Differences between early- and late-onset forms. *British Journal of Psychiatry, 134,* 463–466.

Mennemeier, M., Garner, R., & Heilman, K. (1993). Memory, mood and measurement in hypothyroidism. *Journal of Clinical and Experimental Neuropsychology, 15,* 882–831.

Menza, M., Golbe, L., Cody, R., & Forman, N. (1993). Dopamine-related personality traits in Parkinson's disease. *Neurology, 43,* 505–508.

Merello, M., Sabe, L., Teson, A., Migliorelli, R., Petracchi, M., Leiguarda, R., & Starkstein, S. (1994). Extrapyramidalism in Alzheimer's disease: Prevalence, psychiatric and neuropsychological correlates. *Journal of Neurology, Neurosurgery and Psychiatry, 57,* 1503–1509.

Mesulam, M., Mufson, E., Levey, A., & Wainer, B. (1983). Cholinergic innervation of cortex by the basal forebrain: Cytochemistry and cortical connections of the septal area, diagonal band nuclei, nucleus basalis (substantia innominata), and hypothalamus in the rhesus monkey. *Journal of Comparative Neurology, 214,* 170–197.

Mesulam, M., & Weintraub, S. (1992). Primary progressive aphasia. In F. Boller (Ed.), *Heterogeneity of Alzheimer's Disease* (pp. 43–66). Berlin: Springer-Verlag.

Mesulam, M.-M. (1985). *Principles of Behavioral Neurology.* Philadelphia: F.A. Davis.

Meyer, J., McClintic, K., Rogers, R., Sims, P., & Mortel, K. (1988). Aetiological considerations and risk factors for multi-infarct dementia. *Journal of Neurology, Neurosurgery, and Psychiatry, 51,* 1489–1497.

Michon, A., Deweer, B., Pillon, B., Agid, Y., & Dubois, B. (1992). Anosognosia and frontal dysfunction in SDAT. *Neurology, 42,* 221.

Milberg, W., & Albert, M. (1989). Cognitive differences between patients with progressive supranuclear palsy and Alzheimer's disease. *Journal of Clinical and Experimental Neuropsychology, 11,* 605–614.

Milberg, W., Hebben, N., & Kaplan, E. (1986). The Boston Process Approach to neuropsychological assessment. In I. Grant & K. Adams (Eds.), *Neuropsychological Assessment of Neuropsychiatric Disorders* (2nd ed., pp. 58–80). New York: Oxford University Press.

Miller, B., Cummings, J., Villanueva-Meyer, J., Boone, K., Mehringer, C., Lesser, I., & Mena, I. (1991). Frontal lobe degeneration: Clinical, neuropsychological and SPECT characteristics. *Neurology, 41,* 1374–1382.

Miller, B., Ikonte, C., Ponton, M., Levy, M., Boone, K., Darby, A., Berman, N., Mena, I., & Cummings, J. (1997). A study of the Lund-Manchester research criteria for frontotemporal dementia: Clinical and single-photon emission CT correlations. *Neurology, 48,* 937–942.

Miller, B., Lesser, I., Boone, K., Goldberg, M., Hill, E., Miller, M., Benson, D., & Mehringer, M. (1989). Brain white-matter lesions and psychosis. *British Journal of Psychiatry, 155,* 73–78.

Milner, B. (1963). Effects of different lesions on card sorting. *Archives of Neurology, 9,* 100–110.

Milner, B. (1968). Disorders of memory after brain lesions in man: Preface: Material-specific and generalized memory loss. *Neuropsychologia, 6,* 175–179.

Milner, B. (1970). Memory and the medial temporal regions of the brain. In K. Pribram & D. Broadbent (Eds.), *Biological Bases of Memory.* New York: Academic Press.

Mirra, S., Heyman, A., & McKeel, D. (1991). The Consortium to Establish a Registry for Alzheimer's Disease (CERAD), II: Standardization of the neuropathologic assessment of Alzheimer's disease. *Neurology, 41,* 479–486.

Mittenberg, W., Seidenberg, M., O'Leary, D., & DiGiulio, D. (1989). Changes in cerebral functioning associated with normal aging. *Journal of Clinical and Experimental Neuropsychology, 11,* 918–932.

Mohr, E., Juncos, J., Cox, C., Litvan, I., Fedio, P., & Chase, T. (1990). Selective deficits in cognition and memory in high-functioning parkinsonian patients. *Journal of Neurology, Neurosurgery and Psychiatry, 53,* 603–606.

Monsch, A., Bondi, M., Butters, N., Paulsen, J., Salmon, D., Brugger, P., & Swenson, M. (1994). A comparison of category and letter fluency in Alzheimer's disease and Huntington's disease. *Neuropsychology, 8,* 25–30.

Monsch, A., Bondi, M., Butters, N., Salmon, D., Katzman, R., & Thal, L. (1992). Comparisons of verbal fluency task in the detection of dementia of the Alzheimer type. *Archives of Neurology, 49,* 1253–1258.

Monsch, A., Bondi, M., Salmon, D., Butters, N., Thal, L., Hansen, L., Wiederholt, W., Cahn, D., & Klauber, M. (1995). Clinical validity of the Mattis Dementia Rating Scale in detecting dementia of the Alzheimer' type. *Archives of Neurology, 52,* 899–904.

Mooradian, A., Perryman, K., Fitten, J., Kavonian, G., & Morley, J. (1988). Cortical function in elderly non-insulin dependent diabetic patients. *Archives of Neurology, 148,* 2369–2372.

Moray, N. (1970). *Attention: Selective Processes in Vision and Hearing.* New York: Academic Press.

Mortensen, E., Gade, A., & Reinisch, J. (1991). A critical note on Lezak's "best performance method" in clinical neuropsychology. *Journal of Clinical and Experimental Neuropsychology, 13,* 361–371.

Mortimer, J., Ebbitt, B., Jun, S., & Finch, M. (1992). Predictors of cognitive and functional decline in patients with probable Alzheimer's disease. *Neurology, 42,* 1689–1696.

Mortimer, J., van Duijn, C., Chandra, V., Fratiglioni, L., Graves, A., Heyman, A., Jorm, A., Kokmen, E., Kondo, K., Rocca, W., Shalat, S., Soinenen, H., & Hofman, A. (1991). Head trauma as a risk factor for Alzheimer's disease: A collaborative re-analysis of case-control studies. *International Journal of Epidemiology, 20 (Suppl 2),* S28–S35.

Moss, H., Tarter, R., Yao, J., & VanThiel, D. (1992). Subclinical hepatic encephalopathy: Relationship between neuropsychological deficits and standard laboratory tests assessing hepatic status. *Archives of Clinical Neuropsychology, 7,* 419–429.

Moss, M., Albert, M., Butters, N., & Payne, M. (1986). Differential patterns of memory loss among patients with Alzheimer's disease, Huntington's disease and alcoholic Korsakoff's syndrome. *Archives of Neurology, 43,* 239–246.

Myers, R., Sax, D., Koroshetz, W., Mastromauro, C., Cupples, L., Kiely, D., Pettengill, F., & Bird, E. (1991). Factors associated with slow progression in Huntington's disease. *Archives of Neurology, 48,* 800–804.

National Institutes of Health Consensus Development Conference (1993). Diagnosis and treatment of depression in late life. *Psychopharmacology Bulletin, 29,* 87–95.

Naugle, R. (1990). Epidemiology of traumatic brain injury in adults. In E. Bigler (Ed.), *Traumatic Brain Injury* (pp. 69–103). Austin, TX: Pro-Ed.

Naugle, R., Chelune, G., Cheek, R., Luders, H., & Awad, I. (1993). Detection of changes in material-specific memory following temporal lobectomy using the Wechsler Memory Scale–Revised. *Archives of Clinical Neuropsychology, 8,* 381–395.

Naugle, R., Chelune, G., Schuster, J., Luders, H., & Comair, Y. (1994). Recognition memory for words and faces before and after temporal lobectomy. *Assessment, 1,* 373–381.

Neary, D., & Snowden, J. (1996). Fronto-temporal dementia: Nosology, neuropsychology, and neuropathology. *Brain and Cognition, 31,* 176–187.

Neary, D., Snowden, J., Gustafson, L., Passant, U., Stuss, D., Black, S., Freeman, M., Kertesz, A., Robert, P., Albert, M., Boone, K., Miller, B., Cummings, J., & Benson, D. (1998). Frontotemporal lobar degeneration: A consensus on clinical diagnostic criteria. *Neurology, 51,* 1546–1554.

Neary, D., Snowden, J., Mann, D., Northen, B., Goulding, P., & Mcdermott, N. (1990). Frontal lobe dementia and motor neuron disease. *Journal of Neurology, Neurosurgery and Psychiatry, 53,* 23–32.

Neary, D., Snowden, J., Northen, B., & Goulding, P. (1988). Dementia of the frontal lobe type. *Journal of Neurology, Neurosurgery and Psychiatry, 51,* 353–361.

Neary, D., Snowden, J., Shields, R., Burjan, A., Northen, B., MacDermott, N., Prescott, M., & Testa, H. (1987). Single photon emission tomography using 99mTc-HMPAO in the investigation of dementia. *Journal of Neurology, Neurosurgery and Psychiatry, 50,* 1101–1109.

Nelson, H. (1976). A modified card sorting test sensitive to frontal deficits. *Cortex, 12,* 313–324.

Nelson, H. (1982). *National Adult Reading Test.* Windsor, England: The NFER-Nelson Publishing Company, Ltd.

Nelson, H., & O'Connell, A. (1978). Dementia: The estimation of premorbid intelligence levels using the New Adult Reading Test. *Cortex, 14,* 234–244.

Netter, F. (1989). *Atlas of Human Anatomy.* Summit, NJ: CIBA-GEIGY Corporation.

Newcombe, F. (1969). *Missile Wounds of the Brain.* London: Oxford University Press.

Niederehe, G. (1986). Depression and memory impairment in the aged. In L. Poon (Ed.), *Handbook for Clinical Memory Assessment of Older Adults.* Washington, DC: American Psychological Association.

Norman, D. (1968). *Memory and Attention: An Introduction to Human Information Processing.* New York: Wiley.

Norris, J., Gallagher, D., Wilson, A., & Winograd, C. (1987). Assessment of depression in geriatric medical outpatients: The validity of two screening measures. *Journal of the American Geriatrics Society, 35,* 989–995.

Numann, P., Torppa, A., & Blumetti, A. (1984). Neuropsychologic deficits associated with primary hyperparathyroidism. *Surgery, 96,* 1119–1123.

Nussbaum, P. (1997). Late-life depression: A neuropsychological perspective. In P. Nussbaum (Ed.), *Handbook of Neuropsychology and Aging* (pp. 260–270). New York: Plenum Press.

Nussbaum, P., Kaszniak, A., Allender, J., & Rapcsak, S. (1995). Depression and cognitive decline in the elderly: A follow-up study. *The Clinical Neuropsychologist, 9,* 101–111.

Nussbaum, P., Kaszniak, A., Swanda, R., & Allender, J. (1988). Quantitative and qualitative aspects of memory performance in older depressed versus probable Alzheimer's disease patients. *Journal of Clinical and Experimental Neuropsychology, 10,* 63.

Ogden, J., Growdon, J., & Corkin, S. (1990). Deficits in visuospatial test involving forward planning in high-functioning parkinsonians. *Neuropsychiatry, Neuropsychology and Behavioral Neurology, 3,* 125–139.

Olin, J., Schneider, L., Eaton, E., Zemansky, M., & Pollock, V. (1992). The Geriatric Depression Scale and the Beck Depression Inventory as screening instruments in an older adult outpatient population. *Psychological Assessment, 4,* 190–192.

Olton, D., Wenk, G., Church, R., & Meck, W. (1988). Attention and the frontal cortex as examined by simultaneous temporal processing. *Neuropsychologia, 26,* 307–318.

O'Rourke, N., Tuokko, H., Hayden, S., & Beattie, B. (1997). Early identification of dementia: Predictive validity of the clock test. *Archives of Clinical Neuropsychology, 12,* 257–267.

Osterrieth, P. (1944). Le test de copie d'une figure complexe. *Archives de Psychologie, 30,* 206–356.

Osterweil, D., Syndulko, K., Cohen, S., Pettler-Jennings, P., Hershman, J., Cummings, J., Toutellotte, W., & Solomon, D. (1992). Cognitive function in non-demented older adults with hypothyroidism. *Journal of the American Geriatrics Society, 40,* 325–335.

Ouslander, J. (1981). Drug therapy in the elderly. *Annals of Internal Medicine, 95,* 711–722.

Owsley, C., Ball, K., Sloane, M., Roenker, D., & Bruni, J. (1991). Visual/cognitive correlates of vehicle accidents in older drivers. *Psychology and Aging, 6,* 403–415.

Pachana, N., Boone, K., Miller, B., Cummings, J., & Berman, N. (1996). Comparison of neuropsychological functioning in Alzheimer's disease and frontotemporal dementia. *Journal of the International Neuropsychological Society, 2,* 505–510.

Pan, G., Stern, Y., Sano, M., & Mayeux, R. (1989). Clock-drawing in neurological disorders. *Behavioral Neurology, 2,* 39–48.

Paolo, A., Axelrod, B., & Ryan, J. (1994). Administration accuracy of the Wisconsin Card Sorting Test. *The Clinical Neuropsychologist, 8,* 112–116.

Paolo, A., Axelrod, B., Troster, A., Blackwell, K., & Koller, W. (1996). Utility of the Wisconsin Card Sorting Test short form in persons with Alzheimer's and Parkinson's disease. *Journal of Clinical and Experimental Neuropsychology, 18,* 892–897.

Paolo, A., Troster, A., Glatt, S., Hubble, J., & Koller, W. (1995). Differentiation of the dementias of Alzheimer's and Parkinson's disease with the Dementia Rating Scale. *Journal of Geriatric Psychiatry and Neurology, 8,* 184–188.

Paque, L., & Warrington, E. (1995). A longitudinal study of reading ability in patients suffering from dementia. *Journal of the International Neuropsychological Society, 1,* 517–524.

Parasuraman, R., & Nestor, P. (1991). Attention and driving skills in aging and Alzheimer's disease. *Human Factors, 33,* 539–557.

Parasuraman, R., & Nestor, P. (1993). Attention and driving. Assessment in elderly individuals with dementia. *Clinics in Geriatric Medicine, 9,* 377–387.

Parkin, A., Blunden, J., Rees, J., & Hunkin, N. (1991). Wernicke-Korsakoff syndrome of nonalcoholic origin. *Brain and Cognition, 15,* 69–82.

Parkinson, J. (1817). *An Essay on the Shaking Palsy.* London: Sherwood, Neely and Jones.

Parks, R., Loewenstein, D., Dodrill, K., Barker, W., Yoshii, F., Chang, J., Emran, A., Apicella, A., Sheramata, W., & Duara, R. (1988). Cerebral metabolic effects of a verbal fluency test: A PET scan study. *Journal of Clinical and Experimental Neuropsychology, 10,* 565–575.

Parsons, O., Butters, N., & Nathan, P. (1987). *Neuropsychology of Alcoholism: Implications for Diagnosis and Treatment.* New York: Guilford Press.

Parsons, O., & Leber, W. (1981). The relationship between cognitive dysfunction and brain damage in alcoholics: Causal, interactive or epiphenomenal? *Alcoholism: Clinical and Experimental Research, 5,* 326–343.

Patterson, A., & Zangwill, O. (1944). Disorders of visual space perception associated with lesions of the right cerebral hemsiphere. *Brain, 67,* 331–358.

Patterson, K., Graham, N., & Hodges, J. (1994). Reading in Alzheimer's type dementia: A preserved ability? *Neuropsychology, 8,* 395–407.

Paulesu, E., Frith, C., & Frackowiak, R. (1993). The neural correlates of the verbal components of working memory. *Nature, 362,* 342–345.

Paulson, H., & Stern, M. (1997). Clinical manifestations of Parkinson's disease. In R. Watts & W. Koller (Eds.), *Movement Disorders: Neurologic Principles and Practice* (pp. 183–199). New York: McGraw-Hill.

Paulson, J., Butters, N., Salmon, D., Heindel, W., & Swenson, M. (1993). Prism adaptation in Alzheimer's and Huntington's disease. *Neuropsychology, 7,* 73–81.

Pearson, J., Teri, L., Reifler, B., & Raskind, M. (1989). Functional status and cognitive impairment in Alzheimer's patients with and without depression. *Journal of the American Geriatrics Society, 37,* 1117–1121.

Perez, J., Rivera, V., Meyer, J., Gay, J., Taylor, R., & Mather, N. (1975). Analysis of intellectual and cognitive performance in patients with multi-infarct dementia, vertebro-basilar insufficiency with dementia and Alzheimer's disease. *Journal of Neurology, Neurosurgery and Psychiatry, 38,* 533–540.

Peterson, R., Mokri, B., & Laws, E. (1985). Surgical treatment of idiopathic hydrocephalus in elderly patients. *Neurology, 35,* 307–311.

Peterson, R., Smith, G., Ivnik, R., Tangalos, E., Schaid, D., Thibodeau, S., Kokmen, E., Waring, S., & Kurland, L. (1995). Apolipoprotein E status as a predictor of the development of Alzheimer's disease in memory-impaired individuals. *Journal of the American Medical Association, 273,* 1274–1278.

Petracca, G., Teson, A., Chemerinski, E., Leiguarda, R., & Starkstein, S. (1996). A double-blind placebo-controlled study of clomipramine in depressed patients. *Journal of Neuropsychiatry and Clinical Neurosciences, 8,* 270–275.

Pettinati, H., & Rosenberg, J. (1984). Memory self-ratings before and after electroconvulsive therapy: Depression- versus ECT induced. *Biological Psychiatry, 19,* 539–548.

Pfefferbaum, A., Lim, K., Zipursky, R., Mathalon, D., Rosenbloom, M., Lane, B., Ha, C., & Sullivan, E. (1992). Brain gray and white matter volume loss accelerates with aging in chronic alcoholics: A quantitative study. *Alcoholism: Clinical and Experimental Research, 16,* 1078–1089.

Pfefferbaum, A., Rosenbloom, M., Crusan, K., & Jernigan, T. (1988). Brain CT changes in alcoholics: Effects of age and alcohol consumption. *Alcoholism: Clinical and Experimental Research, 12,* 81–87.

Physician's Desk Reference. (1999). Montvale, NJ: Medical Economics Company.

Pick, A. (1977). On the relationship between aphasia and senile atrophy of the brain (1892). In D. Rottenberg & F. Hochberg (Eds.), *Neurological Classics in Modern Translation* (pp. 35–40). New York: Hafner Press.

Pillon, B., Blin, J., Vidailhet, M., Deweer, B., Sirigu, A., Dubois, B., & Agid, Y. (1995a). The neuropsychological pattern of corticobasal degeneration: Comparison with progressive supranuclear palsy and Alzheimer's disease. *Neurology, 45,* 1477–1483.

Pillon, B., Dubois, B., Cusimano, G., Bonnet, A.-M., Lhermitte, F., & Agid, Y. (1989). Does cognitive impairment in Parkinson's disease result from non-dopaminergic lesions? *Journal of Neurology, Neurosurgery and Psychiatry, 52,* 201–206.

Pillon, B., Dubois, B., Lhermitte, F., & Agid, Y. (1986). Heterogeneity of cognitive impairment in progressive supranuclear palsy, Parkinson's disease and Alzheimer's disease. *Neurology, 36,* 1179–1185.

Pillon, B., Dubois, B., & Ploska, A. (1991). Severity and specificity of cognitive impairment in Alzheimer's, Huntington's, Parkinson's disease and progressive supranuclear palsy. *Neurology, 41,* 634–643.

Pillon, B., Gouider-Khouja, N., Deweer, B., Vadailhet, M., Malapani, C., Dubois, B., & Agid, Y. (1995b). Neuropsychological pattern of striatonigral degeneration: Comparison with Parkinson's disease and progressive supranuclear palsy. *Journal of Neurology, Neurosurgery, and Psychiatry, 58,* 174–179.

Poewe, W., Daramat, E., Kemmler, G., & Gerstenbrand, F. (1990). The premorbid personality of patients with Parkinson's disease: A comparative study with healthy controls and patients with essential tremor. *Parkinson's Disease: Anatomy, Pathology and Therapy. Advances in Neurology* (Vol. 53, pp. 339–342). New York: Raven Press.

Pomara, N., Stanley, B., Block, R., Berchou, R., Stanley, M., Greenblatt, D., Newton, R., & Gershon, S. (1985). Increased sensitivity of the elderly to the central depressant effects of diazepam. *Journal of Clinical Psychiatry, 46,* 185–187.

Pomara, N., Stanley, B., Block, R., Guido, J., Russ, D., Berchou, R., Stanley, M., Greenblatt, D., Newton, R., & Gershon, S. (1984). Adverse effects of single therapeutic doses of diazepam on performance in normal geriatric subjects: Relationship to plasma concentrations. *Psychopharmacology, 84,* 342–346.

Pomara, N., Tun, H., DaSilva, D., Hernando, R., Deptula, D., & Greenblatt, D. (1998). The acute and chronic performance effects of alprazolam and lorazepam in the elderly: Relationship to duration of treatment and self-rated sedation. *Psychopharmacology Bulletin, 34,* 139–153.

Portin, R., & Rinne, U. (1986). Predictive factors for cognitive deterioration and dementia in Parkinson's disease. In M. Yahr & K. Bergmann (Eds.), *Advances in Neurology* (Vol. 45, pp. 413–416). New York: Raven Press.

Posner, M.I., & Peterson, S.E. (1990). The attention system of the human brain. *Annual Review of Neuroscience, 13,* 25–42.

Postle, B., Jonides, J., Smith, E., Corkin, S., & Growdon, J. (1997). Spatial, but not object, delayed response is impaired in early Parkinson's disease. *Neuropsychology, 11,* 171–179.

Pramming, S., Thorsteinsson, B., Theilgaard, A., Pinner, E., & Binder, C. (1986). Cognitive function during hypoglycemia in type I diabetes mellitus. *British Medical Journal, 292,* 647–650.

Preskorn, S., & Jerkovich, G. (1990). Central nervous system toxicity of tricyclic antidepressants: Phenomenology, risk factors and role of therapeutic drug monitoring. *Journal of Clinical Psychopharmacology, 10,* 88–95.

Price, T., & Tucker, G. (1977). Psychiatric and behavioral manifestations of normal pressure hydrocephalus. *Journal of Nervous and Mental Disease, 164,* 51–55.

Prigatano, G.P., & Schacter, D.L. (1991). *Awareness of Deficit after Brain Injury.* New York: Oxford University Press.

Prinz, P., Scanlan, J., Vitaliano, P., Moe, K., Borson, S., Toivola, B., Merriam, G., Larsen, L., & Reed, H. (1999). Thyroid hormones: Positive relationships with cognition in healthy, euthyroid older men. *Journals of Gerontology. Series A, Biological Sciences and Medical Sciences, 54,* M111–116.

Prohovnik, I., Smith, G., Sackeim, H., Mayeux, R., & Stern, Y. (1989). Gray-matter degeneration in presenile Alzheimer's disease. *Annals of Neurology, 25,* 117–124.

Pujol, J., Leal, S., Fluvia, X., & Conde, C. (1989). Psychiatric aspects of normal pressure hydrocephalus: A report of 5 cases. *British Journal of Psychiatry, 154,* 77–80.

Quinn, N. (1989). Multiple system atrophy—the nature of the beast. *Journal of Neurology, Neurosurgery and Psychiatry (Suppl),* 78–89.

Quinn, N., Critchley, P., & Marsden, C. (1987). Young onset Parkinson's disease. *Movement Disorders, 2,* 73–91.

Rabins, P., Merchant, A., & Nestadt, G. (1984). Criteria for diagnosing reversible dementia caused by depression: Validation by 2-year follow-up. *British Journal of Psychiatry, 144,* 488.

Rabins, P., Starkstein, S., & Robinson, R. (1991). Risk factors for developing atypical (schizophreniform) psychosis following stroke. *Journal of Neuropsychiatry and Clinical Neuroscience, 3,* 6–9.

Rajput, A., Offord, K., Beard, C., & Durland, L. (1984). Epidemiology of parkinsonism: Incidence, classification and mortality. *Annals of Neurology, 16,* 278–282.

Rajput, A.H. (1992). Prevalence of dementia in Parkinson's disease. In S.J. Huber & J.L. Cummings (Eds.), *Parkinson's Disease: Neurobehavioral Aspects* (pp. 119–131). New York: Oxford University Press.

Randolph, C., Braun, A., Goldberg, T., & Chase, T. (1993). Semantic fluency in Alzheimer's, Parkinson's and Huntington's disease: Dissociation of storage and retrieval failures. *Neuropsychology, 7,* 82–88.

Rao, S. (1990). Neuroimaging correlates of cognitive dysfunction. In S. Rao (Ed.), *Neurobehavioral Aspects of Multiple Sclerosis.* New York: Oxford University Press.

Rao, S., Mittenberg, W., Bernardin, L., Haughton, V., & Leo, G. (1989). Neuropsychological test findings in subjects with leukoaraiosis. *Archives of Neurology, 46,* 40–44.

Rapp, S., Parisi, S., Walsh, D., & Wallace, C. (1988). Detecting depression in elderly medical outpatients. *Journal of Consulting and Clinical Psychology, 56,* 509–513.

Rapport, L., Webster, J., & Dutra, R. (1994). Digit span performance and unilateral neglect. *Neuropsychologia, 32,* 517–525.

Raskin, A. (1986). Partialing out the effects of depression and age on cognitive functions: Experimental data and methodologic issues. In L. Poon (Ed.), *Handbook for Clinical Memory Assessment of Older Adults* (pp. 244–256). Washington, DC: American Psychological Association.

Rasmussen, D., Brandt, J., Martin, D., & Folstein, M. (1995). Head injury as a risk factor for Alzheimer's disease. *Brain Injury, 9,* 213–219.

Rasmussen, K., & Abrams, R. (1992). The role of electroconvulsive therapy in Parkinson's disease. In S. Huber & J. Cummings (Eds.), *Parkinson's Disease: Neurobehavioral Aspects* (pp. 255–270). New York: Oxford University Press.

Rasmusson, D., Carson, K., Brookmeye, R., Kawas, C., & Brandt, J. (1996). Predicting rate of cognitive decline in probable Alzheimer's disease. *Brain and Cognition, 31,* 133–147.

Reaven, G., Thompson, L., Nahum, D., & Haskins, E. (1990). Relationship between hyperglycemia and cognitive function in older NIDDM patients. *Diabetes Care, 13,* 16–21.

Rebeck, G., Perls, T., West, H., Sodhi, P., Lipsitz, L., & Hyman, B. (1994). Reduced apolipoprotein e4 allele frequency in the oldest old Alzheimer's patients and cognitively normal individuals. *Neurology, 44,* 1513–1516.

Rebok, G., Brandt, J., & Folstein, M. (1990). Longitudinal decline in patients with Alzheimer's disease. *Journal of Geriatric Psychiatry and Neurology, 3,* 91–97.

Rebok, G., Bylsma, F., Keyl, P., Brandt, J., & Folstein, S. (1995). Automobile driving in Huntington's disease. *Movement Disorders, 10,* 778–787.

Reed, B.R., Jagust, W.J., & Coulter, L. (1993). Anosognosia in Alzheimer's disease: Relationships to depression, cognitive function, and cerebral perfusion. *Journal of Clinical and Experimental Neuropsychology, 15,* 321–244.

Regier, D., Boyd, J., Burke, J., Jr, Rae, D., Myers, J., Kramer, K., Robins, M., George, L., Karno, L., & Locke, B. (1988). One-month prevalence rates of mental disorders in the United States. *Archives of General Psychiatry,* 977–986.

Reifler, B., Larson, E., & Hanley, R. (1982). Coexistence of cognitive impairment and depression in geriatric outpatients. *American Journal of Psychiatry, 139,* 623.

Reifler, B., Larson, E., Teri, L., & Poulsen, M. (1986). Dementia of the Alzheimer's type and depression. *Journal of the American Geriatrics Society, 34,* 855–859.

Reifler, B., Teri, L., Raskind, M., Veith, R., Barnes, R., White, E., & McLean, P. (1989). Double-blind trial of imipramine in Alzheimer's disease patients with and without depression. *American Journal of Psychiatry, 146,* 45–49.

Reiman, E., Caselli, R., Yun, L., Chen, K., Bandy, D., Minoshima, S., Thibodeau, S., & Osborne, D. (1996). Preclinical evidence of Alzheimer's disease in persons homozygous for the e4 allele for apolipoprotein E. *New England Journal of Medicine, 334,* 752–758.

Reitan, R., & Wolfson, D. (1995). Category Test and Trail-Making Test as measures of frontal lobe functions. *The Clinical Neuropsychologist, 9,* 50–56.

Rey, A. (1941). Psychological examination of traumatic encephalopathy. *Archives de Psychologie, 28,* 286–340.

Rezai, K., Andreasen, N., Alliger, R., Cohen, G., Swayze, V., & O'Leary, D. (1993). The neuropsychology of prefrontal cortex. *Archives of Neurology, 50,* 636–642.

Richards, M., Bell, K., Dooneief, G., Marder, K., Sano, M., Mayeux, R., & Stern, Y. (1993a). Patterns of neuropsychological performance in Alzheimer's disease patients with and without extrapyramidal signs. *Neurology, 43,* 1708–1711.

Richards, M., Cote, L., & Stern, Y. (1993b). The relationship between visuospatial ability and perceptual motor function in Parkinson's disease. *Journal of Neurology, Neurosurgery and Psychiatry, 56,* 400–406.

Richards, M., Stern, Y., Marder, K., Cote, L., & Mayeux, R. (1993c). Relationships between extrapyramidal signs and cognitive function in a community-dwelling cohort of patients with Parkinson's disease and normal elderly individuals. *Annals of Neurology, 33,* 267–274.

Richards, M., Stern, Y., & Mayeux, R. (1993d). Subtle extrapyramidal signs can predict the development of dementia in elderly individuals. *Neurology, 43,* 2184–2188.

Richardson, J. (1991). Cognitive performance following rupture and repair of intracranial aneurysm. *Acta Neurologica Scandinavica, 83,* 110–122.

Ricker, J., Axelrod, B., & Houtler, B. (1996). Clinical validation of the oral Trail-Making Test. *Neuropsychiatry, Neuropsychology and Behavioral Neurology, 9,* 50–53.

Riley, D., Lang, A., Lewis, A., Resch, L., Ashby, P., Hornykiewicz, O., & Black, S. (1990). Cortical-basal ganglionic degeneration. *Neurology, 40,* 1203–1212.

Robbins, T., James, M., Lange, K., Owen, A., Quinn, N., & Marsden, C. (1992). Cognitive dysfunction in multiple system atrophy. *Brain, 115,* 271–291.

Robinson, A., Heaton, R., Lehman, R., & Stilson, D. (1980). The utility of the Wisconsin Card Sorting Test in detecting and localizing frontal lesions. *Journal of Clinical and Consulting Psychology, 48,* 605–614.

Robinson, L., Kester, D., Saykin, A., Kaplan, E., & Gur, R. (1991). Comparison of two short forms of the Wisconsin Card Sorting Test. *Archives of Clinical Neuropsychology, 6,* 27–33.

Robinson, R., Kubos, K., Starr, L., Rao, K., & Price, T. (1984). Mood disorders in stroke patients: Importance of location of lesion. *Brain, 107,* 81–93.

Robinson, R., Starr, L., Kubos, K., & Price, T. (1983). A two-year longitudinal study of poststroke mood disorders: Findings during the initial evaluation. *Stroke, 14,* 736–744.

Robinson, R., & Szetela, B. (1981). Mood change following left hemisphere brain injury. *Neurology, 9,* 447–453.

Rocca, W., Amaducci, L., & Schoenberg, B. (1986). Epidemiology of clinically diagnosed Alzheimer's disease. *Annals of Neurology, 19,* 415–424.

Roman, G. (1987). Senile dementia of the Binswanger type: A vascular form of dementia in the elderly. *Journal of the American Medical Association, 258,* 1782–1788.

Roman, G. (1991). The epidemiology of vascular dementia. In A. Hartmann, W. Kuschinsky, & S. Hoyer (Eds.), *Cerebral Ischemia and Dementia* (pp. 9–15). Berlin: Springer-Verlag.

Roman, G., Tatemichi, T., Erkinjuntti, T., Cummings, J., Masdeu, J., Garcia, J., Amaducci, L., Orgogozo, J.-M., Brun, A., Hofman, A., Moody, D., O'Brien, M., Yamaguchi, T., Grafman, J.,

Drayer, B., Bennett, D., Fisher, M., Ogata, J., Kokmen, E., Bermejo, F., A., Korczyn, A., Bougousslavsky, J., Hartmann, A., & Scheinberg, P. (1993). Vascular dementia: Diagnostic criteria for research studies. Report of the NINDS-AIREN International Workshop. *Neurology, 43,* 250–260.

Rosen, W., Terry, R., Fuld, P., Katzman, R., & Peck, A. (1980). Pathological verification of ischemic scores in differentiation of dementias. *Annals of Neurology, 7,* 486–488.

Ross, H., Glaser, F., & Germanson, T. (1988). The prevalence of psychiatric disorders in patients with alcohol and other drug problems. *Archives of General Psychiatry, 45,* 1023–1031.

Ross, R., Lichtenberg, P., & Christensen, K. (1995). Normative data on the Boston Naming Test for elderly adults in a demographically diverse medical sample. *The Clinical Neuropsychologist, 9,* 321–325.

Ross, T., & Lichtenberg, P. (1998). Expanded normative data for the Boston Naming Test for use with urban, elderly medical patients. *The Clinical Neuropsychologist, 12,* 475–481.

Rosser, A., & Hodges, J. (1994). The dementia rating scale in Alzheimer's disease, Huntington's disease and progressive suprenuclear palsy. *Journal of Neurology, 241,* 531–536.

Rothweiler, B., Temkin, N., & Dikmen, S. (1998). Aging effect on psychosocial outcome in traumatic brain injury. *Archives of Physical Medicine and Rehabilitation, 79,* 881–887.

Rouleau, I., Salmon, D., & Butters, N. (1996). Longitudinal analysis of clock drawing in Alzheimer's disease patients. *Brain & Cognition, 31,* 17–34.

Rouleau, I., Salmon, D., Butters, N., Kennedy, N., & McGuire, K. (1992). Quantitative and qualitative analyses of clock drawings in Alzheimer's and Huntington's disease. *Brain and Cognition, 18,* 70–87.

Rourke, S., & Grant, I. (1999). The interactive effects of age and length of abstinence on the recovery of neuropsychological functioning in chronic male alcoholics: A 2-year follow-up study. *Journal of the International Neuropsychological Society, 5,* 234–246.

Rourke, S., & Loberg, T. (1996). The Neurobehavioral Correlates of Alcoholism. In I. Grant & K. Adams (Eds.), *Neuropsychological Assessment of Neuropsychiatric Disorders* (pp. 423–485). New York: Oxford University Press.

Rovner, B., Broadbent, J., Spencer, M., Carson, K., & Folstein, M. (1989). Depression and Alzheimer's disease. *American Journal of Psychiatry, 146,* 350–353.

Ruff, R., Light, R., & Parker, S. (1996). Benton Controlled Oral Word Association Test: Reliability and Updated Norms. *Archives of Clinical Neuropsychology, 11,* 329–338.

Rummans, T., Davis, L., Morse, R., & Ivnik, R. (1993). Learning and memory impairment in older, detoxified, benzodiazepine-dependent patients. *Mayo Clinic Proceedings, 68,* 731–737.

Ryan, C., & Butters, N. (1986). The neuropsychology of alcoholism. In D. Wedding, A.J. Horton, & J. Webster (Eds.), *The Neuropsychology Handbook: Behavioral and Clinical Perspectives* (pp. 376–409). New York: Springer.

Ryan, C., & Williams, T. (1993). Effects of insulin-dependent diabetes on learning and memory efficiency in adults. *Journal of Clinical and Experimental Neuropsychology, 15,* 685–700.

Sackheim, H. (1992). The cognitive effects of electroconvulsive therapy. In W. Moos, E. Gamzu, & L. Thal (Eds.), *Cognitive disorders: Pathophysiology and Treatment.* New York: Marcel Dekker.

Sackheim, H., Prudic, J., Devanand, D., Kiersky, J., Fitzsimons, L., Moody, B., McElhiney, M., Coleman, E., & Settembrino, J. (1993). Effects of stimulus intensity and electrode placement on the efficacy and cognitive effects of electroconvulsive therapy. *New England Journal of Medicine, 32,* 839–846.

Sagar, H., Sullivan, E., Cooper, J., & Jordan, N. (1991). Normal release from proactive interference in untreated patients with Parkinson's disease. *Neuropsychologia, 29,* 1033–1044.

Sagar, H., Sullivan, E., Gabrieli, J., Corkin, S., & Growdon, J. (1988). Temporal ordering and short-term memory deficits in Parkinson's disease. *Brain, 111,* 525–539.

Saint-Cyr, J., Taylor, A., & Lang, A. (1988). Procedural learning and neostriatal dysfunction in man. *Brain, 111,* 941–959.

Saint-Cyr, J., Taylor, A., & Lang, A. (1993). Neuropsychological and psychiatric side effects in the treatment of Parkinson's disease. *Neurology, 43*(6), S47–S52.

Sala, D., Spinnler, H., & Venneri, A. (1997). Persistent global amnesia following right thalamic stroke: An 11-year longitudinal study. *Neuropsychology, 11,* 90–103.

Salloway, S., Malloy, P., Kohn, R., Gillard, E., Duffy, J., Rogg, J., Rung, G., Richardson, E., Thomas, C., & Westlake, R. (1996). MRI and neuropsychological differences in early- and late-life-onset geriatric depression. *Neurology, 46,* 1567–1574.

Salmon, D., Butters, N., & Heindel, W. (1993). Alcoholic dementias and related disorders. In R. Parks, R. Zec, & R. Wilson (Eds.), *Neuropsychology of Alzheimer's Disease and Other Dementias* (pp. 186–209). New York: Oxford University Press.

Salmon, D., Butters, N., & Schuckit, M. (1986). Memory for temporal order and frequency of occurrence in detoxified alcoholics. *Alcohol, 3,* 323–329.

Salmon, D., & Galasko, D. (1996). Neuropsychological aspects of Lewy body dementia. In R. Perry, I. McKeith, & E. Perry (Eds.), *Dementia with Lewy Bodies* (pp. 99–113). New York: Cambridge University Press.

Salmon, D., Galasko, D., Hansen, L., Masliah, E., Butters, N., Thal, L., & Katzman, R. (1996). Neuropsychological deficits associated with diffuse Lewy body disease. *Brain and Cognition, 31,* 148–165.

Salmon, D., Kwo-on-Yuen, P., Heindel, W., Butters, N., & Thal, L. (1989). Differentiation of Alzheimer's disease and Huntington's disease with the Dementia Rating Scale. *Archives of Neurology, 46,* 1204–1208.

Sanchez-Ramos, J., Ortoll, R., & Paulson, G. (1996). Visual hallucinations associated with Parkinson disease. *Archives of Neurology, 53,* 1265–1268.

Sano, M., & Mayeux, R. (1992). Biochemistry of depression in Parkinson's disease. In S. Huber & J. Cummings (Eds.), *Parkinson's Disease: Neurobehavioral Aspects* (pp. 229–239). New York: Oxford University Press.

Santamaria, J., & Tolosa, E. (1992). Clinical subtypes of Parkinson's disease and depression. In S. Huber & J. Cummings (Eds.), *Parkinson's Disease: Neurobehavioral Aspects* (pp. 217–228). New York: Oxford University Press.

Satz, P. (1993). Brain reserve capacity on symptom onset after brain injury: A formulation and review of evidence for threshold theory. *Neuropsychology, 7,* 273–295.

Saunders, A.M., Strittmatter, W.J., Schmechel, D., St. George-Hyslop, P.H., Pericak-Vance, M.A., Joo, S.H., Rosi, B.L., Gusella, J.F., Crapper-MacLachlan, D.R., Alberts, M.J., Hulette, C., Crain, B., Goldgaber, D., & Roses, A.D. (1993). Association of apolipoprotein E allele ε4 with late-onset familial and sporadic Alzheimer's disease. *Neurology, 43,* 1467–1472.

Scatton, B., Javoy-Agid, F., Rouquier, L., Dubois, B., & Agid, Y. (1983). Reduction of cortical dopamine, noradrenalin, and serotonin and their metabolites in Parkinson's disease. *Brain Research, 275,* 321–328.

Scatton, B., Rouquier, L., Javoy-Agid, F., & Agid, Y. (1982). Dopamine deficiency in the cerebral cortex in Parkinson's disease. *Neurology, 32,* 1039–1040.

Schacter, D., & Chiu, C.-Y.P. (1993). Implicit memory: A selective review. *Annual Review of Neuroscience, 16,* 159–182.

Schear, J., & Sato, S. (1989). Effects of visual acuity and visual motor speed and dexterity on cognitive test performance. *Archives of Clinical Neuropsychology, 4,* 25–32.

Schenkenberg, T., Bradford, D., & Ajax, E. (1980). Line bisection and unilateral visual neglect in patients with neurologic impairment. *Neurology, 30,* 509–517.

Schmidt, R., Fazekas, F., Offenbacher, H., Dusek, T., Zach, E., Reinhart, B., Grieshofer, P., Freidel, W., Schumaker, M., Koch, M., & Lechner, H. (1993). Neuropsychologic correlates of MRI white matter hyperintensities: A study of 150 normal volunteers. *Neurology, 43,* 2490–2494.

Schmidt, R., Fazekas, F., Offenbacher, H., Lytwyn, H., Blematl, B., Niederkorn, K., Horner, S., Payer, F., & Friedl, W. (1991). Magnetic resonance imaging white matter lesions and cognitive impairment in hypertensive individuals. *Archives of Neurology, 48,* 417–420.

Schmidt, R., Freidl, W., Faxekas, F., Reinhart, B., Grieshofer, P., Koch, M., Eber, B., Schumacher, M., Polmin, K., & Lechner, H. (1994). The Mattis Dementia Rating Scale: Normative data from 1001 healthy volunteers. *Neurology, 44,* 964–966.

Schneider, J., Watts, R., Gearing, M., Brewer, R., & Mirra, S. (1997). Corticobasal degeneration: Neuropathological and clinical heterogeneity. *Neurology, 48,* 959–969.

Schneider, W., & Shiffrin, R. (1977). Controlled and automatic information processing: I. Detection, search and attention. *Psychological Review, 84,* 1–66.

Schoenberg, B. (1986). Epidemiology of Alzheimer's disease and other dementing disorders. *Journal of Chronic Disease, 39,* 1095–1104.

Schofield, P., Tang, M., Marder, K., Bell, K., Dooneief, G., Chun, M., Sano, M., Stern, Y., & Mayeux, R. (1997). Alzheimer's disease after remote head injury. *Journal of Neurology, Neurosurgery and Psychiatry, 62,* 119–124.

Schonfeld, L., & Dupree, L. (1991). Antecedents of drinking for early- and late-onset elderly alcohol abusers. *Journal of Studies on Alcohol, 52,* 587–592.

Schretlen, D., Brandt, J., & Bobholz, J. (1996). Validation of the Brief Test of Attention in patients with Huntington's disease and amnesia. *The Clinical Neuropsychologist, 10,* 80–89.

Schwartz, M., & Saffran, E. (1987). The American-NART: Replication and extension of the British findings on the persistence of word pronunciation skills in patients with dementia. Unpublished manuscript, Philadelphia.

Schweinberger, R., Buse, C., Freeman, R., Jr., Schonle, P., & Sommer, W. (1992). Memory search for faces and digits in patients with unilateral brain lesions. *Journal of Clinical and Experimental Neuropsychology, 14,* 839–856.

Scogin, F., Hamblin, D., Beutler, L., & Corbishley, A. (1988). Reliability and validity of the short-form Beck Depression Inventory with older adults. *Journal of Clinical Psychology, 44,* 853–857.

Scoville, W., & Milner, B. (1957). Loss of recent memory after bilateral hippocampal lesions. *Journal of Neurology, Neurosurgery and Psychiatry, 20,* 11–21.

Segalowitz, S., Unsal, A., & Dywan, J. (1992). CNV evidence for the distinctiveness of frontal and posterior neural processes in a traumatic brain-injured population. *Journal of Clinical and Experimental Neuropsychology, 14,* 545–565.

Selzer, M. (1971). The Michigan Alcoholism Screening Test: The quest for a new diagnostic instrument. *American Journal of Psychiatry, 127,* 1653–1658.

Shallice, T, Fletcher, P., Frith, C., Grasby, P., Frackowik, R., & Dolan, R. (1994). Brain regions associated with acquisition and retrieval of verbal episodic memory. *Nature, 368,* 633–635.

Shay, K.A., Duke, L.W., Conboy, T., Harrell, L.E., Callaway, R., & Folks, D.G. (1991). The clinical validity of the Mattis Dementia Rating Scale in staging Alzheimer's disease. *Journal of Geriatric Psychiatry and Neurology, 4,* 18–25.

Sheikh, J., & Yesavage, J. (1986). Geriatric Depression Scale (GDS): Recent evidence and development of a shorter version. In T. Brink (Ed.), *Clinical Gerontology: A Guide to Assessment and Intervention* (pp. 165–173). New York: Haworth Press.

Shenkin, H., Greenberg, J., Bouzarth, W., Gutterman, P., & Morales, J. (1973). Ventricular shunting for relief of senile symptoms. *Journal of the American Medical Association, 225,* 1486–1489.

Sherrington, R., Rogaev, E., Liang, Y., Rogaeva, E., Levesque, G., Ikeda, M., Chi, H., Lin, C., Li, G., Holman, K., Tsuda, T., Mar, L., Fonci, J.-F., Bruni, A., Montesi, M., Srobi, S., Rainero, I., Pinessi, L., Nee, L., I, Pollen, D., Brookes, A., Sanseau, P., Polinsky, R., Wasco, W., DaSliva, H., Haines, J., Pericak-Vance, M., Tanzi, R., Roses, A., Fraser, P., Rommens, J., & St George-Hyslop, P. (1995). Cloning of a gene bearing missense mutations in early-onset familiar Alzheimer's disease. *Nature, 375,* 754–760.

Shibayama, H., Kasahara, Y., & Kobayshi, H. (1986). Prevalence of dementia in a Japanese elderly population. *Acta Psychiatrica Scandinavica, 74,* 144–151.

Shimomura, T., Mori, E., Hirono, N., Imamura, T., & Yamashita, H. (1998a). Development of Wernicke-Korsakoff syndrome after long intervals following gastrectomy. *Archives of Neurology, 55,* 1242–1245.

Shimomura, T., Mori, E., Yamashit, H., Imamura, T., Hirono, N., Hashimoto, M., Tanimukai, S., Hazui, H., & Hanihara, T. (1998b). Cognitive loss in dementia with Lewy bodies and Alzheimer disease. *Archives of Neurology, 55,* 1547–1552.

Shoenberg, B., Anderson, D., & Haerer, A. (1985). Prevalence of Parkinson's disease in the biracial population of Copiah County, Mississippi. *Neurology, 35,* 841–845.

Shoulson, I. (1990). Huntington's disease: Cognitive and psychiatric features. *Neuropsychiatry, Neuropsychology and Behavioral Neurology, 3,* 15–22.

Shulman, K., Gold, D., Cohen, C., & Zucchero, C. (1993). Clock-drawing and dementia in the community: A longitudinal study. *International Journal of Geriatric Psychiatry, 8,* 487–496.

Shulman, L., & Weiner, W. (1997). Multiple-system atrophy. In R. Watts & K. Koller (Eds.), *Movement Disorders.* New York: McGraw-Hill.

Shuttleworth, E., & Huber, S. (1988). The naming disorder of dementia of the Alzheimer type. *Brain and Language, 34,* 222–234.

Shy, G., & Drager, G. (1960). A neurological syndrome associated with orthostatic hypotension. *Archives of Neurology, 2,* 511–527.

Siegel, B., & Gershon, S. (1986). Dementia, depression, and pseudodementia. In H. Altman (Ed.), *Alzheimer's Disease: Problems, Prospects and Perspectives* (pp. 29–44). New York: Plenum Press.

Siegfried, K., & O'Connolly, M. (1986). Cognitive and psychomotor effects of different antidepressants in the treatment of old age depression. *International Clinical Psychopharmacology, 1,* 231–243.

Silver, J., & Yudofsky, S. (1992). Drug treatment of depression in Parkinson's disease. In S. Huber & J. Cummings (Eds.), *Parkinson's Disease: Neurobehavioral Aspects* (pp. 240–254). New York: Oxford University Press.

Ska, B., Poissant, A., & Joanette, Y. (1990). Line orientation judgment in normal elderly and subjects with dementia of the Alzheimer's type. *Journal of Clinical and Experimental Neuropsychology, 12,* 695–702.

Skoog, I., Nilsson, L., Palmertz, B., Andreasson, L., & Svanborg, A. (1993). A population-based study of dementia in 85-year-olds. *New England Journal of Medicine, 328,* 153–158.

Smith, G.E., Ivnik, R.J., Malec, J.F., Kokmen, E., Tangalos, E., & Petersen, R.C. (1994). Psychometric properties of the Mattis Dementia Rating Scale. *Psychological Assessment, 2,* 123–131.

Smith, J., & Kiloh, L. (1981). The investigation of dementia: results in 200 consecutive admissions. *Lancet, 1,* 824–827.

Smith-Seemiller, L., Franzen, M., & Bowers, D. (1997). Use of the Wisconsin Card Sorting Test short forms in clinical samples. *The Clinical Neuropsychologist, 4,* 421–427.

Snow, B., & Calne, D. (1992). The etiology of Parkinson's disease. In A. Joseph & R. Young (Eds.), *Movement Disorders in Neurology and Neuropsychiatry* (pp. 230–235). Oxford: Blackwell Scientific.

Snowdon, D., Kemper, S., Mortimer, J., Greiner, L., Wekstein, D., & Markesbery, W. (1996). Linguistic ability in early life and cognitive function and Alzheimer's disease in late life: findings from the nun study. *Journal of the American Medical Association, 275,* 528–532.

Snowdon, J., Goulding, P., & Neary, D. (1989). Semantic dementia: a form of circumscribed cerebral atrophy. *Behavioral Neurology, 2,* 167–182.

Sobin, C., Sackeim, H., Prudic, J., Devanand, D., Moody, B., & McElhiney, M. (1995). Predictors of retrograde amnesia following ECT. *American Journal of Psychiatry, 152,* 995–1001.

Soininen, H., Helkala, E.-L., Laulumaa, V., Soikkeli, R., Hartikainen, P., & Riekkinen, P. (1992). Cognitive profile of Alzheimer patients with extrapyramidal signs: A longitudinal study. *Journal of Neural Transmission, 4,* 241–254.

Sorbi, S., Nacmias, B., Forleo, P., Piacentini, S., Sherrington, R., & St. George-Hyslop, P. (1995). Missense mutation of S182 gene in Italian families with early-onset Alzheimer's disease. *Lancet, 346,* 439–440.

Sotrel, A., Paskevich, P., Kiely, D., Bird, E., Williams, R., & Myers, R. (1991). Morphometric analysis of the prefrontal cortex in Huntington's disease. *Neurology, 41,* 1117–1123.

Souheaver, G., Ryan, J., & DeWolfe, A. (1982). Neuropsychological patterns in uremia. *Journal of Clinical Psychology, 38,* 490–496.

Spicer, K., Roberts, R., & LeWitt, P. (1988). Neuropsychological performance in lateralized parkinsonism. *Archives of Neurology, 45,* 429–432.

Spielberger, C., Gorsuch, R., & Lushene, R. (1970). *STAI Manual.* Palo Alto, CA: Consulting Psychologists Press, Inc.

Spreen, O., & Benton, A. (1977). *Neurosensory Center Comprehensive Examination for Aphasia.* Victoria, BC: University of Victoria Neuropsychology Laboratory.

Spreen, O., & Strauss, E. (1998). *A Compendium of Neuropsychological Tests Second Edition.* New York: Oxford University Press.

Squire, L. (1982). Comparisons between forms of amnesia: Some deficits are unique to Korsakoff's syndrome. *Journal of Experimental Psychology: Learning, Memory and Cognition, 8,* 560–571.

Squire, L. (1986). Memory functions as affected by electroconvulsive therapy. *Annals of the New York Academy of Science, 462,* 307–314.

Squire, L. (1992). Memory and the hippocampus: a synthesis from findings with rats, monkeys and humans. *Psychological Review, 99,* 195–231.

Squire, L. (1994). Declarative and nondeclarative memory: Multiple brain systems support learning and memory. In D. Schacter & E. Tulving (Eds.), *Advances in the Study of Memory and Memory Systems* (pp. 203–231). Cambridge: MIT Press.

Squire, L., Ojemann, J., Mesiqin, S., Peterson, S., Videen, T., & Raichle, M. (1992). Activation of the hippocampus in normal humans: A functional anatomical study of human memory. *Proceedings of the National Academy of Sciences, 89,* 1837–41.

Stacy, M., & Jankovic, J. (1992). Clinical and neurobiological aspects of Parkinson's disease. In S. Huber & J. Cummings (Eds.), *Parkinson's Disease: Neurobehavioral Aspects* (pp. 10–31). New York: Oxford University Press.

Stambrook, M., Cardoso, E., Hawryluk, G., Erikson, P., Piatek, D., & Sicz, G. (1988). Neuropsychological changes following the neurosurgical treatment of normal pressure hydrocephalus. *Archives of Clinical Neuropsychology, 3,* 323–330.

Stambrook, M., Gill, D., Cardoso, E., & Moore, A. (1993). Communicating (normal-pressure) hydrocephalus. In R. Parks, R. Zec, & R. Wilson (Eds.), *Neuropsychology of Alzheimer's Disease and Other Dementias* (pp. 283–307). New York: Oxford University Press.

Starkman, M., Gebarski, S., Berent, S., & Schteingart, D. (1992). Hippocampal formation volume, memory dysfunction, and cortisol levels in patient's with Cushing's syndrome. *Biological Psychiatry, 32,* 756–765.

Starkstein, S., Brandt, J., Folstein, S., Strauss, M., Berthier, M., Pearlson, G., Wong, D., McDonnel, A., & Folstein, M. (1988). Neuropsychological and neuroradiological correlates in Huntington's disease. *Journal of Neurology, Neurosurgery and Psychiatry, 51,* 1259–1263.

Starkstein, S., Fedoroff, J., Price, T., Leiguarda, R., & Robinson, R. (1992a). Anosognosia in patients with cerbrovascular lesions: a study of causative factors. *Stroke, 23,* 1446–1453.

Starkstein, S., Fedoroff, J., Price, T., Leiguarda, R., & Robinson, R. (1993a). Apathy following cerebrovascular lesions. *Journal of Neurology, Neurosurgery, and Psychiatry, 24,* 1625–1630.

Starkstein, S., Fedoroff, J., Price, T., Leiguarda, R., & Robinson, R. (1993b). Catastrophic reactions after cerebrovascular lesions: Frequency, correlates and validation of a scale. *Journal of Neuropsychiatry and Clinical Neuroscience, 5,* 189–194.

Starkstein, S., Leiguarda, R., Gershanik, O., & Berthier, M. (1987). Neuropsychological disturbances in hemiparkinson's disease. *Neurology, 37,* 1762–1764.

Starkstein, S., Mayberg, H., Leiguarda, R., Preziosi, T., & Robinson, R. (1992b). A prospective longitudinal study of depression, cognitive decline, and physical impairments in patients with Parkinson's disease. *Journal of Neurology, Neurosurgery, and Psychiatry, 55,* 377–382.

Starkstein, S., Migliorelli, R., Teson, A., Sabe, L., Vazuez, S., Turjanski, M., Robinson, R., & Leiguarda, R. (1994). Specificity of changes in cerebral blood in patients with frontal lobe dementia. *Journal of Neurology, Neurosurgery, and Psychiatry, 57,* 790–796.

Starkstein, S., Preziosi, T., Bolduc, P., & Robinson, R. (1990). Depression in Parkinson's disease. *Journal of Nervous and Mental Disorders, 178,* 27–31.

Starkstein, S., Rabins, P., Berthier, M., Cohen, B., Folstein, M., & Robinson, R. (1989a). Dementia of depression among patients with neurological disorders and functional depression. *Journal of Neuropsychiatry and Clinical Neurosciences, 1,* 263–268.

Starkstein, S., & Robinson, R. (1989). Affective disorders and cerebral vascular disease. *British Journal of Psychiatry, 154,* 170–182.

Starkstein, S., & Robinson, R. (1994). Neuropsychiatric aspects of stroke. In C. Coffey & J. Cummings (Eds.), *Textbook of Geriatric Neuropsychiatry* (pp. 458–477). Washington, DC: American Psychiatric Press, Inc.

Starkstein, S., Robinson, R., Honig, M., Parikh, R., Joselyn, J., & Price, T. (1989b). Mood changes after right hemisphere lesions. *British Journal of Psychiatry, 155,* 79–85.

Starkstein, S., Sabe, L., Vazquez, S., DiLorenzo, G., Martinez, A., Petracca, G., Teson, A., Chemerinski, E., & Leiguarda, R. (1997). Neuropsychological, psychiatric and cerebral perfusion correlates of leukoarasiosis in Alzheimer's disease. *Journal of Neurology, Neurosurgery, and Psychiatry, 63,* 66–73.

Starkstein, S., Sabe, L., Vazquez, S., Teson, A., Petracca, G., Chemerinski, E., DiLorenzo, G., & Leiguarda, R. (1996). Neuropsychological, psychiatric, and cerebral blood flow findings in vascular dementia and Alzheimer's disease. *Stroke, 27,* 408–414.

Starkstein, S.E., Vasquez, S., Migliorelli, R., Teson, A., Sabe, L., & Leiguarda, R. (1995). A single-photon emission computed tomographic study of anosognosia in Alzheimer's disease. *Archives of Neurology, 52,* 415–420.

Stebbins, G., Gilley, D., Wilson, R., Bernard, B., & Fox, J. (1990). Effects of language disturbances on premorbid estimates of IQ in mild dementia. *The Clinical Neuropsychologist, 4,* 64–68.

Steele, J., Richardson, J., & Olszewski, J. (1964). Progressive supranuclear palsy. *Archives of Neurology, 10,* 333–359.

Steif, B., Sackheim, H., Portnoy, S., Decina, P., & Malitz, S. (1986). Effects of depression and ECT on anterograde memory. *Biological Psychiatry, 21,* 921–930.

Stein, M., Heuser, I., & Vade, T. (1990). Anxiety disorders in patients with Parkinson's disease. *American Journal of Psychiatry, 147,* 217–220.

Steingart, A., Hachinski, V., Lau, C., Fox, A., Fox, H., Lee, D., Inzitari, D., & Merskey, H. (1987). Cognitive and neurologic findings in demented patients with diffuse white matter lucencies on computed tomographic scan (leuko-araiosis). *Archives of Neurology, 44,* 36–39.

Steingart, A., Lau, K., Fox, A., Diaz, F., Fisman, M., Hachinski, V., & Merskey, H. (1986). The significance of white matter lucencies on CT scan in relation to cognitive impairment. *Canadian Journal of Neurological Sciences, 13,* 383–384.

Stern, Y., Albert, M., Brandt, J., Jacobs, D., Tang, M., Marder, K., Bell, K., Sano, M., Devanand, D., Bylsma, F., & Lafleche, G. (1994a). Utility of extrapyramidal signs and psychosis as predictors of cognitive and functional decline, nursing home admission, and death in Alzheimer's disease: Prospective analyses from the Predictors Study. *Neurology, 44,* 2300–2307.

Stern, Y., Alexander, G., Prohovnik, I., & Mayeux, R. (1992). Inverse relationship between education and parietotemporal perfusion deficit in Alzheimer's disease. *Annals of Neurology, 32,* 371–375.

Stern, Y., Gurland, B., Tatemichi, T., Tang, M., Wilder, D., & Mayeux, R. (1994b). Influence of education and occupation on the incidence of Alzheimer's disease. *Journal of the American Medical Association, 271,* 1004–1010.

Stern, Y., Liu, X., Albert, M., Brandt, J., Jacobs, D., Del Castillo-Castaneda, C., Marder, K., Bell, K., Sano, M., & Bylsma, F. (1996). Modeling the influence of extrapyramidal signs on the progression of Alzheimer disease. *Archives of Neurology, 53,* 1121–1126.

Stern, Y., Marder, K., Tang, M., & Mayeux, R. (1993). Antecedent clinical features associated with dementia in Parkinson's disease. *Neurology, 43,* 1690–1692.

Stern, Y., Tang, M.-X., Jacobs, D., Sano, M., Marder, K., Bell, K., Dooneief, G., Schofield, P., & Cote, L. (1998). Prospective comparative study of the evolution of probable Alzheimer's disease and Parkinson's disease dementia. *Journal of the International Neuropsychological Society, 4,* 279–284.

Stern, Y., Tang, M., Denaro, J., & Mayeux, R. (1995). Increased risk of mortality in Alzheimer's disease patients with more advanced education and occupational attainment. *Annals of Neurology, 37*, 590–595.

Stevens, M., Van Duijn, C., Kamphorst, W., de Knijff, P., Heutink, P., vanGool, W., Scheltens, P., Ravid, R., Oostra, B., Niermeijer, M., & vanSwieten, J. (1998). Familial aggregation in frontotemporal dementia. *Neurology, 50*, 1541–1545.

Stewart, S., Rioux, G., Connolly, J., Dunphy, S., & Teehan, M. (1996). Effects of oxazepam and lorazepam on implicit and explicit memory: Evidence for possible influences of time course. *Psychopharmacology, 128*, 139–149.

Storandt, M., Botwinick, J., & Danziger, W. (1986). Longitudinal changes: Patients with mild SDAT and matched healthy controls. In L. Poon (Ed.), *Handbook for Clinical Memory Assessment of Older Adults* (pp. 277–284). Washington, DC: American Psychological Association.

Storandt, M., Botwinick, J., Danziger, W., Berg, L., & Hughes, C. (1984). Psychometric differentiation of mild senile dementia of the Alzheimer type. *Archives of Neurology, 41*, 497–499.

Storandt, M., Stone, K., & LaBarge, E. (1995). Deficits in reading performance in very mild dementia of the Alzheimer type. *Neuropsychology, 9*, 174–176.

Stoudemire, A., Hill, C., Gulley, L., & Morris, R. (1989). Neuropsychological and biomedical assessment of depression-dementia syndromes. *Journal of Neuropsychiatry and Clinical Neurosciences, 1*, 347–361.

Stoudemire, A., Hill, C., Morris, R., & Dalton, S. (1995). Improvement in depression-related cognitive dysfunction following ECT. *Journal of Neuropsychiatry and Clinical Neurosciences, 7*, 31–34.

Strittmatter, W., Saunders, A., Schmechel, D., Pericakvance, M., Enghild, J., Salvesen, G., & Roses, A. (1993). Apolipoprotein E: high-avidity binding to b-amyloid and increased frequency of type 4 allele in late-onset familial Alzheimer disease. *Proceedings of the National Academy of Sciences, 90*, 1977–1981.

Strub, R., & Black, F. (1988). *Neurobehavioral Disorders: A Clinical Approach*. Philadelphia: FA Davis Company.

Strub, R., & Geschwind, N. (1983). Localization in Gerstmann syndrome. In A. Kertesz (Ed.), *Localization in Neuropsychology* (pp. 295–321). New York: Academic Press.

Stuerenburg, H., Hansen, H., Thie, A., & Kunze, K. (1996). Reversible dementia in idiopathic hypoparathyroidism associated with normocalcemia. *Neurology, 47*, 474–476.

Stuss, D., Alexander, M., Hamer, L., Palumbo, C., Dempster, R., Binns, M., Levine, B., & Izukawa, D. (1998). The effects of focal anterior and posterior brain lesions on verbal fluency. *Journal of the International Neuropsychological Society, 4*, 265–278.

Stuss, D., & Benson, D. (1986). *The Frontal Lobes*. New York: Raven Press.

Stutts, J., Stewart, J., & Martell, C. (1998). Cognitive test performance and crash risk in an older driver population. *Accident Analysis and Prevention, 30*, 337–346.

Suhr, J., Grace, J., Allen, J., Nadler, J., & McKenna, M. (1998). Quantitative and qualitative performance of stroke versus normal elderly on six clock drawing systems. *Archives of Clinical Neuropsychology, 13*, 495–502.

Sullivan, E., Sagar, H., Gabrieli, J., Corkin, S., & Growdon, J. (1989). Different cognitive profiles on standard behavioral tests in Parkinson's disease and Alzheimer's disease. *Journal of Clinical and Experimental Neuropsychology, 11*, 799–820.

Sunderland, T., Hill, J., Mellow, A., Lawlor, B., Gundersheimer, J., Newhouse, P., & Grafman, J. (1989). Clock drawing in Alzheimer's disease: A novel measure of dementia severity. *Journal of the American Geriatrics Society, 3*, 725–729.

Taillia, H., Chabriat, H., Kurtz, A., Verin, M., Levy, C., Vahedi, K., Tournier-Lasserve, E., & Bousser, M. (1998). Cognitive alterations in non-demented CADASIL patients. *Cerebrovascular Disease, 8*, 97–101.

Tanner, C., Hubble, J., & Chan, P. (1997). Epidemiology and genetics of Parkinson's disease. In R. Watts & W. Koller (Eds.), *Movement Disorders: Neurologic Principles and Practice* (pp. 137–152). New York: McGraw Hill.

Tanner, C., Vogel, C., Goetz, C., & Klawans, H. (1983). Hallucinations in Parkinson's disease: A population study. *Annals of Neurology, 14,* 136–144.

Tarter, R., Hegedus, A., Van Thiel, D., Gavaler, J., & Schade, R. (1986). Hepatic dysfunction and neuropsychological test performance in alcoholics with cirrhosis. *Journal of Studies of Alcohol, 47,* 74–77.

Tata, P., Rollings, J., Collins, M., Pickering, A., & Jacobson, R. (1994). Lack of cognitive recovery following withdrawal from long-term benzodiazepine use. *Psychological Medicine, 24,* 203–213.

Taylor, A., & Saint-Cyr, J. (1992). Executive function. In S. Huber & J. Cummings (Eds.), *Parkinson's Disease: Neurobehavioral Aspects* (pp. 75–85). New York: Oxford University Press.

Taylor, A., Saint-Cyr, J., & Lang, A. (1986a). Frontal lobe dysfunction in Parkinson's disease: The cortical focus of neostrial outflow. *Brain, 109,* 845–883.

Taylor, A., Saint-Cyr, J., & Lang, A. (1987). Parkinson's disease: Cognitive change in relation to treatment response. *Brain, 110,* 35–51.

Taylor, A., Saint-Cyr, J., & Lang, A. (1990). Memory and learning in early Parkinson's disease: evidence for a "frontal lobe syndrome". *Brain and Cognition, 13,* 211–232.

Taylor, A., Saint-Cyr, J., Lang, A., & Kenny, F. (1986b). Parkinson's disease and depression: A critical re-evaluation. *Brain, 109,* 279–292.

Taylor, C., Fields, R., Starratt, G., Russo, B., & Diamond, D. (1993). *Neuropsychiatric complaints following traumatic brain injury: Head injured versus non-head-injured trauma patients.* Paper presented at the American Neuropsychiatric Association, San Antonio, Texas.

Taylor, K., Salmon, D., Rice, V., Bondi, M., Hill, L., Ernesto, C., & Butters, N. (1996). Longitudinal examination of American National Adult Reading Test (AMNART) performance in dementia of the Alzheimer' type (DAT): Validation and correction based on degree of cognitive decline. *Journal of Clinical and Experimental Neuropsychology, 18,* 883–891.

Teasdale, G., & Jennett, B. (1974). Assessment of coma and impaired consciousness: A practical scale. *Lancet, 2,* 81–84.

Teri, L., & Wagner, A. (1992). Alzheimer's disease and depression. *Journal of Consulting and Clinical Psychology, 60,* 379–391.

Terry, R., & Katzman, R. (1983). Senile dementia of the Alzheimer type. *Annals of Neurology, 14,* 497–506.

Thal, L., Grundman, M., & Klauber, M. (1988). Dementia. Characteristics of a referral population and factors associated with progression. *Neurology, 38,* 1083–1090.

Thompson, R. (1986). The neurobiology of learning and memory. *Science, 233,* 941–947.

Thompson, R., Moran, M., & Neis, A. (1983). Psychotropic drug use in the elderly, Part 1. *New England Journal of Medicine, 308,* 134–138.

Thomsen, A., Borgesen, S., Bruhn, S., & Gjerras, F. (1986). Prognosis of dementia in normal pressure hydrocephalus after a shunt operation. *Annals of Neurology, 20,* 304–310.

Tierney, M., Szalai, J., Snow, W., Fisher, R., Tsuda, T., Chi, H., McLachlan, D., & St. George-Hyslop, P. (1996). A prospective study of the clinical utility of ApoE genotype in the prediction of outcome in patients with memory impairment. *Neurology, 46,* 149–154.

Tombaugh, T., & Hubley, A. (1997). The 60-item Boston Naming Test: Norms for cognitively intact adults aged 25 to 88 years. *Journal of Clinical and Experimental Neuropsychology, 19,* 922–932.

Tomer, R., & Levin, B. (1993). Differential effects of aging on two verbal fluency tasks. *Perceptual and Motor Skills, 76,* 465–466.

Tomlinson, B., Blessed, G., & Roth, M. (1970). Observations on the brains of demented old people. *Journal of Neurological Sciences, 11,* 205–242.

Trobe, J., Waller, P., Cook-Flannagan, C., Teshima, S., & Bieliauskas, L. (1996). Crashes and violations among drivers with Alzheimer's disease. *Archives of Neurology, 53,* 411–416.

Troster, A., Paolo, A., Lyons, K., Glatt, S., Hubble, J., & Koller, W. (1995a). The influence of depression on cognition in Parkinson's disease: A pattern of impairment distinguishable from Alzheimer's disease. *Neurology, 45,* 672–676.

Troster, A., Stalp, L., Paolo, A., Fields, J., & Koller, W. (1995b). Neuropsychological impairments in Parkinson's disease with and without depression. *Archives of Neurology, 52,* 1164–1169.

Tulving, E. (1972). Episodic and semantic memory. In E. Tulving & W. Donaldson (Eds.), *Organization of Memory.* New York: Academic Press.

Tulving, E., Kapur, S., Craik, F., Moscovitch, M., & Houle, S. (1994). Hemispheric encoding/retrieval asymmetry in episodic memory: Positron emission tomography findings. *Proceedings of the National Academy of Science, 91,* 2016–2020.

Tulving, E., & Schacter, D. (1990). Priming and human memory systems. *Science, 247,* 301–306.

Tulving, E., & Thomson, D. (1973). Encoding specificity and retrieval processes in episodic memory. *Psychological Review, 80,* 352–737.

Tuokko, H., Hadjistavropoulos, T., Miller, J., & Beattie, B. (1992). The Clock Test: A sensitive measure to differentiate normal elderly from those with Alzheimer disease. *Journal of the American Geriatrics Society, 40,* 575–584.

Tuokko, H., Hadjistavropoulos, T., Miller, J., Horton, A., & Beattie, B. (1995a). *The Clock Drawing Test: Administration and Scoring Manual.* Toronto: Multi-Health Systems.

Tuokko, H., Tallman, K., Beattie, B., Cooper, P., & Weir, J. (1995b). An examination of driving records in a dementia clinic. *Journals of Gerontology: Psychological Sciences and Social Sciences, 50,* S173–181.

Tyrrell, P., Warrington, E., Frackowiak, R., & Rossor, M. (1990). Heterogeneity in progressive aphasia due to focal cortical atrophy. *Brain, 113,* 1321–1336.

Ungerleider, L., & Mishkin, M. (1982). Two cortical visual systems. In D. Ingle, M. Goodale, & R. Mansfield (Eds.), *Analysis of Visual Behavior.* Cambridge, MA: MIT Press.

Vallar, G., & Baddeley, A. (1984a). Fractionation of working memory: Neuropsychological evidence for a short-term store. *Journal of Verbal Learning and Verbal Behavior, 23,* 151–161.

Vallar, G., & Baddeley, A. (1984b). Phonological short-term store, phonological processing and sentence comprehension: A neuropsychological case study. *Cognitive Neuropsychology, 1,* 121–141.

Van der Does, A., & Van den Bosch, R. (1992). What determines Wisconsin Card Sorting Performance in schizophrenia? *Clinical Psychology Review, 12,* 567–583.

Van der Eecken, H., Adams, R., & van Bogaert, L. (1960). Striopallidal-nigral degeneration: A hitherto undescribed lesion in paralysis agitans. *Journal of Neuropathology and Experimental Neurology, 19,* 159–161.

Van Gorp, W., Satz, P., Kiersch, M., & Henry, R. (1986). Normative data on the Boston Naming Test for a group of normal older adults. *Journal of Clinical and Experimental Neuropsychology, 8,* 702–705.

Van Zagten, M., Lodder, J., & Kessels, F. (1998). Gait disorder and parkinsonian signs in patients with stroke related to small deep infarcts and white matter lesions. *Movement Disorders, 13,* 89–95.

Vanderploeg, R. (1994). *Clinician's Guide to Neuropsychological Assessment.* Hillsdale, NJ: Lawrence Erlbaum Associates.

Vanderploeg, R., Schinka, J., & Axelrod, B. (1996). Estimation of WAIS-R premorbid intelligence: Current ability and demographic data used in a best-performance fashion. *Psychological Assessment, 8,* 404–411.

Vangel, S.J., & Lichtenberg, P.Q. (1995). Mattis Dementia Rating Scale: Clinical utility and relationship with demographic variables. *The Clinical Neuropsychologist, 9,* 209–213.

Veselis, R., Reinsel, R., Feshchenko, V., & Wronski, M. (1997). The comparative amnestic effects of midazolam, propofol, thiopental and fentanyl at equi-sedative concentrations. *Anesthesiology, 87,* 749–764.

Victor, M., & Adams, R. (1985). The alcoholic dementias. In J. Fredericks (Ed.), *Handbook of Clinical Neurology: Neurobehavioral Disorders* (Vol. 2, pp. 335–352). New York: Elsevier Press.

Victor, M., Adams, R., & Collins, G. (1989). *The Wernicke-Korsakoff Syndrome.* Philadelphia: FA Davis.

Victoroff, J., Mack, W., Lyness, S., & Chui, H. (1995). Multicenter clinicopathological correlation in dementia. *American Journal of Psychiatry, 152,* 1476–1484.

Vitaliano, P., Breen, A., Russo, J., Albert, M., Vitiello, M., & Prinz, P. (1984). The clinical utility of the Dementia Rating Scale for assessing Alzheimer patients. *Journal of Chronic Diseases, 37,* 743–753.

Volkow, N., Hitzemann, R., Wang, G., Fowler, J., Burr, G., Pascani, K., Dewey, S., & Wolf, A. (1992). Decreased brain metabolism in neurologically intact healthy alcoholics. *American Journal of Psychiatry, 149,* 1016–1022.

Vonsattel, J., Myers, R., Stevens, T., Ferrante, J., Bird, E., & Richardson, E., Jr. (1985). Neuropathological classification of Huntington's disease. *Journal of Neuropathology and Experimental Neurology, 44,* 559–577.

WAIS-III WMS-III Technical Manual. (1997). San Antonio: The Psychological Corporation.

Waldstein, S., Manuck, S., Ryan, C., & Muldoon, M. (1991). Neuropsychological correlates of hypertension: Review and methodologic considerations. *Psychological Bulletin, 110,* 451–468.

Wallesch, C., Kornhuber, H., Kunz, T., & Brunner, R. (1983). Neuropsychological deficits associated with small unilateral thalamic lesions. *Brain, 106,* 141–152.

Waltimo, O., & Putkonen, A.-R. (1974). Intellectual performance of patients with intracranial arteriovenous malformations. *Brain, 97,* 511–520.

Ward, C., Duvoisin, R., Ince, S., Nutt, J., Eldridge, R., & Calne, D. (1983). Parkinson's disease in 65 pairs of twins and in a set of quadruplets. *Neurology, 33,* 815–824.

Warrington, E., James, M., & Maciejewski, C. (1986). The WAIS as a lateralizing and localizing diagnostic instrument. *Neuropsychologia, 24,* 223–239.

WASI Manual. (1999). San Antonio: The Psychological Corporation.

Watts, R., Brewer, R., Schneider, J., & Mirra, S. (1997). Corticobasal degeneration. In R. Watts & W. Koller (Eds.), *Movement Disorders* (pp. 611–621). New York: McGraw-Hill.

Watts, R., & Koller, K. (1997). *Movement Disorders.* New York: McGraw-Hill.

Wechsler, D. (1981). *WAIS-R Manual.* San Antonio: The Psychological Corporation.

Wechsler, D. (1997a). *WAIS-III Administration and Scoring Manual.* San Antonio: The Psychological Corporation.

Wechsler, D. (1997b). *WMS-III Administration and Scoring Manual.* San Antonio: The Psychological Corporation.

Weiner, R., Rogers, H., Davidson, J., & Squire, L. (1986). Effects of stimulus parameters on cognitive side effects. *Annals of the New York Academy of Science, 482,* 315–325.

Weingartner, H., Grafman, J., Boutelle, W., Kaye, W., & Martin, P. (1983). Forms of memory failure. *Science, 221,* 380–382.

Weintraub, S., & Mesulam, M.-M. (1993). Four neuropsychological profiles in dementia. In F. Boller & H. Spinnler (Eds.), *Handbook of Neuropsychology* (Vol. 8, pp. 253–282). Amsterdam: Elsevier Science Publishers.

Weintraub, S., & Mesulam, M.-M. (1996). From neuronal networks to dementia: Four clinical profiles. In F. Foret, Y. Christen, & F. Boller (Eds.), *La Démence: Pourquoi?* (pp. 75–97). Paris: Fondation Nationale de Gérontologie.

Welch, L., Doineau, D., Johnson, S., & King, D. (1996). Educational and gender normative data for the Boston Naming Test in a group of older adults. *Brain and Language, 53,* 260–266.

Welsh, K., Butters, N., Hughes, J., Mohs, R., & Heyman, A. (1991). Detection of abnormal memory decline in mild cases of Alzheimer's disease using CERAD neuropsychological measures. *Archives of Neurology, 48,* 278–281.

Welsh, K., Butters, N., Hughes, J., Mohs, R., & Heyman, A. (1992). Detection and staging of dementia in Alzheimer's disease: Use of the neuropsychological measures developed for the Consortium to Establish a Registry for Alzheimer's disease. *Archives of Neurology, 49,* 448–452.

Welsh, K., Fillenbaum, G., Wilkinson, W., Heyman, A., Mohs, R., Stern, Y., Harrell, L., Edland, S., & Beekly, D. (1995a). Neuropsychological test performance in African-American and white patients with Alzheimer's disease. *Neurology, 45,* 2207–2211.

Welsh, K., Watson, M., Hoffman, J., Lowe, V., Earl, N., & Rubin, D. (1995b). The neural basis of visual naming errors in Alzheimer's disease: A positron emission study. *Archives of Clinical Neuropsychology, 10,* 403.

Welsh-Bohmer, K., Gearing, M., Saunders, A., Roses, A., & Mirra, S. (1997). Apolipoprotein E genotypes in a neuropathological series from the Consortium to Establish a Registry for Alzheimer's Disease. *Annals of Neurology, 42,* 319–325.

Whelihan, W., & Lesher, E. (1985). Neuropsychological changes in frontal functions with aging. *Developmental Neuropsychology, 1,* 371–380.

White, R., Feldman, R., & Travers, P. (1990). Neurobehavioral effects of toxicity due to metals, solvents and insecticides. *Clinical Neuropharmacology, 5,* 392–412.

White, R., & Proctor, S. (1993). Solvent encephalopathy. In R. Parks, R. Zec, & R. Wilson (Eds.), *Neuropsychology of Alzheimer's Disease and Other Dementias* (pp. 350–374). New York: Oxford University Press.

Whitehouse, P. (1986). The concept of cortical and subcortical dementia: Another look. *Annals of Neurology, 19,* 1–6.

Whitehouse, P., Price, D., Clark, A., Coyle, J., & DeLong, M. (1981). Alzheimer disease: evidence of selective loss of cholinergic neurons in the nucleus basalis. *Annals of Neurology, 10,* 122–126.

Whitehouse, P., Price, D., Struble, R., Clark, A., Coyle, J., & DeLong, M. (1982). Alzheimer's disease and senile dementia: Loss of neurons in the basal forebrain. *Science, 215,* 1237–1239.

Wiggins, S., Whyte, P., Huggins, M., Adam, S., Theilmann, J., Bloch, M., Sheps, S., Schecter, M., & Hayden, M. (1992). The psychological consequences of predictive testing for Huntington's disease. Canadian Collaborative Study of Predictive Testing. *New England Journal of Medicine, 327,* 1401–1405.

Williams, B., Mack, W., & Henderson, V. (1989). Boston Naming Test in Alzheimer's disease. *Neuropsychologia, 27,* 1073–1079.

Wilson, F., Scalaidhe, S., & Goldman-Rakic, P. (1993b). Dissociation of object and spatial processing domains in primate prefrontal cortex. *Science, 260,* 1955–1958.

Wilson, R., Sullivan, M., deToledo Morrell, L., Stebbins, G., Bennett, C., & Morrell, F. (1996). Association of memory and cognition in Alzheimer's disease with volumetric estimates of temporal lobe structures. *Neuropsychology, 10,* 459–463.

Wolf, P., Kannel, W., & Verter, J. (1984). Cerebrovascular disease in the elderly: Epidemiology. In M. Albert (Ed.), *Clinical Neurology of Aging* (pp. 458–477). New York: Oxford University Press.

Wolfe, N., Linn, R., Babikian, V., Knoefel, J., & Albert, M. (1990). Frontal systems impairment following multiple lacunar infarcts. *Archives of Neurology, 47,* 129–132.

Wolf-Klein, G., Silverstone, F., Levy, A., & Brod, M. (1989). Screening for Alzheimer's disease by clock drawing. *Journal of the American Geriatrics Society, 37,* 730–736.

Woodard, J.L., Benedict, R., Roberts, V., Goldstein, F., Kinner, K., Capruso, D., & Clark, A. (1996a). Short-form alternatives to the Judgment of Line Orientation. *Journal of Clinical and Experimental Neuropsychology, 18,* 898–904.

Woodard, J.L., Salthouse, T.A., Godsall, R.E., & Green, R.C. (1996b). Confirmatory factor analysis of the Mattis Dementia Rating Scale in patients with Alzheimer's disease. *Psychological Assessment, 8,* 85–91.

Woods, J., & Winger, G. (1995). Current benzodiazepine issues. *Psychopharmacology, 118,* 107–115.

Worrall, L., Yiu, E.-L., Hickson, L., & Barnett, H. (1995). Normative data for the Boston Naming Test for Australian elderly. *Aphasiology, 9,* 541–551.

Wragg, R., & Jeste, D. (1989). Overview of depression and psychosis in Alzheimer's disease. *American Journal of Psychiatry, 146,* 577–587.

Wredling, R., Levander, S., Adamson, U., & Lins, P. (1990). Permanent neuropsychological impairment after recurrent episodes of severe hypoglycaemia in man. *Diabetologia, 33,* 152–157.

Yesavage, J., Brink, T., Rose, T., Lum, O., Huang, O., Adey, V., & Leirer, V. (1983). Development and validation of a geriatric depression screening scale: A preliminary report. *Journal of Psychiatric Research, 17,* 37–49.

Ylikoski, R., Ykikoski, A., Erkinjuntti, T., Sulkava, R., Raininko, R., & Tilvis, R. (1993). White matter changes in healthy elderly persons correlate with attention and speed of mental processing. *Archives of Neurology, 50,* 818–824.

Young, L., Fields, R., & Lovell, M. (1995). Neuropsychological differentiation of geriatric head injury from dementia (abstract). *Journal of Neuropsychiatry, 7,* 414.

Zarit, S., Reever, K., & Back-Peterson, J. (1980). Relatives of the impaired elderly: Correlates of feeling of burden. *Gerontologist, 20,* 649–655.

Zarit, S., Tood, P., & Zarit, J. (1986). Subjective burden of husbands and wives as caregivers. *Gerontologist, 26,* 260–266.

Zervas, I., Calev, A., Jandorf, L., Schwartz, J., Gaudino, E., Tubi, N., Lerer, B., & Shapira, B. (1993). Age-dependent effects of electroconvulsive therapy on memory. *Convulsive Therapy, 9,* 39–42.

Zola-Morgan, S., & Squire, L. (1993). Neuroanatomy of memory. *Annual Review of Neuroscience, 16,* 547–563.

Zomeran, A. (1994). *Clinical Neuropsychology of Attention.* New York: Oxford University Press.

Zubenko, G., Rifai, A., Mulsant, B., Swett, R., & Pasternak, R. (1996). Premorbid history of major depression and the depressive syndrome of Alzheimer's disease. *American Journal of Geriatric Psychiatry, 4,* 85–90.

Zubenko, G., Stiffler, S., Stabler, S., Kopp, U., Hughes, H., Cohen, B., & Moossy, J. (1994). Association of the apolipoprotein E e4 allele with clinical subtypes of autopsy-confirmed Alzheimer's disease. *American Journal of Medical Genetics, 54,* 199–205.

Zweig, R., Cardillo, J., Cohen, M., Giere, S., & Hedreen, J. (1993). The locus ceruleus and dementia in Parkinson's disease. *Neurology, 43,* 986–991.

INDEX